D1757286

MRI Atlas
Orthopedics and Neurosurgery
The Spine

Martin Weyreuther
Christoph E. Heyde
Michael Westphal
Jan Zierski
Ulrich Weber

MRI Atlas
Orthopedics and Neurosurgery The Spine

Foreword by
Prof. Dr. med. Dr. h.c. Karl-Jürgen Wolf

Translated by Bettina Herwig

With 524 Figures in 575 Separate Illustrations

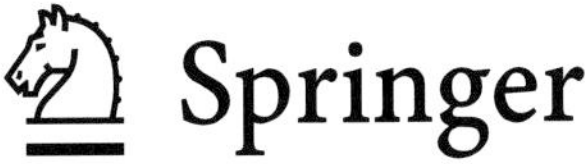
Springer

Authors:
Dr. Martin Weyreuther
Röntgenabteilung, HELIOS Klinik Emil von Behring
Walterhöferstr. 11, 14165 Berlin

Dr. Christoph E. Heyde
Unfallchirurgische Universitätsklinik
Charité Campus Benjamin Franklin
Hindenburgdamm 30, 12200 Berlin

Prof. Dr. Michael Westphal
Bonhoefferufer 13, 10589 Berlin

Prof. Dr. Jan Zierski
Neurochirurgische Klinik
Vivantes Klinikum Neukölln
Rudower Str. 48, 12351 Berlin

Prof. Dr. Ulrich Weber
Orthopädische Universitäts-Klinik,
Charité Campus Benjamin Franklin
Hindenburgdamm 30, 12200 Berlin

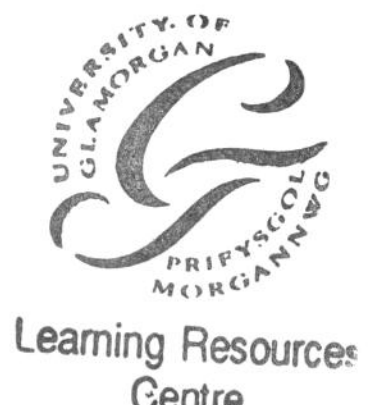

Translator:
Bettina Herwig
Hauptstraße 4H
10317 Berlin

Title of the Original German Edition:
MRT-Atlas Orthopädie und Neurochirurgie. Wirbelsäule
© Springer-Verlag Berlin Heidelberg 2006
ISBN 10 3-540-40285-3

ISBN 10 3-540-33533-1 Springer-Verlag Berlin Heidelberg New York
ISBN 13 978-3-540-33533-7 Springer-Verlag Berlin Heidelberg New York

Library of Congress Control Number: 2006929607

Springer is a part of Springer Science+Business Media
springer.com

Editor: Dr. Ute Heilmann, Heidelberg
Desk Editor: Wilma McHugh, Heidelberg
Cover design: Frido Steinen-Broo, Pau, Spain
Typesetting: Satz-Druck-Service, Leimen
Image Editing: AM-productions GmbH, Wiesloch
Production: LE-TEX Jelonek, Schmidt & Vöckler GbR, Leipzig

Printed on acid-free paper 21/3100/YL 5 4 3 2 1 0

Foreword

Though a fairly recent development in the field of radiology, MRI has successfully established itself in the spectrum of imaging modalities. Insights into the body that, until recently, were inconceivable and that have paved the way for devising new diagnostic and therapeutic options have been made possible by the constant improvement in spatial and anatomic detail resolution and advances in data processing that include improved image reconstruction algorithms. On the other hand, the amount of image information now obtainable with state-of-the-art MR scanners makes it ever more important to provide guidance for radiologists, orthopedic surgeons, traumatologists, and other interested specialists, so that they can find their way through the plethora of details. This is the intention of the atlas presented here: it is a practically oriented guide offering a concise overview of the important aspects of normal spinal anatomy and pathology, MR findings in spinal disease and the postoperative spine as well as therapeutic and surgical approaches. Such a guide is especially important for the spine with its unique and complex anatomic structure and function. The rigorous and uniform organization of the book is the work of a group of dedicated authors from different specialties who offer the reader a systematic overview based on their own vast experience and skills.

An invaluable asset of this book is its concise presentation of important interdisciplinary aspects in dealing with spinal disorders. With its unique format, this atlas guides readers through the fundamentals of spinal anatomy and disease states to better establish diagnostic strategies and surgical management.

In the interest of high-quality patient care, our hope is that many readers will find this atlas a vital source of information in the diagnosis and treatment of their patients.

Professor Dr. med. Dr. h.c. Karl-Jürgen Wolf
Berlin, June 2006

Preface

Magnetic resonance imaging is a computer-assisted diagnostic tool that is well established for numerous indications involving the skeleton and its associated structures. Soon after its clinical introduction in the early 1980's, it became apparent that the application of MRI in the evaluation of normal and abnormal conditions yields widely varying qualitative and quantitative results for different anatomic regions of the locomotor system. The most common indications for MRI in this area are diseases and injuries of the spine and joints, in particular the knee. The significance of MRI for these two skeletal areas is reflected by the fact that knee MRI has largely replaced invasive techniques such as diagnostic arthrography and arthroscopy, while spinal MRI has assumed an important place in therapeutic decision-making, especially in surgical planning.

Inspired by the great interest that the MRI atlas of the knee created in 2003, we decided to compile a similar atlas for the spine. Like its predecessor, the MRI atlas of the spine is the result of interdisciplinary cooperation. Many disorders and injuries of the spine and associated structures are treated by orthopedic surgeons, traumatologists, and neurosurgeons alike, while others are predominantly treated in just one of these specialties. Thus, the decision was made to have orthopedic surgeons/traumatologists, MRI radiologists, and neurosurgeons jointly write this atlas in order to comprehensively discuss all aspects of spinal MRI, particularly its benefits and limitations. As always with such a complex field, the choice of conditions (e.g. tumors or vascular malformations) had to be limited. This may appear arbitrary to some readers, but our selection was necessary to illustrate the role of MRI in exemplary cases and to avoid exceeding the scope of this atlas by including rare diseases.

The presentation of the material should help the reader to quickly identify the most important spinal structures on MR images as a basis for rapidly and efficiently detecting abnormal changes and differentiating them from the normal appearance. Thus, as with the MRI atlas of the knee, the focus is again on the presentation of a carefully selected series of images ranging from the normal appearance to abnormal changes combined with concise information on specific MR sequences and parameters as well as pitfalls. Basic background information on anatomy and pathophysiology is presented here, and the clinical significance of MR findings is discussed in relation to the individual spinal diseases and injuries.

The authors hope that our cooperative approach to spinal MRI successfully reconciles the different aspects of our specialties for a unified approach that enables our readers to make the most effective use of MR findings in treating their patients with spinal disorders.

We thank the staff of our publisher, Springer-Verlag, for their excellent support. Particular gratitude is owed to our secretaries, Miriam Ziegler and

Brigitte Seyd, for their contribution. Finally, our thanks go to Dr. S. Stein, Dr. P. Teller, and in particular Dr. M.C. Dulce, who provided many of the images and helped arrange them systematically.

The Authors
Berlin, June 2006

Table of Contents

1 Normal Anatomy and Variants 1
1.1 Normal Anatomy 1
1.2 Conjoined Nerve Roots 1
1.3 Transitional Vertebra 1

2 Congenital and Developmental Anomalies 11
2.1 Spinal Meningeal Cysts 11
2.2 Bony Malformations 12
2.3 Hemivertebra, Wedge Vertebra, Butterfly Vertebra, and Hemimetameric Segmental Shift 12
2.4 Klippel-Feil Syndrome 13
2.5 Atlantoaxial Instability and Basilar Impression 14
2.6 Os Odontoideum 14
2.7 Block Vertebra with Disc Atresia 15
2.8 Split Cord Malformations (Diastematomyelia) 15
2.9 Syringohydromyelia 16
2.10 Spinal Dysraphism 17
2.11 Tethered Cord 18
2.12 Scoliosis 19
2.13 Kyphosis 20
2.14 Lipomatosis and Lipoma 21
2.15 Scheuermann's Disease 21
2.16 Hemangioma 22
2.17 Spondylolisthesis 23

3 Trauma and Fractures 61
3.1 Dens Fractures 62
3.2 Axis Fractures 62
3.3 Spinal Contusion 63
3.4 Atlas Fractures 63
3.5 Stable Vertebral Fractures 63
3.6 Unstable Vertebral Fractures 63
3.7 Fractures of Transverse and Spinous Processes 64
3.8 Disc Injuries 64
3.9 Osteoporotic Fractures 64
3.10 Posttraumatic Syrinx 65
3.11 Spinal Cord Injuries 65
3.12 Ligament Injuries 65
3.13 Fractures in Ankylosing Spondylitis 65
3.14 Clinical Significance of MRI in Spinal Injuries 66
3.15 Nerve Root Avulsion 66

4 Degenerative Disorders . . . 99
4.1 Osteochondrosis . . . 99
4.2 Spondyloarthrosis . . . 101
4.3 Synovial Cysts . . . 102
4.4 Spinal Stenosis . . . 102
4.5 Foraminal Stenosis . . . 103
4.6 Atlantoaxial Arthrosis . . . 104
4.7 Disc Herniation . . . 104
4.8 Muscular Dystrophy . . . 107

5 Inflammatory Conditions . . . 143
5.1 Spondylitis/Spondylodiscitis . . . 143
5.2 Chronic Polyarthritis . . . 144
5.3 Ankylosing Spondylitis (Bechterew's Disease) . . . 145
5.4 Myelitis . . . 147
5.5 Multiple Sclerosis . . . 147

6 Tumors and Tumor-like Lesions . . . 195
6.1 Neurinoma, Schwannoma, Neurofibroma, and Meningioma . . . 195
6.2 Astrocytoma . . . 197
6.3 Ependymoma . . . 197
6.4 Hemangioblastoma . . . 198
6.5 Epidermoids and Dermoids . . . 198
6.6 Vascular Lesions . . . 199
6.7 Sarcoidosis . . . 200
6.8 Bone Tumors . . . 200

7 The Postoperative Spine . . . 273
7.1 Scars . . . 273
7.2 Recurrent Disc Herniation . . . 273
7.3 Bone Defects/Fenestration . . . 273
7.4 Seroma/Hematoma . . . 273
7.5 Bone Grafting . . . 273
7.6 Vertebroplasty . . . 273
7.7 Osteosynthesis . . . 273

References . . . 289

Subject Index . . . 293

1 Normal Anatomy and Variants

1.1 Normal Anatomy

MR Technique

The standard MR protocol for a routine evaluation of the spine always comprises imaging in sagittal and axial planes, while coronal images are necessary only to answer specialized questions.

Typical sequences are T1- and T2-weighted sequences, T2-weighted fast spin echo sequences, which may be supplemented by fat-suppressed sequences.

MR Findings

The signal intensity of the marrow in adult vertebrae varies with its fat content and is high relative to muscle on T1- and T2-weighted images. The presence of residual red marrow decreases the signal on T1 and T2. Cortical bone and ligaments have a very low signal intensity on both T1 and T2. The signal intensity of vessels is low or high, depending on the pulse sequence used and the flow velocity of the blood (cervical spine, Figs. 1.1–1.4; thoracic spine, Figs. 1.5–1.8; lumbar spine, Figs. 1.9–1.12).

1.2 Conjoined Nerve Roots

Anatomy

Conjoined nerve roots are a normal anatomic variant.

MR Technique

Most conjoined nerve roots are discovered incidentally on routine sagittal or axial MR images.

MR Findings

Two adjacent intraspinal nerve roots of normal signal intensity. Both roots emerge at the same level and can be traced to their shared origin. The presence of conjoined nerve roots is characterized by an asymmetrical appearance because no nerve root exits the thecal sac at the level above or below on the same side. Conjoined nerve roots have the same MR signal intensity and contrast enhancement pattern as normal nerve roots (Fig. 1.13).

MR Pitfalls

Conjoined nerve roots may easily be mistaken for disc herniations or free disc fragments.

Clinical Significance

Conjoined nerve roots are normal anatomic variants but are nevertheless important because they are quite common and must not be confused with pathology such as disc sequesters or root neurinoma in patients with clinical symptoms.

1.3 Transitional Vertebra

Anatomy

Transitional vertebrae are vertebrae whose structure features some of the characteristics of the adjacent spinal region. Such indeterminate vertebrae can occur at all spinal junctions and are designated as occipitocervical, cervicothoracic, thoracolumbar, or lumbosacral. There may be complete or incomplete assimilation between adjacent vertebrae.

Pathomechanism

Transitional vertebrae are not considered malformations although they are associated with shifts in the vertical segmentation of the spine. The shift involves not only the bony elements but also muscles, nerves, vessels, and other anatomic structures.

Cranial shift is reported to be more common than caudal shift. The normal numerical distribution of vertebrae (seven cranial, twelve thoracic, five lumbar, five sacral, and four coccygeal vertebrae) is present in only two thirds of individuals. Transitional vertebrae are most common at the lumbosacral junction (lumbarization of the first sacral vertebra, sacralization of the fifth lumbar vertebra).

MR Technique

Transitional vertebrae are best identified on sagittal T1- or T2-weighted images (Fig. 1.14).

Most transitional vertebrae are detected incidentally on MR images. Correct identification of the level of a transitional vertebra is possible only on images showing the entire spine. In most patients, a transitional vertebra is already known from prior radiographs.

Whenever the involved segment cannot be clearly identified, it must be mentioned in the report and a choice must then be made and consistently applied.

Clinical Significance

Transitional vertebrae can be entirely asymptomatic or can impair the overall static stability of the spine or the biomechanical function of individual motion segments and thus predispose to degenerative spinal disorders. This is especially the case when there is only partial assimilation (e.g. incomplete sacralization of the fifth lumbar vertebra). Of particular significance are skeletal abnormalities of the occipitocervical junction. So-called atlas assimilation (partial or complete fusion of the atlas to the occiput) is rare but is associated with considerable dysfunction (osseous torticollis or wryneck) and often causes neurologic deficits (disturbance of the pyramidal tract, Arnold-Chiari malformation).

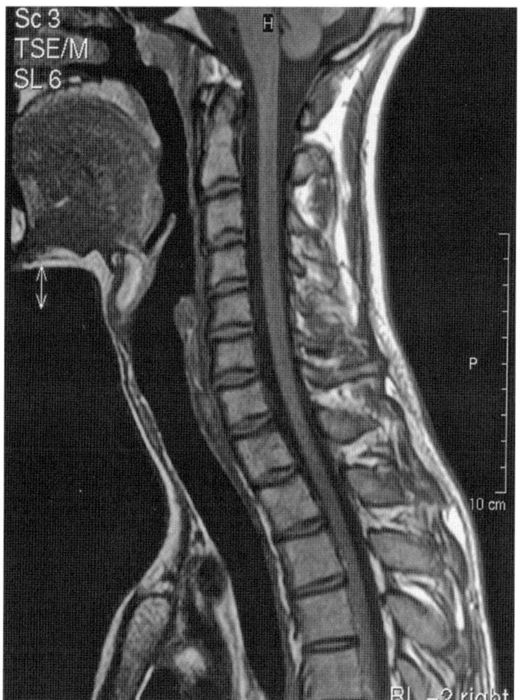

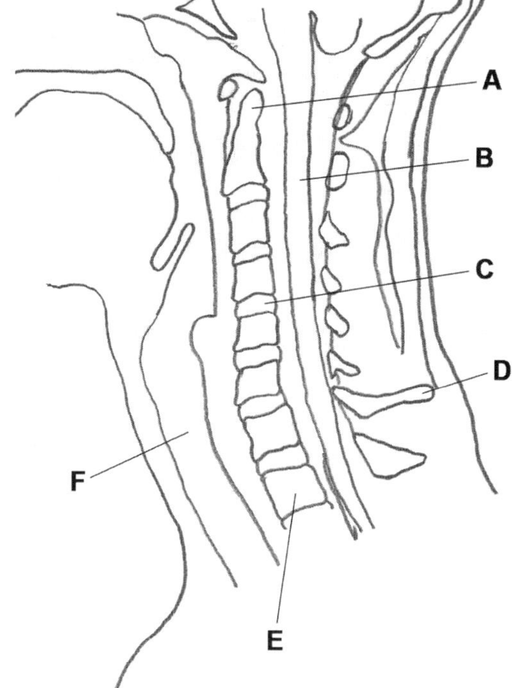

Fig. 1.1. Midline sagittal T1-weighted image of the normal cervical spine obtained with a turbo spin echo (TSE) sequence. Homogeneous appearance of the vertebral marrow. The intervertebral discs are of normal height and nearly isointense to bone. The spinal cord has slightly higher signal intensity relative to the darker cerebrospinal fluid (CSF). A thin layer of soft tissue is depicted anterior to the spine at the level of the epipharynx and pharynx. The soft-tissue-signal structure anterior to the C5 vertebral body represents the proximal portion of the esophagus directly below the glottis. **A** dens axis, **B** spinal cord, **C** C4-5 intervertebral disc, **D** C7 spinous process, **E** T1 vertebral body, **F** trachea

Fig. 1.2. Sagittal T2-weighted TSE image of the normal cervical spine obtained with presaturation of anterior soft tissue structures to eliminate motion artifacts caused by swallowing. The CSF is markedly hyperintense relative to the cord. The vertebral marrow is homogeneous and of similar signal intensity as on T1-weighted images. The CSF appears somewhat inhomogeneous due to pulsation artifacts. The intervertebral discs are of normal height and exhibit some inhomogeneity in signal intensity due to variable fluid content. The posterior neck muscles are clearly seen as low-signal-intensity structures surrounded by fatty tissue

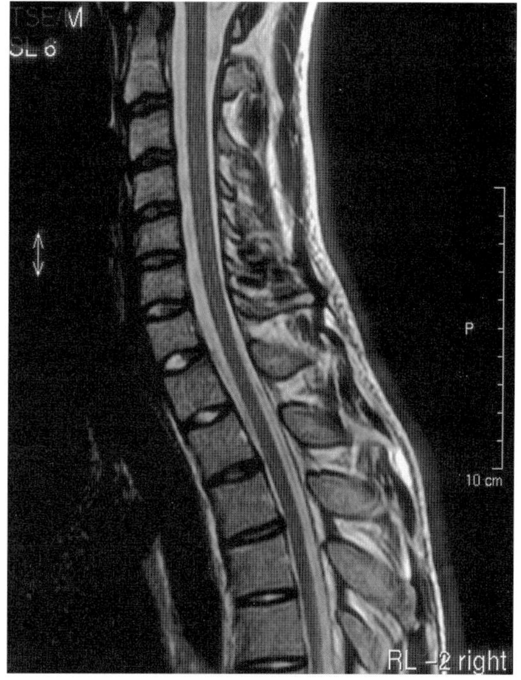

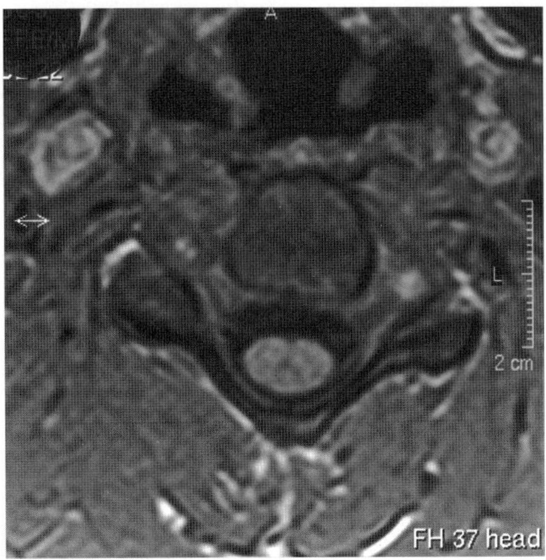

Fig. 1.3. Axial T1-weighted TSE image of the cervical spine through the C4-5 level. There is good visualization of both C5 neural foramina. The spinal nerve roots exiting anteriorly at an angle of about 45° are not very well appreciated on sagittal images. Within the foramina the nerve roots and spinal nerves are seen as low-signal-intensity structures in the bright fatty tissue. The spinal cord has an oval configuration and is well defined by its high signal intensity relative to the surrounding CSF. The posterior portions of the vertebral arch are depicted as delicate bony structures outlined by a dark rim of cortical bone. The vessels are ill-defined relative to surrounding soft tissue

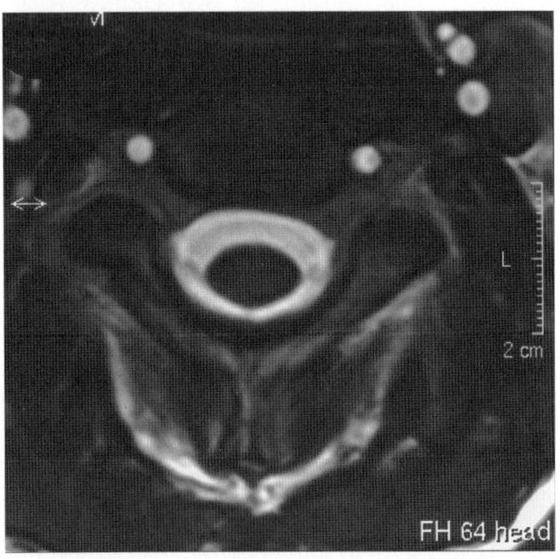

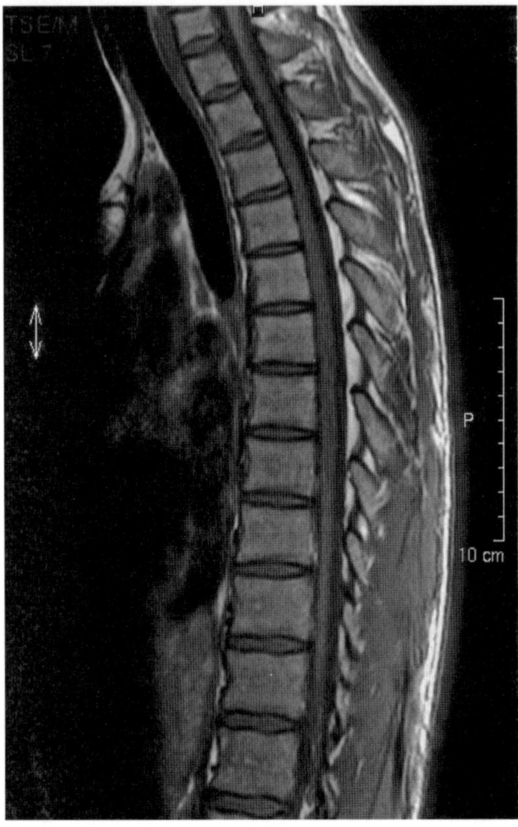

Fig. 1.5. Sagittal T1-weighted image of the thoracic region. Reliable identification of the individual thoracic vertebrae is possible only on images that also visualize portions of the cervical or lumbar spine. The long spinous process at the top is that of C7 (prominent vertebra), thus the spinal region shown extends from C7-T1 to the mid-L2 level. The signal intensities of the different structures are the same as in the cervical region. The epidural fatty tissue posterior to the dural sac is visualized more clearly. The black structure extending down to the T6 level in front of the spine is the air-filled trachea

Fig. 1.4. Axial T2-weighted image of the cervical spine through the C3-4 level obtained with a gradient echo (GRE) sequence. There is good differentiation of the bright CSF and dark, homogeneous spinal cord. Note the bright vessel signal, which is typical of GRE sequences

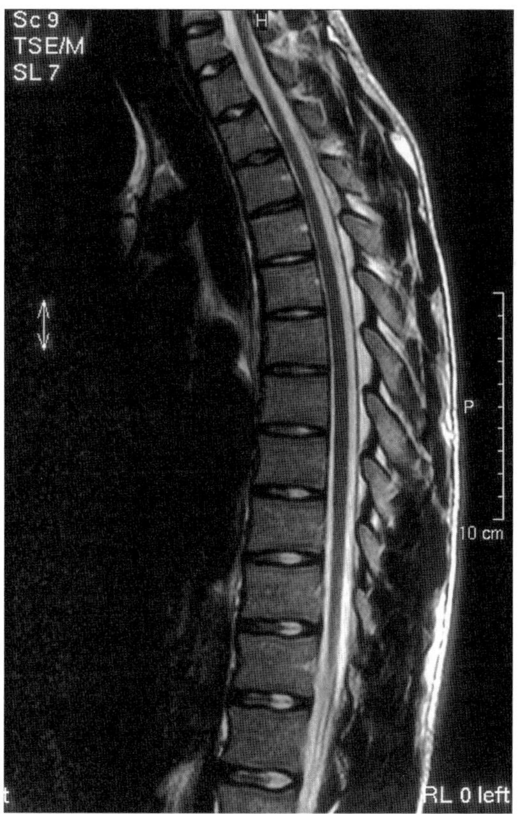

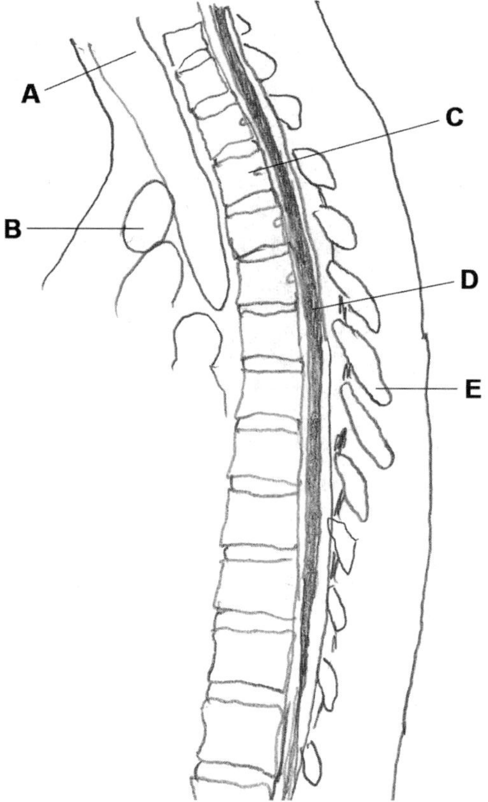

Fig. 1.6. Sagittal T2-weighted image of the thoracic region from C7-T1 to mid-L2. Normal signal intensities of the vertebrae, spinal cord, and soft tissue. Fat and CSF are of the same signal intensity and are separated only by a thin dark line, the dura. **A** trachea, **B** supra-aortic vessels, **C** T3 vertebra, **D** spinal cord, **E** spinous process

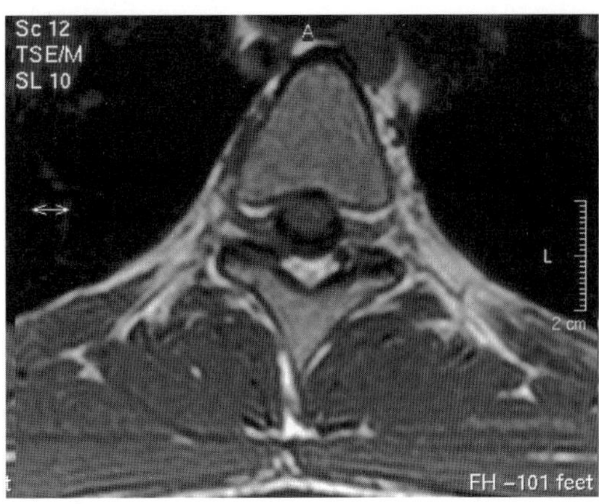

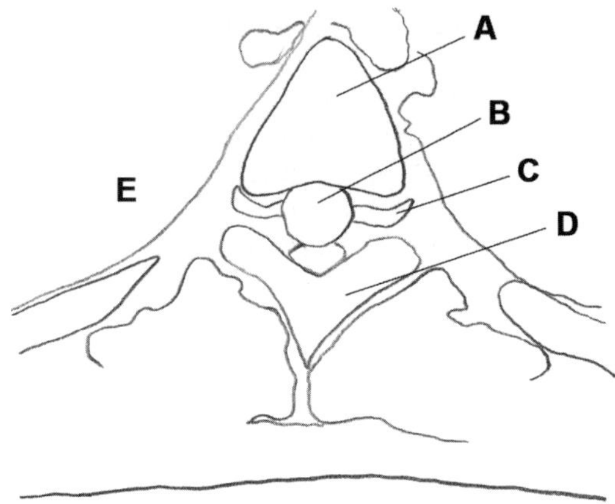

Fig. 1.7. Axial T1-weighted image of the thoracic spine at the level of the T8-9 neural foramina. In relation to the transverse diameter, the anteroposterior diameter of the thoracic vertebral bodies is greater than that of the cervical vertebrae. The nerve roots emerge at an angle of approximately 90°. Within the foramina, the nerve roots are identified by their low signal relative to the bright fatty tissue. The extensor and other back muscles are seen as low-signal-intensity structures relative to fatty tissue in the individual muscle compartments and fasciae. The black areas to the right and left of the vertebral body are the air-filled lungs, which emit no signal. **A** T8 vertebral body, **B** dural sac, **C** left T8 nerve root, **D** vertebral arch/spinous process, **E** lung

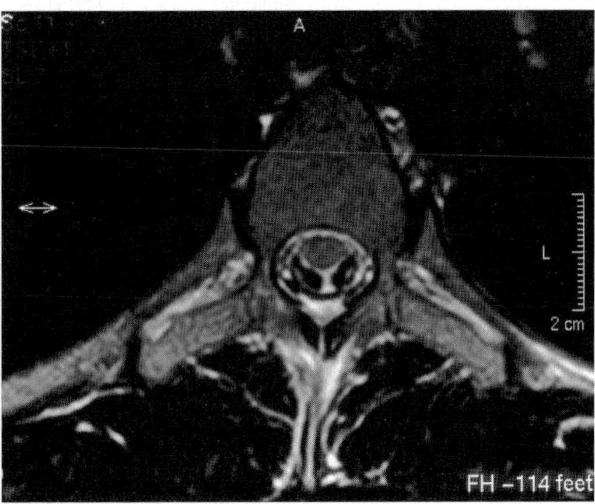

Fig. 1.8. Axial T2-weighted image of the thoracic spine through the T9 level. The pedicles above the neural foramina and the transverse processes are depicted with normal bone signal. The costotransverse joints and portions of the ribs are clearly visible next to the vertebral body and transverse processes. The elongated areas of reduced signal intensity seen in the CSF posterolateral to the cord represent pulsation artifacts

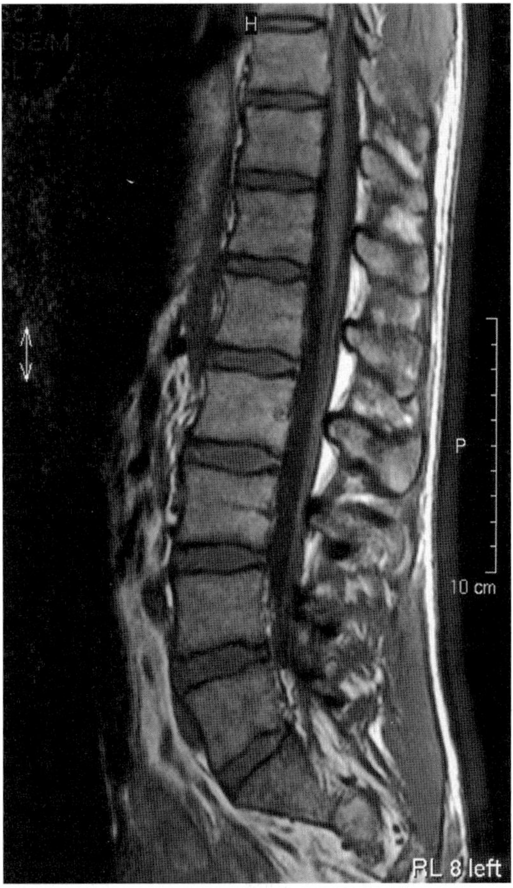

Fig. 1.9. Midline sagittal T1-weighted image of the lumbar spine from T9-10 through S2. The conus medullaris is identified as a slight enlargement of the cord at the T11-12 level. The more delicate nerve fibers of the cauda equina are seen below the conus. Normal appearance and signal intensities of the intervertebral discs and bone

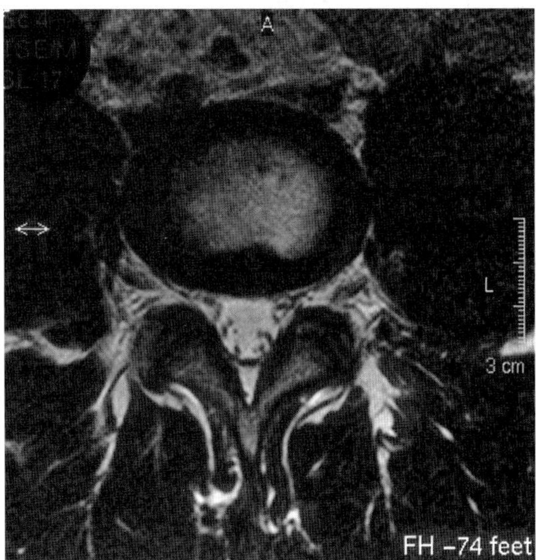

Fig. 1.10. Axial T2-weighted image through the L4-5 level. The neural foramina are oriented anteriorly at an angle of approximately 80°. The facet processes extend posteriorly at an angle of about 45%. The width of the foramina at this level is delimited posteriorly by the facet joints and antero-medially by the disc/L5 endplate. The structures seen posterior to the facet joints are the posterior elements including the spinous process of the L4 vertebra

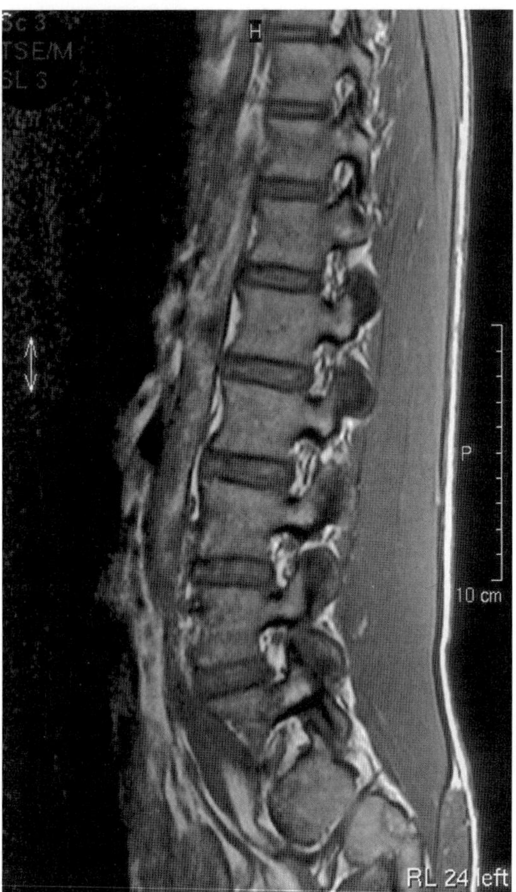

Fig. 1.11. Left parasagittal T1-weighted image of the lumbar spine at the level of the neural foramina. The foramina have an oval configuration with a greater superoinferior diameter. They mostly contain fat in which the spinal nerve roots are discernible as low-signal-intensity punctate structures, typically located in the upper third. The abdominal aorta is seen anterior to the lumbar spine, roughly from T12 through L3-4, as an inhomogeneous vascular structure of mostly high signal intensity. Posterior to the spine, the strong back extensor muscles are depicted as a wide band of intermediate signal intensity beneath the subcutaneous fatty tissue layer

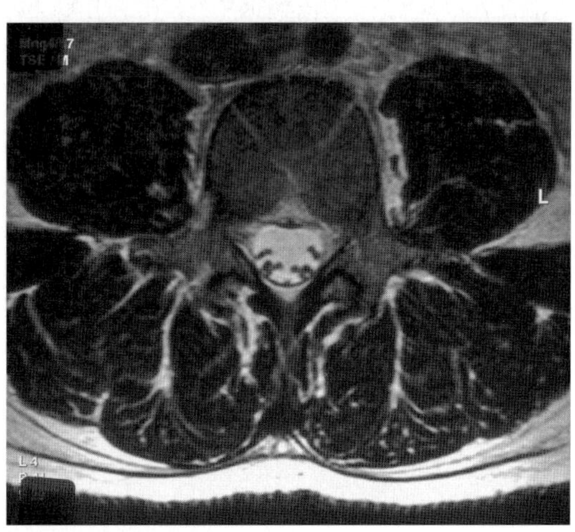

Fig. 1.12. Axial T2-weighted image of the lumbar spine at the L4 level. The Y-shaped hyperintensity in the L4 vertebral body represents venous channels that drain into the epidural veins. The cauda equina fibers are visualized as punctate structures of low signal intensity within the bright CSF. The strong psoas muscle is seen to the right and left of the vertebral body. The inferior vena cava is depicted anterior and to the right of the vertebra adjacent to the two proximal common iliac arteries

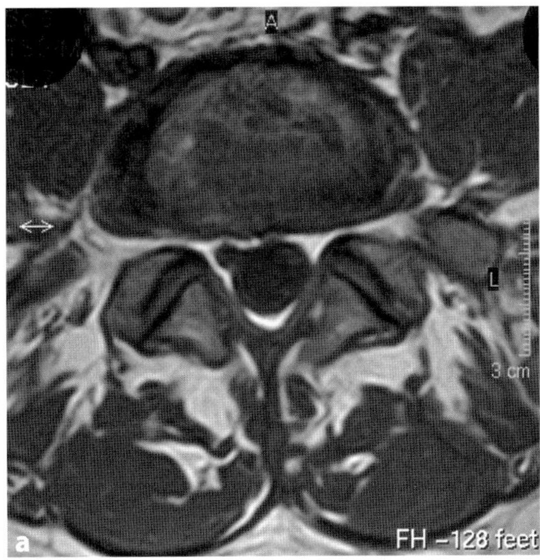

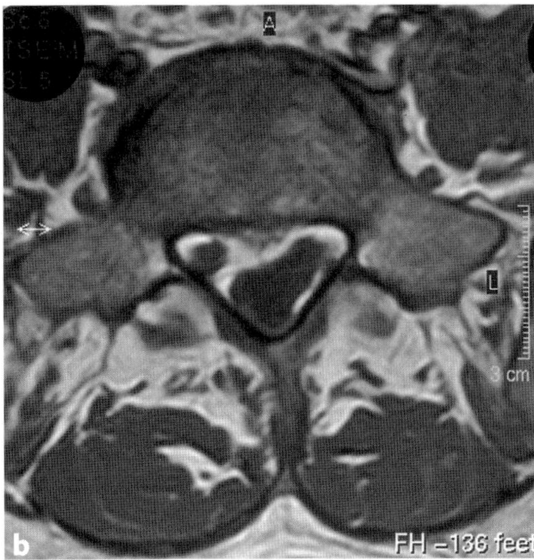

Fig. 1.13a–c. Axial T1-weighted images at the L4-5 and L5 levels. The images illustrate the asymmetrical appearance of the thecal sac resulting from the presence of conjoined L5 and S1 nerve roots on the left

a At this level, only the right L5 nerve root is seen while there is no corresponding root on the left

b The L5 and S1 nerve roots on the left emerge at the same level and are seen as an oval mass

c Both nerve roots are depicted intraspinally to the left of the thecal sac as masses of low signal intensity. On the right, only the L5 nerve root is visualized while the S1 root about to emerge is seen only as an outpouching of the thecal sac

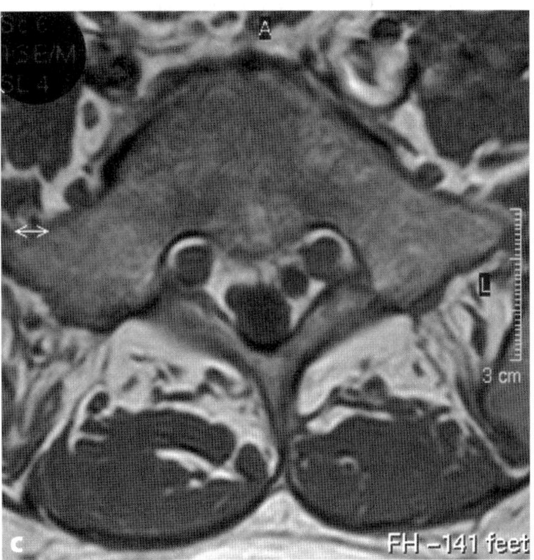

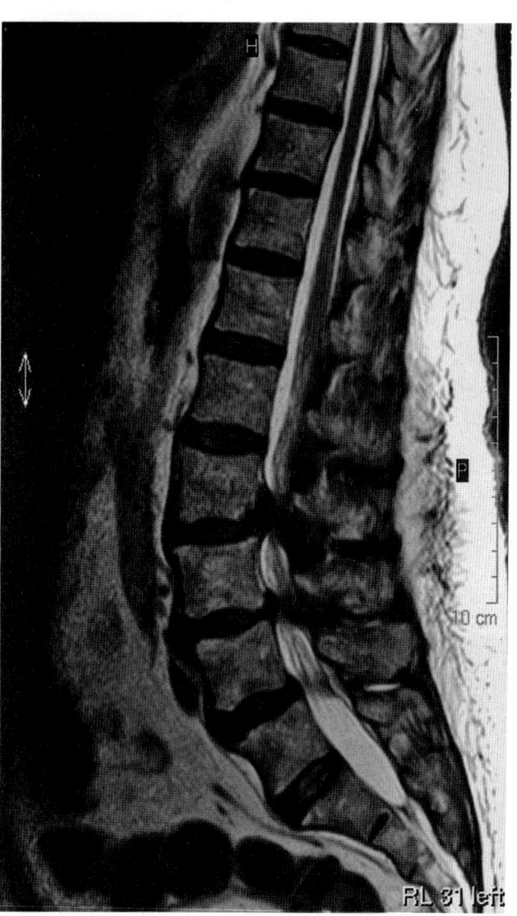

Fig. 1.14. Sagittal T2-weighted image of the lumbar spine and thoracolumbar junction. There is lumbarization of S1 and the lowest intervertebral disc is therefore that of the S1-2 segment. In addition, there are marked degenerative changes of the lower lumbar spine with posterior intervertebral disc herniations at the L3-4 and L4-5 levels

2 Congenital and Developmental Anomalies

2.1 Spinal Meningeal Cysts

The following types are distinguished according to Nabors

Type I	spinal extradural meningeal cysts without spinal nerve root fibers
Type Ia	extradural meningeal cysts
Type Ib	occult intrasacral meningoceles
Type II	spinal extradural meningeal cysts with spinal nerve root fibers
Type III	spinal intradural meningeal cysts (meningeal diverticula)

Pathoanatomy and Pathophysiology

Congenital arachnoid cysts develop from diverticula of the arachnoid mater and communicate with the subarachnoid space. However, a direct communication may not be seen on MRI in all cases. Arachnoid cysts increase in size by a valve mechanism.

Intradural arachnoid cysts most commonly occur in the thoracic spine but may also be found in the lumbar or cervical region. They are lined with arachnoidal cells (type III cysts).

Extradural arachnoid cysts without nerve root elements: type I cysts.

A disorder of secondary neurulation may give rise to a so-called terminal ventricle, a saclike expansion of the central canal of the spinal cord within the conus medullaris.

Extradural meningeal cysts with nerve root fibers (type II, Tarlov cysts) arise from the dorsal ganglion between the arachnoid membrane of the dorsal nerve root (perineurium) and the outer layer of the pia (endoneurium). These cysts are typically multiple and communicate with the subarachnoid space. They often expand the intervertebral foramina and cause smooth erosion of the posterior surface of the vertebral body.

MR Technique

Spinal meningeal cysts can be detected on MR images in all three planes (sagittal, coronal, and axial) and are typically found incidentally (Figs. 2.1–2.14).

MR Findings

Spinal meningeal cysts are depicted on T2-weighted images as sharply demarcated lesions with fluid signal along the course of the spinal nerve roots. The cysts do not enhance after contrast administration. Long-standing cysts may expand the surrounding bony structures (neural foramina).

Clinical Significance

Extradural cysts present with signs of spinal cord compression.

There is controversy about the clinical relevance of Tarlov cysts. Such cysts are often detected incidentally and it is often difficult to establish an association between a patient's clinical symptoms and the cyst. Symptoms are due to other changes in most cases and only very few patients require surgical management.

MR Pitfalls

Meningeal cysts must be differentiated from synovial cysts of the facet joints, which may have the same signal intensity but typically attach to the adjacent articular cavity.

2.2 Bony Malformations

Pathomechanism

Malformations of the bony spine or a spinal segment may be formally classified as:

- segmentation anomalies,
- fusion anomalies,
- defects (formation anomalies), and
- mixed forms (undifferentiated).

The spinal column is derived from the middle layer of the three primary germ layers of the embryo (mesoderm), more specifically from the paraxial mesoderm.

The axial mesoderm develops to form the notochord, thereby defining the longitudinal axis of the body.

So-called somites are paired, blocklike masses that form in the paraxial mesoderm and are arranged segmentally alongside the neural tube, thereby giving rise to a metameric arrangement. Functionally, each somite consists of a so-called dermomyotome (developing into skeletal muscles and connective tissue) and a sclerotome (developing into vertebrae and ribs). Thus, each mesodermal somite gives rise to a spinal motion segment comprising an intervertebral disc and two facet joints (except for the junctional regions) and the adjacent bony structures. The future vertebrae (vertebral body, pedicles, and laminae) form by resegmentation of the somites, which separate into two halves. These original halves then unite with adjacent half segments in such a way that the lower half of one old segment joins with the upper half of the old segment below, forming the primitive vertebra. In this way, the future spinal segments are shifted by half a segment relative to their original metameric arrangement. The development of a normal bony spine relies on both undisturbed horizontal fusion of the paired protovertebral segments (in the regions of the vertebral bodies and arches) and undisturbed vertical fusion.

2.3 Hemivertebra, Wedge Vertebra, Butterfly Vertebra, and Hemimetameric Segmental Shift

Pathoanatomy

Congenital anomalies of the vertebrae may range from mild wedge deformity to complete absence.

Complete absence of a vertebral body is extremely rare, while variable degrees of incomplete development are rather common. There is controversy about the existence of anterior hemivertebrae.

A rudimentary vertebral body may show partial or complete fusion with one or both of its neighbors and the intervening disc may be hypoplastic.

Hemimetameric segmental shift, or segmental displacement, is defined as the presence of two contralateral hemivertebrae which may be separated by one or more normal vertebrae.

As with other vertebral defects, the different forms of rudimentary vertebrae that have just been outlined are often associated with other congenital anomalies (diastema, tethered cord, condylar hyperplasia, basilar impression, and others).

Sagittal cleft vertebral bodies are attributed to the presence of separate ossification centers in the two paired chondrification centers. Similar clefts have also been found in the anterior arch of the atlas.

Sagittal clefts may be complete or incomplete. An incomplete vertebral cleft may affect either the anterior or the posterior portion of the vertebral body. More commonly, there are two notches, one in the superior and one in the inferior endplate, giving rise to the typical butterfly appearance on radiographs.

Pathomechanism

Vertebral anomalies such as hemivertebrae are classified as formation defects while hemimetameric segmental shift, based on current understanding, is attributable to deranged resegmentation of the sclerotomes into vertebrae during early embryonic development.

Butterfly vertebrae result from horizontal fusion defects.

MR Technique

Hemivertebrae and wedge vertebrae are best appreciated on coronal and sagittal images but secondary scoliosis/kyphosis, which is present in the majority of cases, may preclude full evaluation of the spine on a single sagittal image. MRI is performed with T1- and T2-weighted sequences with T2-weighted images often providing a better overview of anatomy in children.

MR Findings

Hemivertebrae/wedge vertebrae have the normal bone marrow signal that varies with the ratio of fat to red marrow. The different vertebral anomalies – hemivertebra, wedge vertebra, and butterfly vertebra – can be distinguished on the basis of their characteristic shapes. Oblique axial images angled parallel to the intervertebral disc space are usually helpful in obtaining true axial images of the vertebral body (Figs. 2.15–2.17).

MR Pitfalls

In most cases, the patient's history will help differentiate congenital vertebral anomalies from posttraumatic vertebral defects. Adequate evaluation of the shape and size of abnormal vertebrae and their arrangement requires careful selection of sagittal and axial slices and images obtained in oblique axial orientation.

Clinical Significance

Abnormal vertebrae may contain large amounts of cartilage due to delayed ossification. In such cases, MRI can diagnose true vertebral deformities even before the completion of growth.

Associated anomalies must be excluded before surgery (basilar impression, diastematomyelia), especially in patients with formation defects of the vertebrae.

Lateral hemivertebrae may lead to congenital mechanical scoliosis, which differs from other forms of scoliosis in that torsion is minimal. Kyphosis may develop when only the posterior portion of a vertebra is present. The smaller the size of the residual vertebral body, the more severe the expected kyphotic or scoliotic deformity. This is why very early surgical correction (in infancy) may be required when the residual vertebral body is reduced to half or less of its normal size. This holds true especially for posterior hemivertebrae since short kyphotic curves (unlike scoliotic deformities) virtually always compromise the spinal canal and bear the risk of later damage to neural structures. In such cases, a wedge vertebra acts as an anterior hypomochlion.

Differentiation of a sagittal cleft vertebra from a sagittal burst fracture is usually straightforward on radiographs and no additional modalities such as MRI are necessary.

The examiner should also look for associated malformations (e.g. abdominal or urogenital).

An isolated sagittal cleft vertebra does not require treatment.

2.4 Klippel-Feil Syndrome

This condition was first described by Klippel and Feil in 1912 and is characterized by shortness of the neck resulting from complete or incomplete fusion of multiple or all cervical vertebrae. The number of cervical vertebrae may also be reduced. The syndrome is typically associated with other anomalies such as Sprengel's deformity, cervical ribs and other rib anomalies, lipoma and angioma in the posterior neck, cervical spina bifida, congenital scoliosis and kyphosis, and basilar impression.

Pathomechanism

Developmental disorder (malsegmentation) inherited as an autosomal dominant trait.

MR Technique

The cervical anomalies associated with Klippel-Feil syndrome are best seen on sagittal and coronal T1- and T2-weighted images. Axial images are less important. Additional sagittal and coronal T2-weighted images with fat saturation are useful to evaluate adjacent discs for signs of osteochondrosis and degenerative changes of the inferior and superior endplates. Fat-suppressed images are more sensitive in demonstrating bone marrow edema typically present in Klippel-Feil syndrome.

MR Findings

MRI shows the extent of fusion of the cervical vertebrae and other changes such as degeneration of preserved disc spaces and disc herniation, which are more common in patients with Klippel-Feil syndrome. Moreover, patients with synostosis of two or more cervical segments also have a higher incidence of other deformities (platybasia, syringomyelia, encephalocele, facial and cranial asymmetry, and Sprengel's deformity in about 25-40% of cases).

Coronal and axial images may fail to show fusion of the posterior elements, which is best appreciated on sagittal images.

MR Pitfalls

Posttraumatic syringomyelia with bony changes may resemble the cervical deformities seen in Klippel-Feil syndrome.

Clinical Significance

In most patients, conventional radiographs are sufficient to diagnose Klippel-Feil syndrome. MRI has a role in identifying the underlying cause in infants presenting with torticollis.

There are no effective therapeutic approaches to correct the unnatural position of the head and limited range of motion. Nevertheless, therapeutic measures may occasionally be indicated if the deformities cause neurologic deficits (cervical spinal canal stenosis, syringomyelia, basilar impression).

2.5 Atlantoaxial Instability and Basilar Impression

MR Technique

Sagittal and axial T1- and T2-weighted images.

MR Findings

Atlantoaxial Instability

Atlantoaxial instability is characterized by increased mobility at the junction between the atlas and the axis. It is defined as an atlantoaxial distance greater than 3 mm in adults and greater than 4 mm in children. Spinal compression myelopathy may occur when the distance is 10 mm or greater.

The atlantoaxial distance can be measured on axial and sagittal images, while concomitant rupture of the annular ligament can only be detected on axial images. Rheumatoid arthritis is characterized by inflammatory tissue in the widened joint space, which shows enhancement on postcontrast images. Erosion of the dens is identified by an altered signal and shape on sagittal T1- and T2-weighted images. Myelomalacia is indicated by areas of increased signal within the spinal cord on T2-weighted images.

The MR appearance of atlantoaxial instability is illustrated in Figs. 2.18 to 2.20. In the example shown, there is marked narrowing of the spinal canal at the C2 level due to anterior displacement of the skull.

Basilar Impression

Projection of the dens tip more than 5 mm above a line connecting the dorsal edge of the hard palate and the posterior border of the foramen magnum (Chamberlain's line) constitutes basilar impression (Figs. 2.21 and 2.22).

MR Pitfalls

Platybasia is also associated with occipitalization of the dens axis (Fig. 2.23) but is a distinct entity. By definition, platybasia exists if the angle between the anterior base of skull and the clivus is greater than 140 degrees (normal range, 125 to 140 degrees).

2.6 Os Odontoideum

Pathoanatomy and Pathophysiology

Os odontoideum is an anomalous bone above a hypoplastic dens that is not attached to the atlas and may occasionally show incomplete fusion with the clivus. It is considered a congenital anomaly, but some authors attribute this condition to a missed dens fracture in infancy.

Os odontoideum may be asymptomatic or present with symptoms in patients with concomitant atlantoaxial instability. This constellation is more common in conjunction with trisomy 21, Klippel-Feil syndrome, or calcifying chondrodystrophy. Instability is due to laxity of the cruciate ligament. Soft tissue forming around an os odontoideum has a similar morphologic appearance on MR images as pannus tissue and may impinge on the spinal cord.

MR Technique

Sagittal and coronal T1- and T2-weighted images and T2 STIR images.

MR Findings

MRI demonstrates an oval or round ossicle with a smooth border. Both the ossicle and dens are imaged with normal bone marrow signal surrounded by a cortical layer of low signal intensity (Fig. 2.24).

MR Pitfalls

Os odontoideum must be differentiated from acute fractures of the dens, which are characterized by the presence of sharp-edged, matching fragments with an altered signal of the fracture margins. In contrast, os odontoideum is typically oval in configuration with smooth borders, and there are no associated soft tissue or spinal cord injuries.

Clinical Significance

Symptoms may first occur after trauma. Patients with incidentally detected os odontoideum and without signs of instability or clinical symptoms should undergo regular clinical follow-up. Posterior instability is treated with C1-2 fusion.

While MRI is not the method of choice for diagnosing os odontoideum, it is indispensable for identifying cervical cord impingement in patients without clinical signs of myelopathy.

2.7 Block Vertebra with Disc Atresia

Pathoanatomy

Congenital block vertebrae are characterized by the partial or complete fusion of two or more adjacent vertebrae due to failure of vertebral segmentation. The intervening disc is rudimentary or absent. When there is incomplete fusion, the affected vertebral bodies are usually normal in shape and height. In complete fusion, deficient growth leads to reduced height, narrow sagittal diameter, and concave anterior configuration. If the corresponding vertebral arches, articular processes, and spinous processes are not fused or if fusion is confined to anterior vertebral portions, affected patients have short kyphotic curves. The rudimentary discs often show calcification on radiographs. In contrast, unilateral failure of segmentation (unilateral unsegmented bar) causes congenital scoliosis.

Pathomechanism

Fusion of one or more vertebrae is attributed to the reduced expression of the Pac-1 gene, a segmentation gene of the family of developmental control genes which is assumed to ascertain the integrity of the discs and spinal segments during spinal development.

MR Technique

Sagittal and coronal T1- and T2-weighted images (Figs. 2.25–2.27).

Clinical Significance

MRI provides important diagnostic information to differentiate congenital vertebral fusion with rudimentary or absent discs from acquired conditions. Normal appearance of the surrounding soft tissue structures, intact endplates, a reduced sagittal diameter of the vertebral bodies, and a concave anterior vertebral surface suggest a congenital defect. Isolated block vertebrae that do not alter the shape of the vertebral column have no clinical relevance. However, as with loss of mobility in individual spinal segments due to other causes, the changes associated with congenital vertebral fusion can also lead to the development of secondary arthrosis resulting from altered stresses at adjacent levels. Surgical treatment may be required for biomechanical reasons if block vertebra is associated with kyphotic deformity or – in rare cases – if there is clinically significant secondary stenosis of the spinal canal due to a short kyphotic curve.

Congenital scoliosis due to unilateral fusion (unilateral bar) tends to have an unfavorable prognosis and may require early surgical management.

2.8 Split Cord Malformations (Diastematomyelia)

Pathoanatomy and Pathophysiology

Diastematomyelia is a congenital anomaly in which the spinal cord is split into halves. Each hemicord has a pair of ventral and dorsal nerve roots and is contained in its own dural sac. The term diplomyelia refers to the complete duplication of the spinal cord with four pairs of nerve roots in a single dural sac. In contrast to earlier assumptions, these two malformations appear to have a similar embryogenesis, which is why the term split cord malformation should be used for both forms with type I denoting diastematomyelia with a bony spur and type II denoting diplomyelia with a thin fibrous septum. A duplicated or split cord develops if there is dorsal migration and herniation of the endomesenchymal tract into the area of the neural tube. This is why type I split cord malformation may be associated with cleft vertebra (bifid vertebra) or neurenteric cysts of endodermal origin. Whether type I or type II malformation develops, depends on whether the cells of the neural tube split into medial or lateral cell clusters. All split cord malformations have a mesenchymal midline component, either a fibrous strand or vessels coursing along the midline. If the endomesenchymal tract migrates all the way to the skin ectoderm, a dermal sinus will develop with a tract extending from the body surface to the bony spur and hypertrichosis in this area. As a result of migration of the endomesenchymal tract, a broad connection persists between the dura and ectoderm, which explains the coexistence of split cord malformation and open myelomeningocele. In addition, many patients with split cord malformation have associated vertebral anomalies with scoliosis.

MR Technique

Axial T1- and T2-weighted images, which may be supplemented by sagittal and coronal images. GRE sequences are more suitable for demonstrating a bony spicule or septum separating the split or doubled cord. In addition, a CT scan of the affected region may be required.

MR Findings

MR images show the typical appearance of a split spinal cord with tethering and hydromyelia (Figs. 2.28–2.33).

MR Pitfalls

Hydromyelia and syringomyelia may be mistaken for diastematomyelia, especially on sagittal and coronal MR images. This is important to bear in mind particularly because there is an association between diastematomyelia and these two entities.

CT is more reliable in evaluating a bony or connective tissue spur or septum. In many cases, however, it is not possible to differentiate type I and II split cord malformations because images will not show whether one or two separate dural sheaths are present.

Clinical Significance

Skin stigmata on the back should always alert the physician to the possibility of split cord malformation. The clinical symptoms are caused by adhesions and tethering of the cord. Even patients with only mild but progressive symptoms should be operated on before irreversible damage occurs.

2.9 Syringohydromyelia

Pathoanatomy and Pathophysiology

Syringomyelia denotes a pathologic condition characterized by longitudinally oriented CSF cavities within the spinal cord. The term is restricted to this condition and should not be used to designate similar entities such as cysts with a high protein content (e.g. tumor cysts), a terminal ventricle, or residues of the central canal occasionally seen on MR images. The term hydromyelia refers to the cystic dilatation of the ependyma-lined central canal by CSF. However, the syrinx may dissect into the parenchyma of the spinal cord and its original connection with the central canal may disappear. Moreover, the type of lining is also not a reliable criterion to distinguish syringomyelia and hydromyelia. Because of these difficulties, the term syringohydromyelia has been introduced as a convenient term to refer to both entities.

A distinction is made between communicating and noncommunicating syringomyelia, depending on whether the syrinx cavity has a connection to the fourth ventricle. Only 10% of the lesions are of the communicating type. Communicating syringomyelia is often associated with hydrocephalus or complex malformations of the posterior cranial fossa such as Chiari II or Dandy-Walker cysts.

The exact pathomechanism underlying the occurrence of syringomyelia is not clear and various theories have been advanced. Two popular explanations are the hydrodynamic theory, proposing that syringomyelia results from a "water hammer"-like transmission of pulsatile CSF pressure, and a theory that assumes a differential between intracranial and spinal pressure caused by a valvelike action at the foramen magnum. The second of these theories does not adequately account for the occurrence of noncommunicating syrinx cavities.

A further mechanism has been proposed to explain syringomyelia associated with malformations at the craniocervical junction. Here it is assumed that CSF is forced into the spinal canal through perivascular spaces as a result of pulsation-related pressure differences in the subarachnoid space. This is also the preferred mechanism to explain syringomyelia developing in the presence of posttraumatic adhesions. In the past, posttraumatic syringomyelia used to be interpreted as residual intramedullary hematoma. Moreover, this mechanism can also account for the development of syrinx cavities after infarction or intramedullary bleeding.

Syringomyelia is present in about 65% of patients with Arnold-Chiari I malformation, and it is assumed that narrowing of the subarachnoid space at the craniocervical junction is responsible for this association. The factors contributing to partial or complete obstruction of the subarachnoid space around the medulla oblongata with subsequent development of a syrinx in patients with Chiari I malformation are platybasia, basilar invagination, and a small bony posterior cranial fossa. Syringobulbia is the extension of syrinx cavities into the medulla oblongata.

MR Technique

Sagittal and axial T1- and T2-weighted images. Contrast-enhanced T1-weighted images should be acquired to exclude a tumor.

MR Findings

Demonstration of a syrinx cavity in the spinal cord – whether in the cervical or the lumbar region – should prompt an MRI examination of the entire CNS. In patients scheduled for surgery, it is recommended to assess CSF flow on an electrocardiography-triggered pulse sequence.

MR images rarely enable differentiation of hydromyelia (dilatation of the central canal by CSF) and syringomyelia (intramedullary fluid collection adjacent to the central canal). Both entities are characterized on MRI by the presence of a longitudinally oriented fluid collection in the spinal cord. The lesion is depicted with CSF signal on axial, sagittal, and coronal images.

Congenital or posttraumatic syringohydromyelia does not show contrast enhancement. Tumor-associated syrinx cavities occur inferior to the tumor. Thus, an intramedullary tumor is suggested if an enhancing lesion is seen at the upper end of a fluid collection on T1-weighted images (Figs. 2.34–2.44).

Clinical Significance

Syringomyelia is characterized by slow clinical progression and the syrinx cavities may exist for years without becoming symptomatic. The aim of surgical management is to correct the assumed underlying mechanism. Decompression of the posterior cranial fossa with enlargement of the cisterna magna is the method of first choice. Attempted correction of the associated deformity with decompression is also the primary operative approach in patients with posttraumatic syringomyelia and adhesions, tethered cord, or spinal deformity. Shunting of the syrinx to the subarachnoid space should only be performed in cases where these surgical measures fail or are not an option. The size and extent of a syrinx cavity do not always correlate with a patient's clinical symptoms.

2.10 Spinal Dysraphism

Classification

A distinction is made between open and occult spinal dysraphism. Myelomeningocele is the most common major form of open spinal dysraphism. The second category encompasses meningocele, dermal sinus, lipoma, thickened filum terminale, split cord malformations, and neurenteric cysts.

Clinically, this heterogeneous group of neural tube defects is characterized by tethering of the cord. A subgroup comprises the different forms of lumbosacral agenesis (e.g. terminal myelocystocele) associated with complex urogenital and intestinal anomalies.

Pathoanatomy and Pathomechanism

Dysraphic malformations result from deranged neurulation. The neural tube fails to close and persists as a neural plate (so-called placode). As a result, the superficial ectoderm cannot separate from the neural ectoderm and remains in the lateral position. The skin therefore also develops laterally, leaving a midline defect. Moreover, the mesenchyma is prevented from migrating around the neural tube, resulting in concomitant midline defects of the vertebral arches, muscles, and ligaments. The placode is surrounded from both sides by an outpouching of the anterior arachnoid membrane. Motor and sensory nerve roots emerge from the ventral surface of the placode. The dura mater is preserved ventrally while its dorsal portion blends into the skin at the edge of the defect. Hence, the meninges and placode are contiguous with the skin. An indentation in the dorsal surface of the placode corresponds to the open central canal at the site of the defect. The central canal above the defect is often widened, and extensive hydromyelia may be present in severe cases.

Over 90% of patients with myelomeningocele have associated deformities of the brain stem, cerebellum, and the upper cervical spinal cord. This complex of deformities is known as Chiari type II malformation and may range from slight rostral displacement of the spinal cord with the upper cervical nerve roots coursing cranially to severe forms with inferior displacement and kinking of the medulla oblongata behind the upper cervical cord, downward displacement of portions of the fourth ventricle and cerebellum into the spinal canal, and deformity of the mesencephalic tectum. By the age of 10, scoliosis is present in about 80% of patients with myelomeningocele, in half of them with a Cobb angle of over 20°. Scoliosis is due to associated vertebral body defects and neuromuscular disorders. Other concurrent conditions include increased lumbar lordosis, thoracic kyphosis, and lumbar kyphosis.

MR Technique

Imaging using T2- and T1-weighted pulse sequences is performed in three planes to determine the site and extent of the deformity. More specifically, MRI serves to evaluate the size and content of the neurocele and to exclude concomitant defects. In patients scheduled for surgery, MR findings provide the basis for planning the surgical approach. In the postoperative follow-up, MRI is performed to exclude retethering and iatrogenic cord ischemia.

MR Findings

MR images show dysraphic lesions of the spinal cord, bony spine, and soft tissues as well as intracranial deformities (Figs. 2.45–2.47).

MR Pitfalls

Confirmation or exclusion of postoperative retethering of the cord may be impaired by the fact that it is often difficult to distinguish strands of scar tissue and nerve roots.

Clinical Significance

Spinal MRI is not required in the primary management of patients with myelomeningocele and merely serves to document the local findings. Patients who show posttherapeutic deterioration of neurologic deficits should undergo repeat MRI to confirm or exclude retethering as a cause of progressive scoliosis. Other lesions that must be excluded are progressive epidermoid tumors, hydromyelia, and arachnoid cysts.

2.11 Tethered Cord

Pathoanatomy and Pathophysiology

Tethered cord is a condition in which the spinal cord is attached to an immobile structure such as the dura, skin, lipoma, or bony vertebral canal.

Between 8 and 25 weeks of gestation, the conus medullaris "ascends" because the bony vertebral column grows faster longitudinally than the spinal cord. As a result of these differences in growth velocity, the conus medullaris terminates at the L2-3 intervertebral disc level at birth and reaches its final height at L1-2 at the age of one.

Pathophysiologically, lesions or dysfunction more commonly affect the spinal cord than the caudal nerve roots. Clinical symptoms are often precipitated by growth spurs in children and activities involving sudden stretching of the spinal column in adults.

MR Technique

Sagittal and axial T1- and T2-weighted images.

MR Findings

MR imaging shows thinning and stretching of the conus medullaris and termination below the L2 level.

Also demonstrated is a conspicuously tense filum terminale, often with thickened fibers (Figs. 2.48–2.51).

Clinical Significance

Tethering of the spinal cord is associated with a very heterogeneous group of congenital anomalies. It presents with characteristic clinical symptoms such as sensory deficits, paresis and muscle atrophy of the legs, pain, urinary and rectal dysfunction, and spinal deformities such as kyphoscoliosis. However, the symptoms differ in children and adults. Concurrent lesions in patients with primary tethered cord are dermal sinus, split cord malformation (diastematomyelia), intraspinal tumors, meningocele and meningomyelocele, intraspinal lipoma, dermoids, and epidermoids.

Patients with cord tethering associated with occult spinal dysraphism have a thick and short filum terminale, often with fat infiltration. A filum terminale lipoma is assumed only if the diameter of the filum terminale is increased to over 2 mm. The mere presence of fatty tissue without tethering or clinical symptoms is a normal variant.

The most common causes of secondary tethering are postinfectious adhesions, trauma, and intradural surgery. Secondary tethering differs from primary tethered cord in that the cord is attached at a different level and not by the filum terminale.

2.12 Scoliosis

Anatomy and Pathoanatomy

Scoliosis is the lateral curvature of the spinal column and is typically associated with spinal torsion due to rotation of vertebrae. Among the few forms of scoliosis without a rotational element is scoliosis secondary to lateral hemivertebrae.

The lateral curve and especially the associated torsion lead to typical changes of the paravertebral structures. In the thoracic region, for example, vertebral rotation also includes the ribs, giving rise to a posterior rib hump on the convex side and an anterior hump on the concave side. Other pathoanatomic changes are specific to the etiology of the different types of scoliosis.

Pathomechanism

The pathogenesis of scoliotic deformities is extremely heterogeneous. A basic distinction can be made between structural and nonstructural forms (functional scoliosis, postural anomalies, improper posture). Structural, or fixed, curves are due to vertebral deformities (wedge vertebra). Typical examples of nonstructural, or mobile, scolioses are reactive forms due to pain (e.g. from disc herniation) and compensatory scoliosis (pelvic tilt).

The pathogenesis of structural scoliosis varies with the age of onset (juvenile versus adult onset). Structural scoliosis in children and young adults is typically due to abnormal growth of the bony spine secondary to vertebral defects (see overview below). In contrast, the underlying pathologic process itself causes the deformity in most forms of adult scoliosis (vertebral destruction due to trauma, inflammation, degenerative lumbar scoliosis). About 95% of the structural scolioses occurring in children and juveniles are of the idiopathic type (right convexity of the thoracic spine).

Forms of Scoliosis

- Neuropathic scoliosis, e.g. meningomyelocele
- Myopathic scoliosis, e.g. muscular dystrophy
- Osteopathic scoliosis, e.g. scoliosis due to formation defects
- Scoliosis due to connective tissue disorders, e.g. Marfan's syndrome
- Other symptomatic scolioses
  - e.g. posttraumatic, postinfectious, and actinogenic scolioses
- Idiopathic scolioses

MR Technique

Coronal and sagittal T1- and T2-weighted images. Full evaluation of the spine in patients with scoliotic curves usually requires sequential imaging of individual regions that are similar in orientation.

MR Findings

Bridging osteophytes on the concave side of the curvature are better appreciated on CT scans. On MR images, osteophytic structures are depicted as thin cortical bands of low signal intensity. In most forms of scoliosis, MRI will show mild to severe asymmetries of the vertebral bodies (hemivertebrae). Osteochondrosis of the endplates predominantly involves the concave side. Osteochondrotic changes are isointense with fluid in the acute stage (Modic type 1) and isointense with fat in the chronic stage (Modic type 2). The chronic sclerotic stage (Modic type 3) is characterized by low signal intensity in all sequences. The abnormal stresses associated with scoliotic curves often cause asymmetric enlargement of the facet joints and may lead to stenosis of the spinal canal.

Scoliosis is also associated with a higher risk of disc herniation (Figs. 2.52–2.56).

Clinical Significance

Radiography is the primary diagnostic modality in evaluating patients with scoliosis. MRI is a supplementary tool and mainly serves to demonstrate or exclude concomitant changes in neural structures or the spinal canal (diastema, basilar impression, spina bifida) including the neural foramina. Therefore, MRI is mainly performed in cases where such changes are likely to be encountered (e.g. congenital scoliosis) and when the scoliotic deformity causes clinical symptoms such as pain (reactive scoliosis secondary to vertebral osteoid osteoma). In patients scheduled for surgery, MRI (or CT) findings are helpful in planning the surgical procedure because they enable exact evaluation of vertebral body rotation and assessment of the shape and size of the pedicles. The latter information is important to assess whether the pedicles are suitable as anchorage sites for transpedicular osteosynthesis. However, MRI has no role in the vast majority of patients with clinically and radiographically diagnosed scoliosis.

2.13 Kyphosis

Pathoanatomy

Kyphosis is defined as an abnormally increased posterior convexity of the vertebral column as viewed from the side. Kyphotic deformities of the spine also include loss of normal cervical and lumbar lordosis (hypolordosis).

Multiple wedge deformities of adjacent vertebral bodies and/or intervertebral discs give rise to a smooth kyphotic curve, which must be distinguished from kyphosis with a sharply angled curve (gibbus deformity). Wedge-shaped deformities are shared by all forms of kyphosis, while additional anatomic abnormalities vary with the underlying cause.

Pathogenesis

Apart from congenital defects, any longer-lasting or permanent instability resulting from the loss of anterior support or posterior tension band function (see overview below) will inevitably cause a kyphotic deformity. In the upright posture, the spine is constantly being pulled forward by the weight of the body, exposing all motion segments to a bending force, which can be converted to axial load only by the posterior tension band in conjunction with intact anterior support.

Causes of Kyphosis

- Congenital anomalies (failure of segmentation)
- Formation defects
- Scheuermann's disease
- Paralysis
- Meningomyelocele
- Traumatic damage
- Inflammatory destruction
- Defects secondary to surgery (laminectomy, spondylectomy) or radiotherapy
- Metabolic bone disease (storage diseases, mucolipidosis, Hurler's syndrome)
- Osteochondrodysplasia
- Collagen diseases
- Tumors
- Neurofibromatosis

Clinical Significance

Spinal stenosis due to narrowing of the bony canal or anterior displacement of the spinal cord is much more common in patients with kyphotic deformities than in patients with scoliosis. MRI is currently the most suitable imaging modality for evaluating the anterior, epidural, and subarachnoid reserve space both in the initial diagnostic work-up and follow-up of patients with kyphotic curves. In addition, MRI provides information on intramedullary abnormalities (myelomalacia, syringomyelia).

2.14 Lipomatosis and Lipoma

Pathoanatomy and Pathophysiology

Spinal lipomas are attributed to a developmental disorder caused by the premature focal disjunction of the epidermal and neural ectoderm before closure of the neural tube. As a result, mesenchymal tissue becomes contiguous with the posterior neural tube, which is assumed to induce subsequent differentiation of the mesenchymal tissue into fatty tissue.

Subdural lipomas found beneath an intact dura are also ensheathed by pia mater. The bulk of the mass is usually located posterior to the spinal cord and impinges on it.

Lipoma of the Filum Terminale

The most common form of lipoma of the filum terminale is a lipomyelomeningocele with the fatty mass arising from the dorsal aspect of the cord and extending below the skin. Terminal lipoma is associated with a defect in the dura mater. The subcutaneous fatty mass is apparent at birth. The lesion is covered by intact skin but skin stigmata are often present. The topographic relationship to the nerve roots is variable – the latter may course directly through the lipoma. There is a nearly 100% association of lipomyelomeningocele with tethered cord and termination of the conus medullaris at an abnormal level.

MR Technique

Multiplanar imaging including fat-suppressed sequences encompassing the lumbar, sacral, and coccygeal regions.

MR Findings

MRI shows the extent of spinal lipoma and concomitant defects.

Clinical Significance

MRI is the method of choice to fully evaluate changes in subcutaneous fatty tissue and the topographic relationship of a lipoma to the vertebral canal and spinal cord.

Surgical removal may also be indicated for prophylactic reasons. Complete removal of a lipoma from the conus medullaris region is almost impossible. The major challenge is to prevent retethering of the cord. Based on morphologic MR criteria, it may be very difficult or even impossible to identify postoperative retethering because there will be adherence of neural structures to the dura in virtually all cases. This is why the diagnosis of retethering primarily relies on a patient's clinical course.

2.15 Scheuermann's Disease

Pathoanatomy

Scheuermann's disease, or adolescent kyphosis, is characterized by wedging of one or more adjacent vertebral bodies, scalloping of vertebral endplates, disturbed anterior vertebral growth, and herniation of intervertebral disc tissue into an adjoining vertebra (Schmorl's node). These changes can occur together or alone and involve the middle and lower thoracic spine and the upper lumbar region. Because the vertebral defects (wedging and scalloping) develop during the growth phase, there may be compensatory molding of adjacent vertebrae.

Pathogenesis

The vertebral changes seen in Scheuermann's disease are due to osteochondrosis of the secondary ossification centers of the vertebral bodies (endplate and anular epiphyses). It is still debated whether Schmorl's nodes represent residues of the cartilaginous endplates resulting from circumscribed developmental defects or whether they actually consist of disc tissue extending through gaps in the cartilaginous endplates. A genetic basis is assumed (dominant trait with low penetrance).

MR Technique

The typical lesions occurring in Scheuermann's disease are evaluated on coronal and sagittal T1- and T2-weighted images. Acute changes of vertebral endplates with concomitant edema of the surrounding bone marrow are best seen on fat-saturated T2-weighted images.

The lesions are less prominent on axial images, which must be angled parallel to the endplates of affected vertebral bodies in patients with kyphotic or scoliotic deformities.

MR Findings

Full-blown spinal osteochondrosis, or juvenile kyphosis, is characterized on MRI by the presence of vertebral defects comprising wedging, contour irregularities of the endplates, and narrowing of the disc spaces. The defects most commonly involve the lower thoracic and upper lumbar regions. The slightly increased anteroposterior diameter of the vertebral bodies is best appreciated on sagittal images, which will also demonstrate the loss of the normal lordotic curvature and the severity of kyphotic deformity. Schmorl's nodes are depicted as gaps with marginal sclerosis in the endplates. The herniated disc material typically has a slightly lower signal intensity on T2-weighted images but the signal intensity may also be slightly higher, depending on the age of the herniation. Bone marrow edema around the herniated tissue suggests an acute process (Figs. 2.57–2.61).

MR Pitfalls

Developmental defects of the anterior vertebral bodies may have a similar appearance as in Scheuermann's disease, while wedge deformities and Schmorl's nodes are absent. Bone dystrophies also involve the extremities, which are unaffected in Scheuermann's disease.

Clinical Significance

In rare cases may it be difficult to distinguish Scheuermann's disease from other entities. For example, large destructive tumors, in particular chondrogenic tumors, may resemble large isolated areas of disturbed ossification in Scheuermann's disease.

In such cases, MRI shows concomitant changes of the adjacent vertebral endplates, pronounced reactive marginal sclerosis around the defect, and signs of reactive growth of adjacent vertebrae.

Disc space narrowing with a concomitant defect in an adjacent inferior endplate is also present in spondylodiscitis. In patients with these MRI findings, Scheuermann's disease is suggested if laboratory testing shows normal inflammatory parameters and only mild clinical symptoms are present. The most important distinguishing feature, however, is the visualization of circumscribed, dense zones of sclerosis around the endplate defects on MR images. Sclerosis is absent in florid inflammation and shows diffuse extension into the vertebral body in the presence of a chronic inflammatory process.

It is open whether conservative therapeutic measures aimed at relieving the spine (e.g. specific exercises or a reclination corset) during florid disease will slow down the progression of vertebral wedging and kyphotic deformity.

MRI performed after the acute stage can identify additional typical lesions, thereby contributing to the differentiation of Scheuermann's disease from posttraumatic wedge vertebrae. Most importantly, the microstructure of the cancellous vertebral bone is preserved in Scheuermann's disease.

2.16 Hemangioma

Pathoanatomy

Hemangiomas are capillary or cavernous tumors that are characterized by proliferation of endothelial cells. Vertebral hemangiomas have a characteristic appearance on conventional radiographs (CT scans) resulting from the presence of vertically oriented trabecular bone structures. MRI (and pathohistologic examinations) has shown that the typical radiographic appearance can be caused by two distinct lesions: intraosseous lipoma (the more common variant) and true intraosseous hemangioma. It is not clear whether a hemangioma diagnosed by MRI must be further differentiated into true angioma or congenital angiectatic nevus.

MR Technique

Vertebral hemangioma can be identified on sagittal, coronal, and axial images. T1- and T2-weighted images with fat saturation should be obtained for lesion characterization and differentiation from lipoma.

MR Findings

Vertebral hemangiomas predominantly occur in the lower thoracic and upper lumbar regions and are seen on T1- and T2-weighted images as well-defined, somewhat inhomogeneous, lesions of high signal intensity. Most hemangiomas do not have a mass effect but may sometimes slightly displace and possibly thin cortical structures without disrupting them. A high signal intensity on T1- and T2-weighted images is typical of a hemangioma; differentiation from a lipoma is more reliable on fat-saturated images (Figs. 2.62-2.65).

Clinical Significance

Vertebral hemangiomas typically affect the bodies of the vertebrae and rarely the vertebral arches. They are asymptomatic and cause pathologic fractures only in exceptional cases. There is only little impairment of vertebral stability and no therapy is required in the vast majority of patients.

2.17 Spondylolisthesis

Anatomy and Pathoanatomy

There is no generally accepted pathoanatomic definition of spondylolisthesis. While some authors use the term to designate any forward displacement of a vertebra (and the vertebral segment above it) over another, others use the term only for those forms of forward displacement that are accompanied by a defect of the pars interarticularis (separation or elongation). Nevertheless, most authors who prefer this restricted definition also postulate a subgroup of degenerative spondylolisthesis in which the affected posterior elements are the facet joints rather than the pars.

Types of Spondylolisthesis

- Dysplastic spondylolisthesis
- Isthmic spondylolisthesis
- Degenerative spondylolisthesis
- Secondary spondylolisthesis: anterior displacement of a vertebra
  1. with defect of the pars interarticularis (symptomatic spondylolisthesis: inflammatory, tumorous, generalized bone diseases, etc.)
  2. without defect of the pars interarticularis (luxation fracture, joint destruction, etc.).

Spondylolisthesis in the narrower sense is characterized by specific pathoanatomic features.

The dysplastic type exclusively occurs at the lumbosacral junction. It decompensates in juveniles and is associated with congenital anomalies of the lumbosacral junction (such as synostoses of the facet joints at L5-S1, dysplasia of the articular processes and vertebral arch, dysraphism). The pars interarticularis is either extremely elongated or separated (spondylolysis). Dysplastic spondylolisthesis is associated with more severe kyphosis than isthmic spondylolisthesis, and L5 (wedge-shaped) and S1 (dome-shaped) are deformed.

Isthmic spondylolisthesis may decompensate in young to middle-aged adults. This type typically affects the L5 or L4 vertebra, but rarely higher vertebral segments. Conspicuous dysplasia of the vertebral arches is absent. The slip is less severe (typically grade I or II) than in dysplastic spondylolisthesis. Two subtypes are distinguished based on the defect of the pars interarticularis: subtype I with separation of the pars, which is the more common form, and elongation of the pars (subtype II). Secondary vertebral deformities are rare, while pronounced secondary intervertebral disc degeneration is quite common.

Degenerative spondylolisthesis (also known as pseudospondylolisthesis) occurs in older individuals (beyond 50 years of age) and exclusively involves the fourth lumbar vertebra. Spondylolysis or excessive elongation of the pars interarticularis is absent. There is considerable narrowing of the L4-5 interspace with degenerative changes in the corresponding facet joints. The slip tends to be less pronounced.

Pathomechanism

Dysplastic or isthmic spondylolisthesis develops secondary to posterior tension band dysfunction resulting from elongation or separation of the pars interarticularis. These pars defects occur on the basis of a disproportion between applied load and loading capacity. Dysplastic spondylolisthesis is most likely due to a reduced loading capacity secondary to congenital vertebral defects while excessive stress, possibly in combination with a reduced loading capacity, tends to be the underlying cause of isthmic spondylolisthesis (fatigue fracture due to chronic overload).

Degenerative spondylolisthesis is caused by longstanding instability due to progressive degeneration and narrowing of the disc space with consecutive displacement of ligaments and other stabilizing structures and secondary arthrosis of the facet joints. As a result of this relative instability, the normal forces acting on the spine induce a self-limiting forward slip in the affected motion segment.

MR Technique

Spondylolisthesis is evaluated on sagittal and axial images. Anterior or posterior displacement of one vertebra over another is best appreciated on sagittal images. Since MRI can only be performed in the supine position, additional radiographs are required to evaluate the increase in vertebral displacement during loading with the patient standing/sitting/bending forward.

MR Findings

Identification and evaluation of spondylolysis is often difficult using MRI, and additional radiographs or CT scans may be required to establish the diagnosis.

Displacement of adjacent vertebrae results in an abnormal oval configuration with a greater transverse diameter of the affected neural foramina, which is nicely depicted on sagittal images. Consecutive narrowing of the passage leads to complete loss of the fatty tissue structures surrounding the nerve root as it traverses the foramen. Marginal sclerosis of affected vertebrae may be seen to a variable extent on T1- and T2-weighted images (Figs. 2.66–2.70).

MR Pitfalls

Spondylolysis may be difficult to differentiate from spinal joint hypertrophy, especially when there is normal alignment of the vertebrae.

Clinical Significance

In most patients with spondylolisthesis, surgical correction or other therapeutic measures are required because of secondary neurologic deficits and not because of direct local symptoms associated with malalignment.

Therefore, the primary diagnostic role of MRI in spondylolisthesis is in evaluating the nonosseous structures in the spinal canal and neural foramina. Moreover, in the preoperative diagnostic work-up, MRI serves to evaluate the relationship to great vessels including the vessels anterior to the spine, especially in patients scheduled for thoracolumbar spinal surgery.

The clinical course of dysplastic spondylolisthesis is characterized by early decompensation (in children or young adults) and rapid progression to higher-grade slippage (spondyloptosis), which is associated with a step-off at the lumbosacral junction, compression of nerve structures, and restricted mobility of the lumbar spine.

Patients with isthmic spondylolisthesis typically present with symptoms caused by irritation of the nerve roots exiting the spinal canal at the affected level. Vertebral displacement alters the configuration of the vertebral foramina, which may additionally be reduced in height by secondary disc degeneration. Moreover, there may be narrowing of the foramen by repair processes in the area of the pars interarticularis (inflammatory and synovial granulation tissue or intercalated bone).

The predominant symptoms in degenerative spondylolisthesis are those associated with stenosis of the spinal canal and of the lateral recess. Factors contributing to stenosis are vertebral slippage, posterior bulging of the annulus fibrosus due to the underlying disc degeneration, and additional high-grade narrowing of the posterior spinal canal secondary to progressive segmental arthrosis of the facet joints.

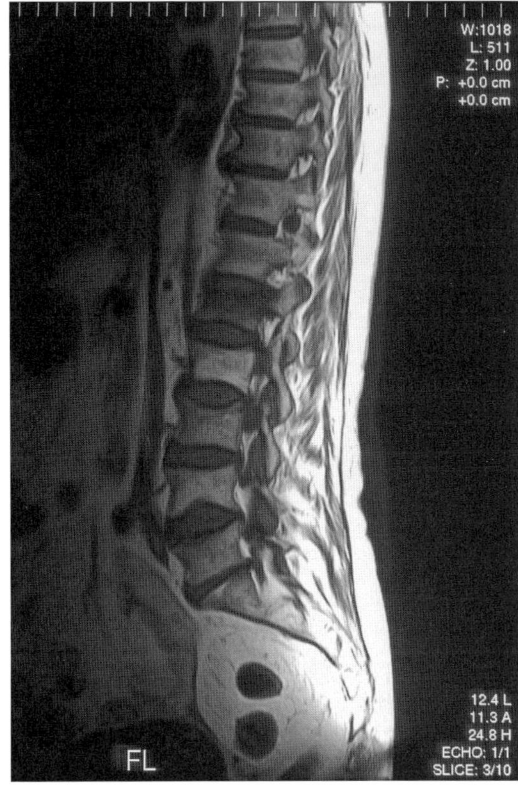

Fig. 2.1. Nerve root cyst. Sagittal T1-weighted image showing a low-signal-intensity lesion in the T11-12 foramen

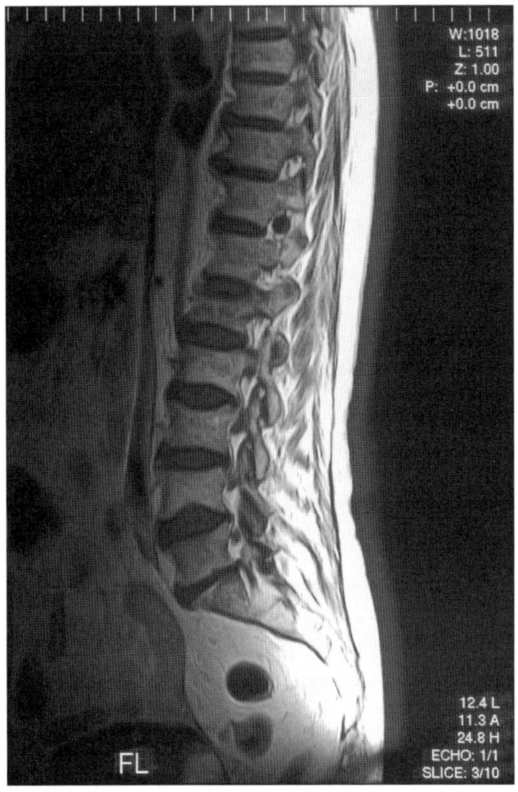

Fig. 2.2. Sagittal T1-weighted image of the cyst after contrast administration. No enhancement of the right intraforaminal cyst

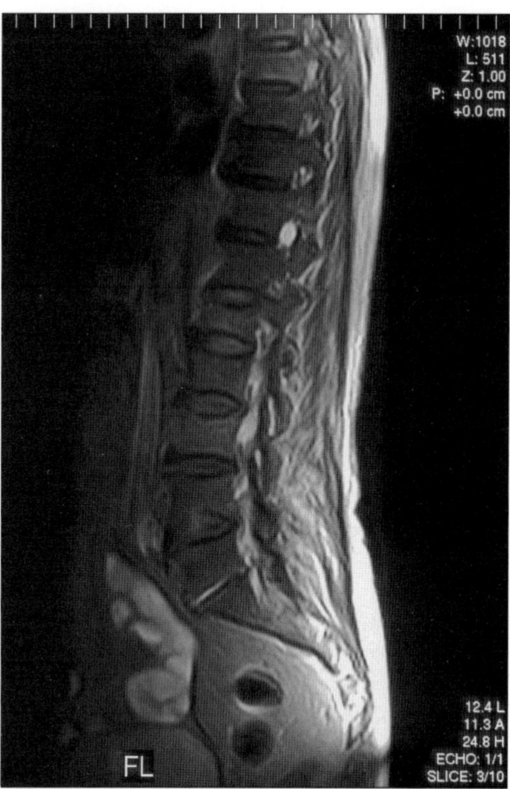

Fig. 2.3. Same patient. Sagittal T2-weighted image with fat saturation showing the nerve root cyst in the right T11-12 foramen with high signal intensity paralleling that of fluid

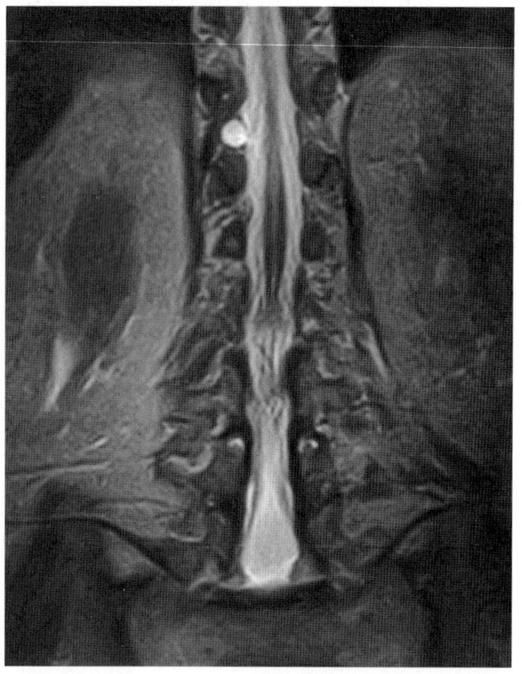

Fig. 2.4. Coronal T2-weighted image with fat saturation depicting the intraforaminal cyst directly below the right T11-12 nerve root

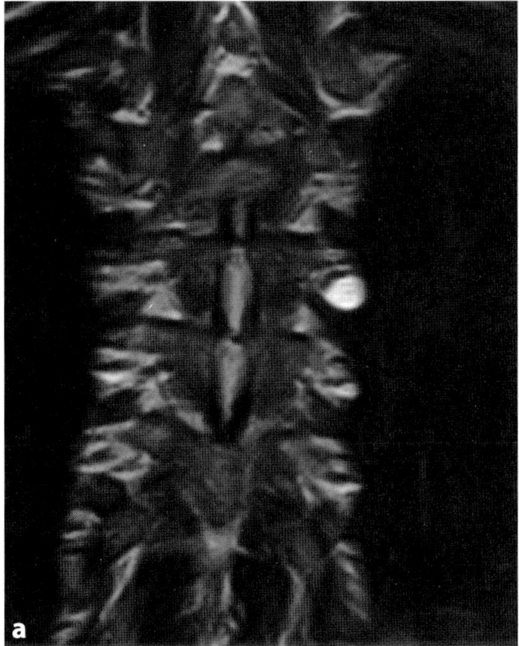

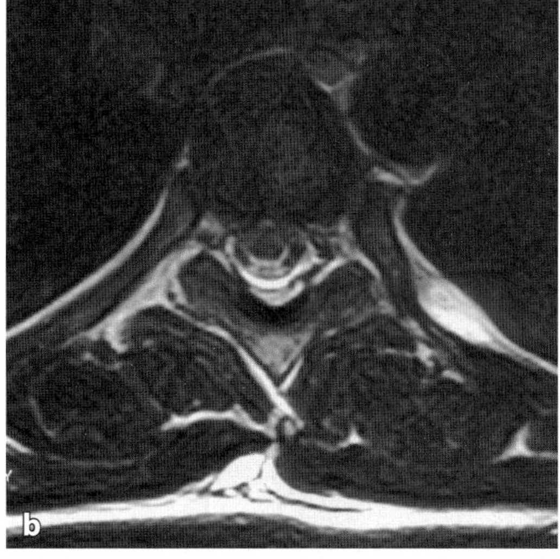

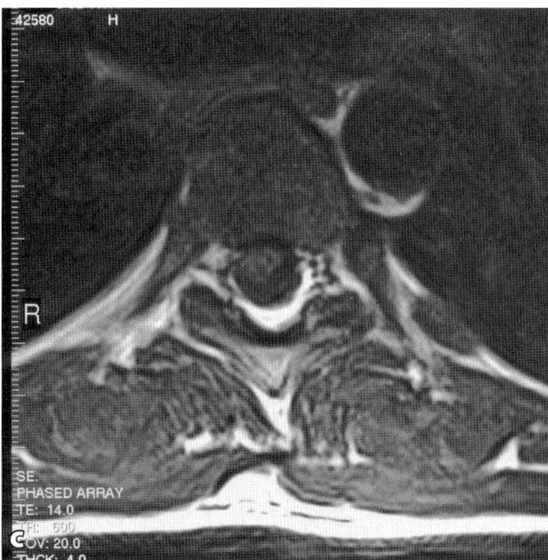

Fig. 2.5a–c. Spinal cyst located more peripherally along the course of the T5 nerve on the left

a T2-weighted image showing a high-signal-intensity lesion with the characteristic appearance of a cyst

b Axial image depicting a spindle-shaped high-signal-intensity lesion along the nerve on the left

c Contrast-enhanced T1-weighted image. Low signal intensity of the spindle-shaped lesion because it does not take up contrast

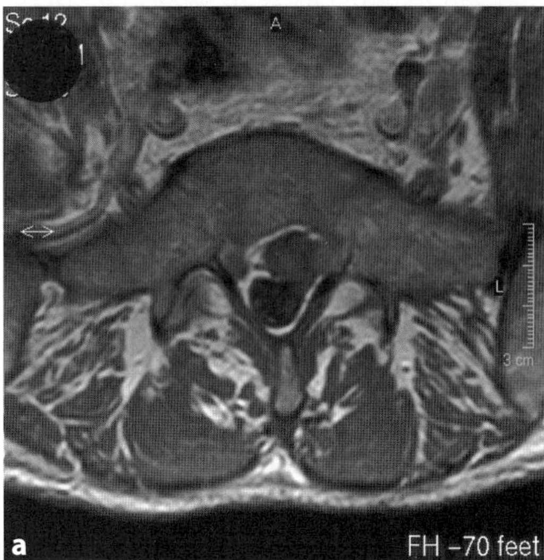

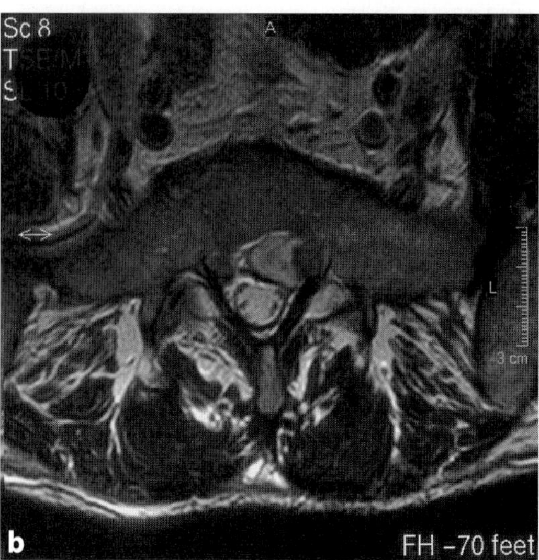

Fig. 2.6a, b. Intraspinal cystic lesion directly adjacent to the S1 nerve root on the left. Low signal intensity of the cyst on T1 (**a**) and high signal intensity on T2 (**b**). Also shown is slight lateral displacement of the nerve root by the cyst

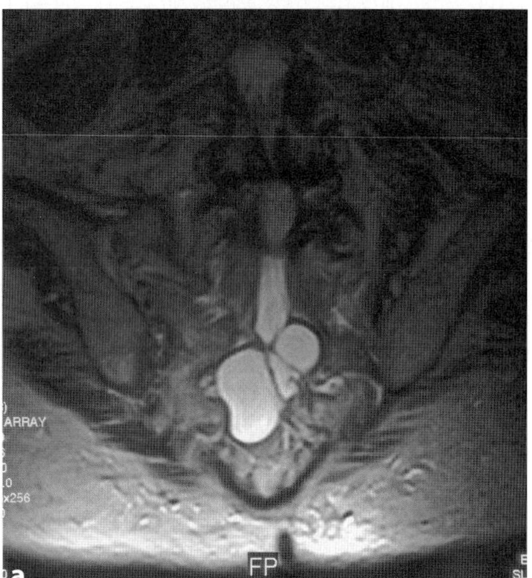

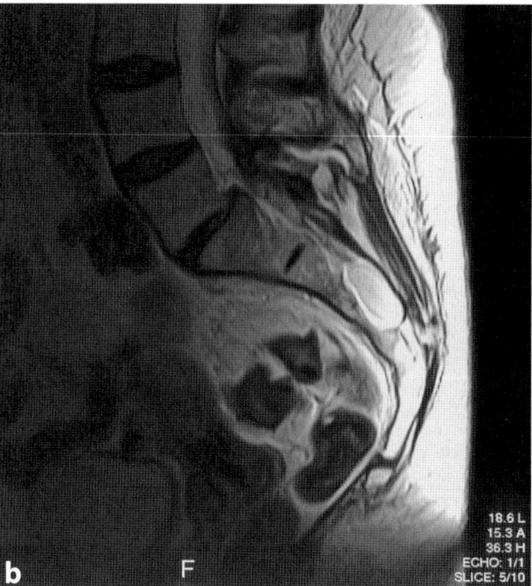

Fig. 2.7a, b. Axial and sagittal T2-weighted images of the sacral region. Well-defined, partially lobulated, lesion at the S2-3 level with cortical thinning and erosion of the posterior aspect of the sacrum. The appearance is consistent with a nerve root cyst (Tarlov cyst)

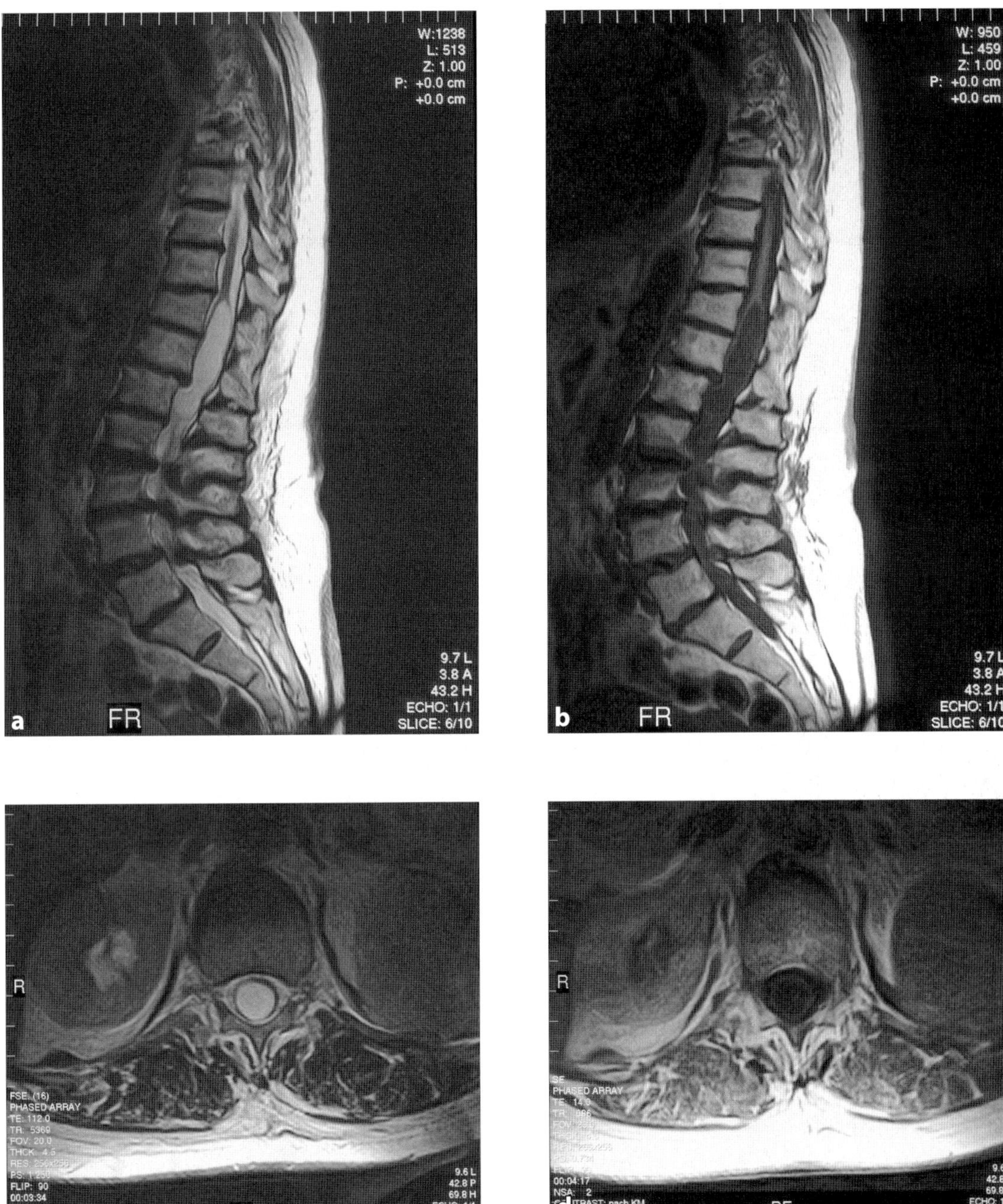

Fig. 2.8a–d. Arachnoid cyst widening the spinal cord in the lower thoracic region

a Sagittal T2-weighted image showing an intramedullary lesion of homogeneous high signal intensity with anterior and posterior displacement and rarefaction of the inferior spinal cord beginning at T10-11

b Sagittal T1-weighted image showing the arachnoid cyst as a homogeneous lesion of low signal intensity

c, d T2- and T1-weighted axial images showing the central intraspinal cyst at about the T12 level. Also seen is pronounced rarefaction of the surrounding cord

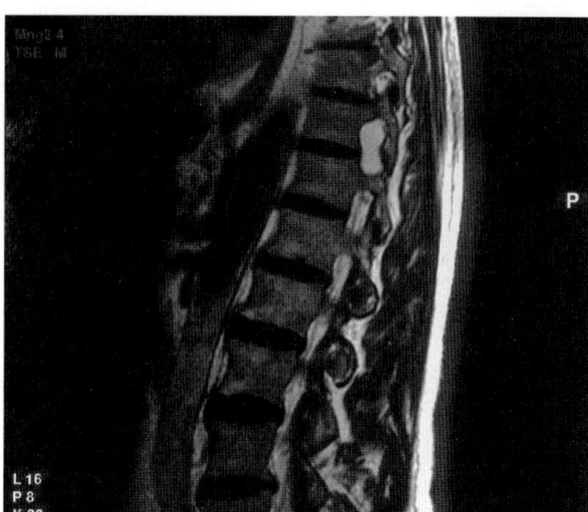

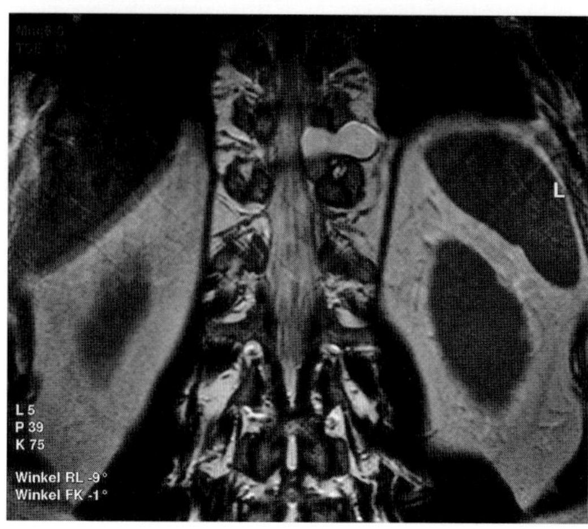

Fig. 2.9. Nerve root cyst in the left T11-12 neural foramen. Sagittal T2-weighted image of the thoracolumbar junction showing expansion of the T11-12 neural foramen on the left. Well-defined, homogeneous intraforaminal lesion with fluid signal

Fig. 2.10. Coronal T2-weighted image of the intraforaminal cyst at T11-12. Characteristic appearance and signal intensity of a nerve root cyst

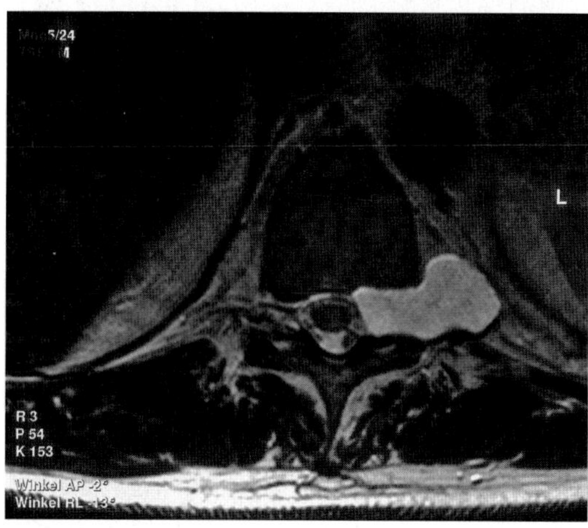

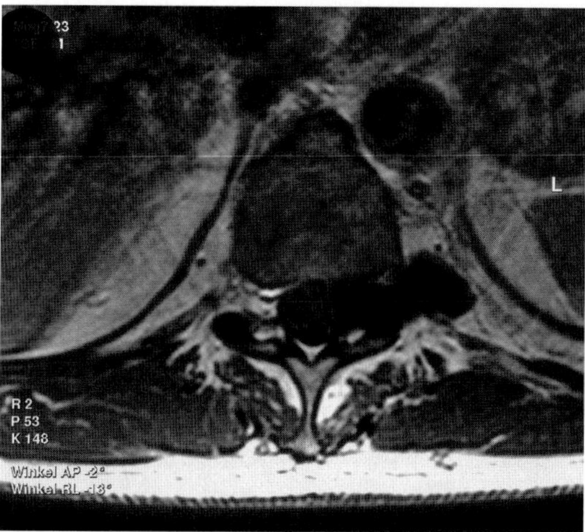

Fig. 2.11. Axial T2-weighted image through the T11-12 level showing the intraforaminal nerve root cyst with moderate expansion of the T11 foramen on the left

Fig. 2.12. Axial T1-weighted image showing the low-signal-intensity nerve root cyst in the left T11-12 foramen

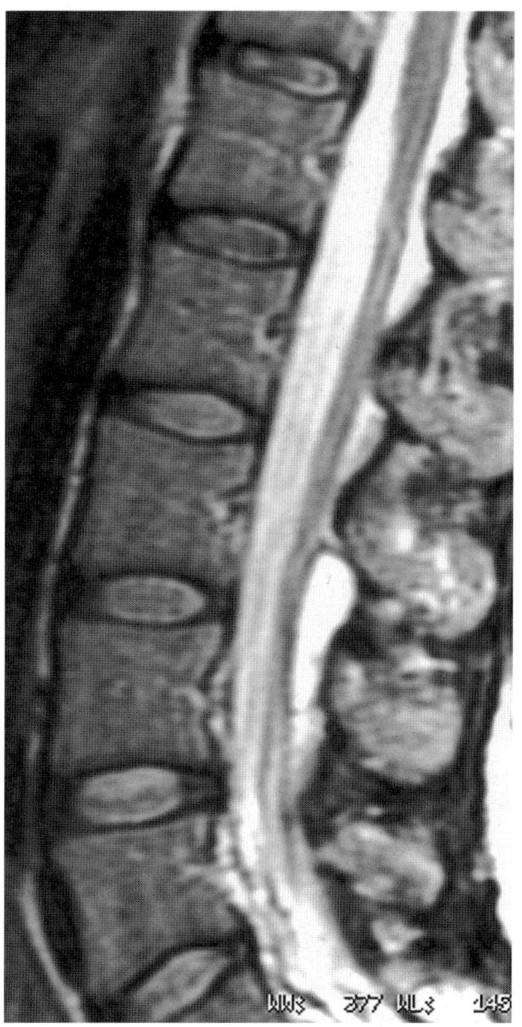

Fig. 2.13. Sagittal T2-weighted image of an extradural type Ia cyst posterior to the nerve roots at the L3-4 level

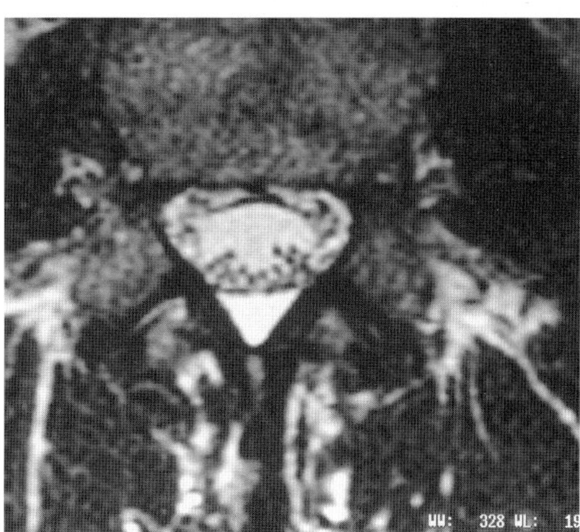

Fig. 2.14. Axial T2-weighted image through the L3-4 level depicting the cyst in the posterior recess

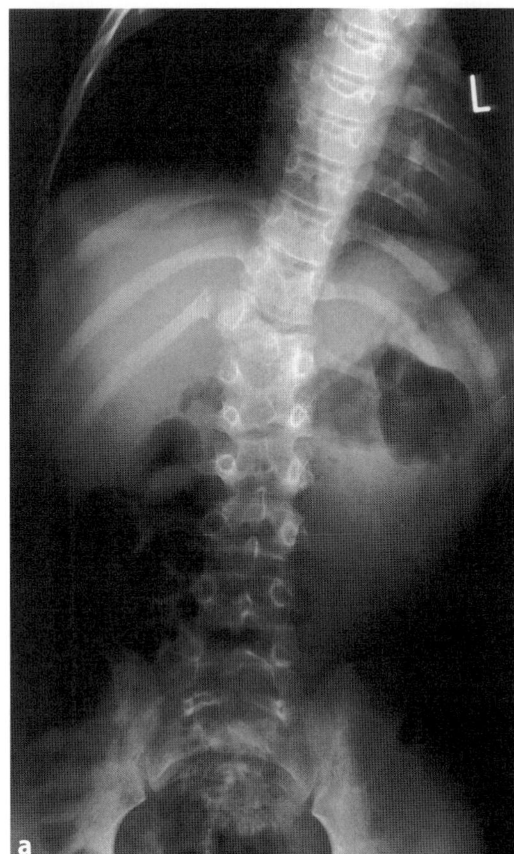

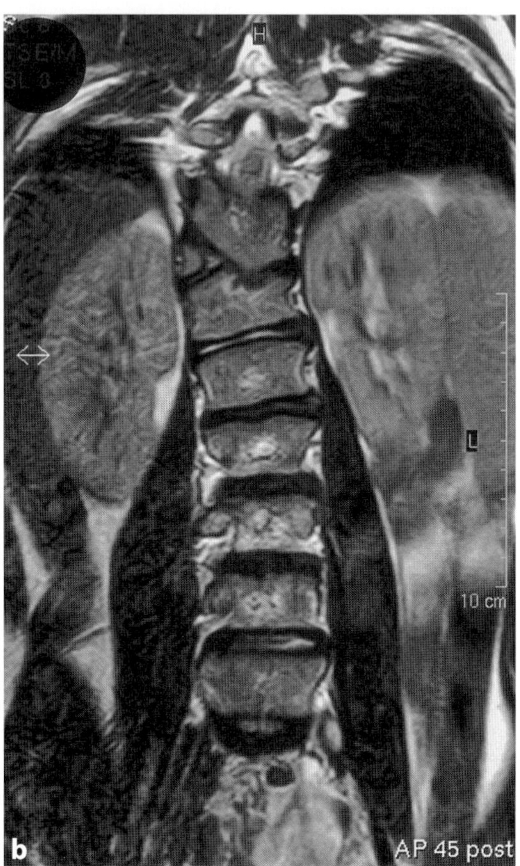

Fig. 2.15a–f. Hemivertebra

a Radiograph of a hemivertebra at T11 with left concavity of the spine and absence/hypoplasia of the 12th rib on the right

Corresponding T2-weighted MR image (**b**) showing the right hemivertebra at T11 with compensatory growth of the vertebrae above and below (T10 and T12). The vertebral abnormalities are more conspicuous on the coronal T1-weighted image (**c**). There are no signs of irritation in the surrounding soft tissue structures and vertebrae

d Sagittal T2-weighted image illustrating poor visualization of the hemivertebra in the sagittal plane

The two axial images - T1-weighted in (**e**) and T2-weighted in (**f**) – visualize the hemivertebra on the right and a portion of the intervertebral disc on the left. The dural sac has a slightly abnormal configuration while surrounding soft tissue structures and the spinal cord appear unremarkable

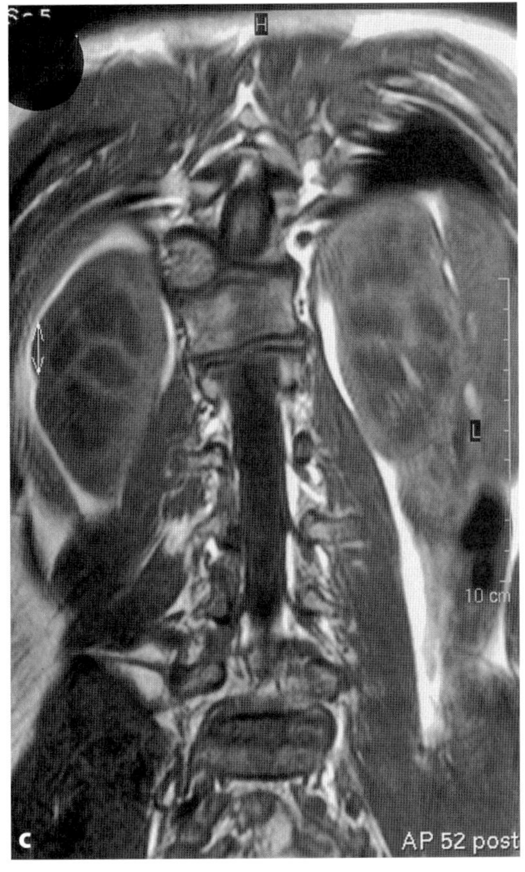
H
L
10 cm
c
AP 52 post

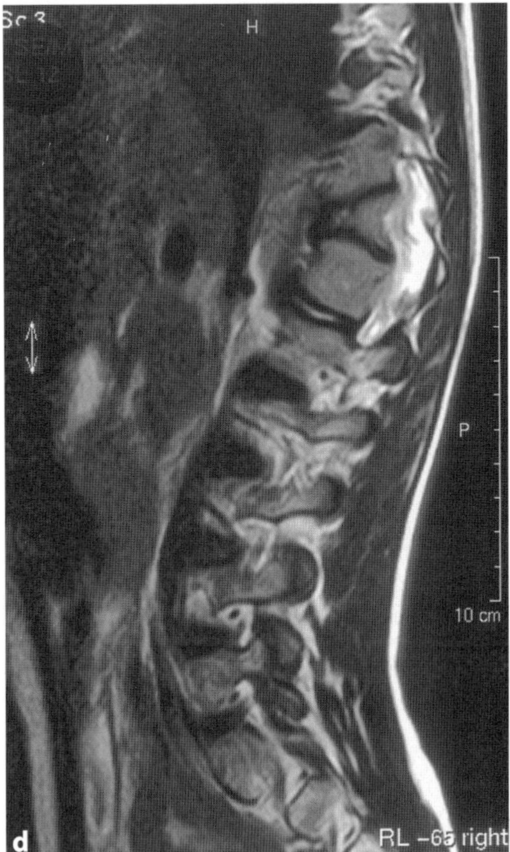
H
P
10 cm
d
RL -65 right

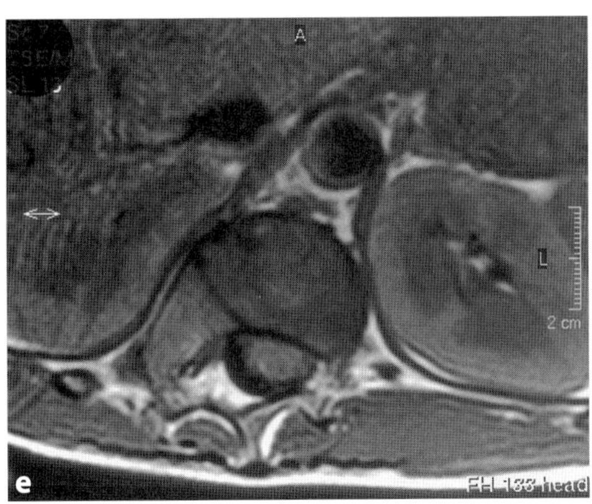
A
L
2 cm
e

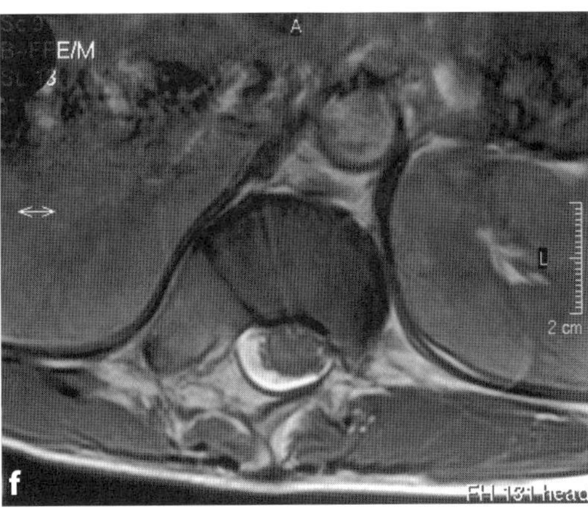
A
L
2 cm
f

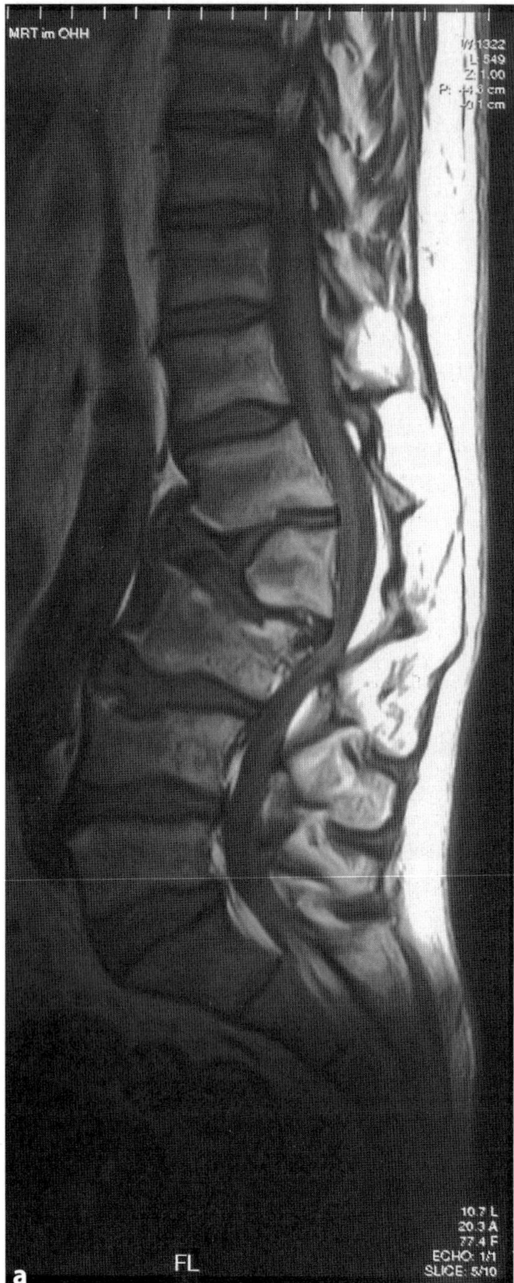

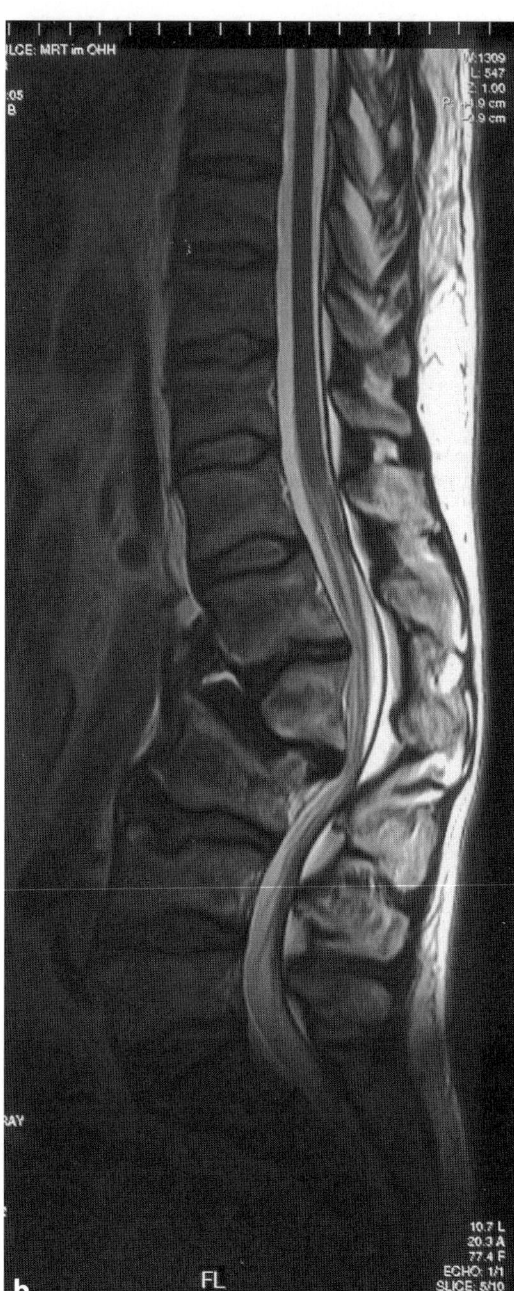

Fig. 2.16a, b. Wedge vertebra

a Sagittal T1-weighted image

b Sagittal T2-weighted image. Wedge deformity at L2. The anterior portion of the L2 vertebral body is absent, while the remainder of the vertebra appears unremarkable. Secondary intervertebral disc degeneration is indicated by an altered signal of L2-3 and less prominent changes also of the L1-2 interspace. Gibbus deformity at L2 and posterior displacement of L2 vertebra with narrowing of the anterior subarachnoid space and displacement of the cauda equina. Slight narrowing of spinal canal also at L2-3

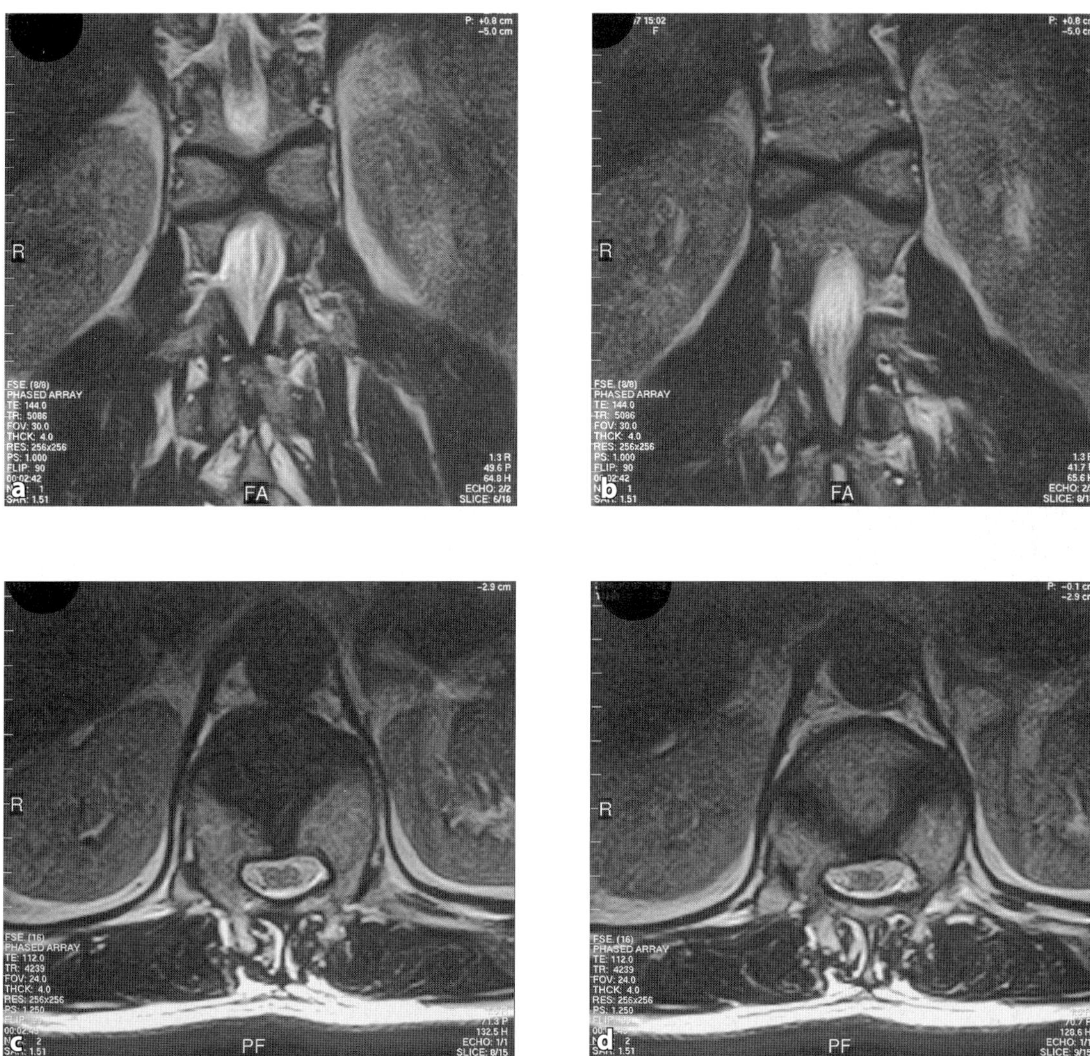

Fig. 2.17a–d. Butterfly vertebra

Typical butterfly appearance of the T12 vertebral body. Nearly symmetrical appearance of the right and left portion of the vertebra. T2-weighted axial images (**c, d**) showing the vertebral deformity in axial orientation

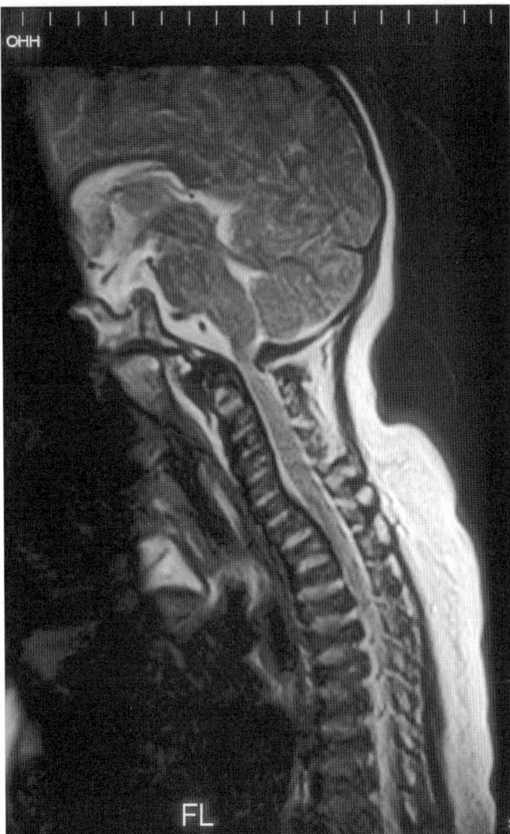

Fig. 2.18. Atlantoaxial instability. Sagittal T2-weighted image of the cervical and upper thoracic regions in an infant. There is a slight signal increase in the spinal cord consistent with myelomalacia

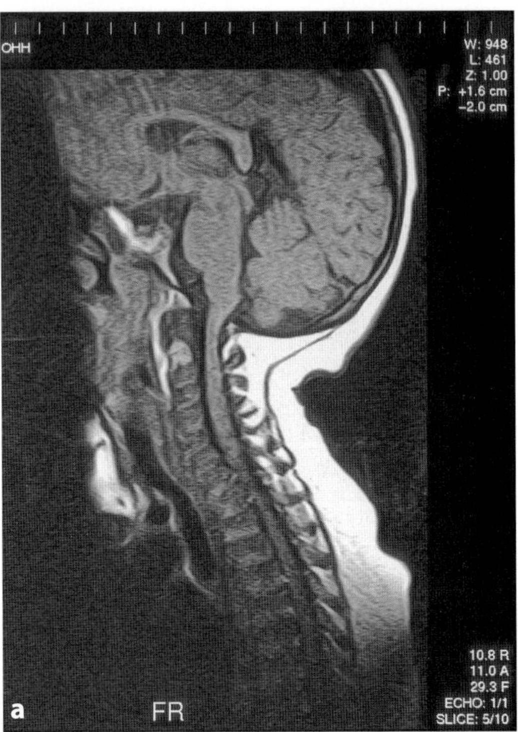

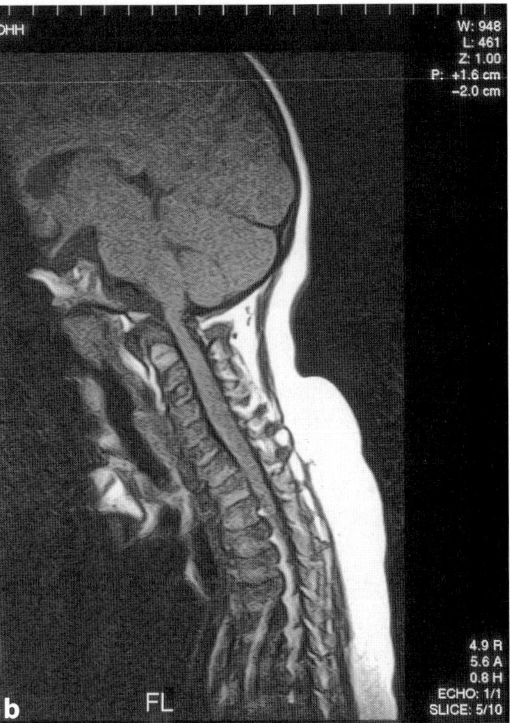

Fig. 2.19a, b. Sagittal T1-weighted flexion and extension views showing the narrowed spinal canal at the C2 level with the head bent backward (**a**) and more pronounced narrowing with the head bent forward (**b**)

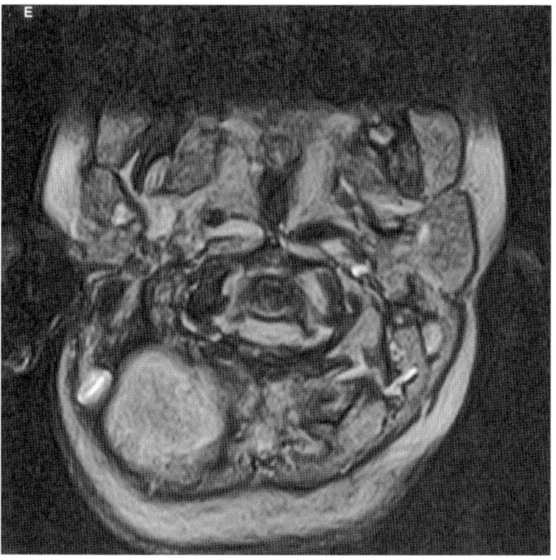

Fig. 2.20. Same patient. Axial T2-weighted image. Conspicuous narrowing of the spinal canal at C1-2

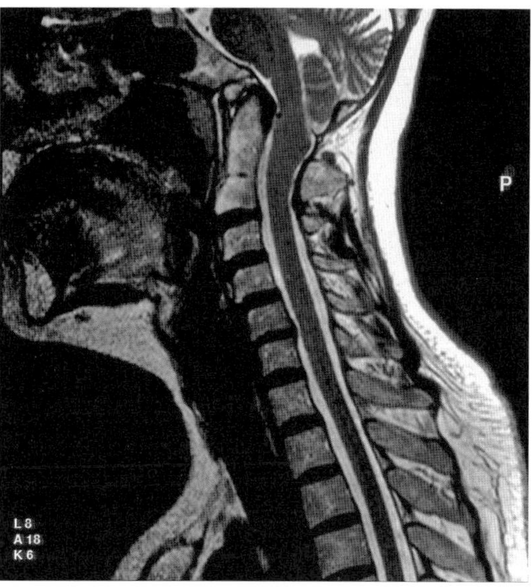

Fig. 2.21. Basilar impression. Sagittal T2-weighted image of the craniocervical junction and cervical spine showing an abnormally high dens axis and flattening of the clivus. Secondary indentation of the medulla oblongata with slight posterior displacement and elevation of the pons but normal signal intensity of neural structures

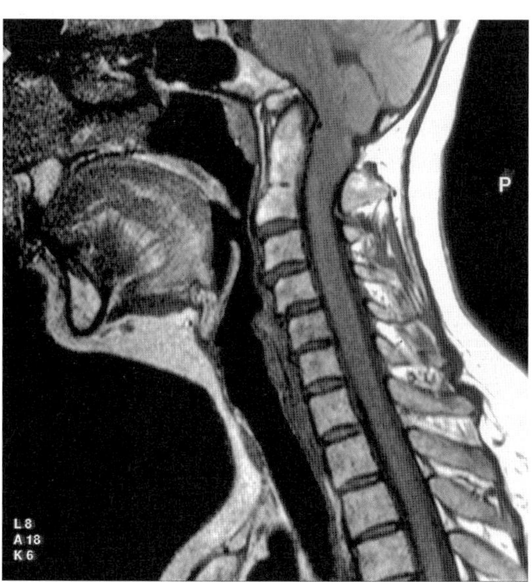

Fig. 2.22. Same patient. Sagittal T1-weighted image of the deformities associated with basilar impression

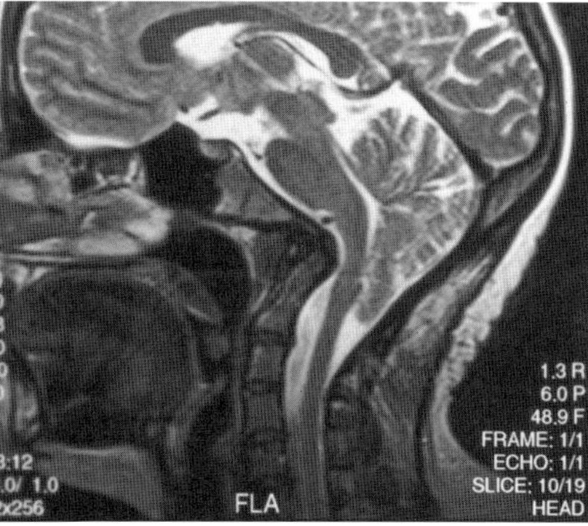

Fig. 2.23. Platybasia. Sagittal T2-weighted image showing flattening of the clivus with invagination of the edge of the foramen magnum. High dens compressing the lower portion of the brainstem and the medulla oblongata

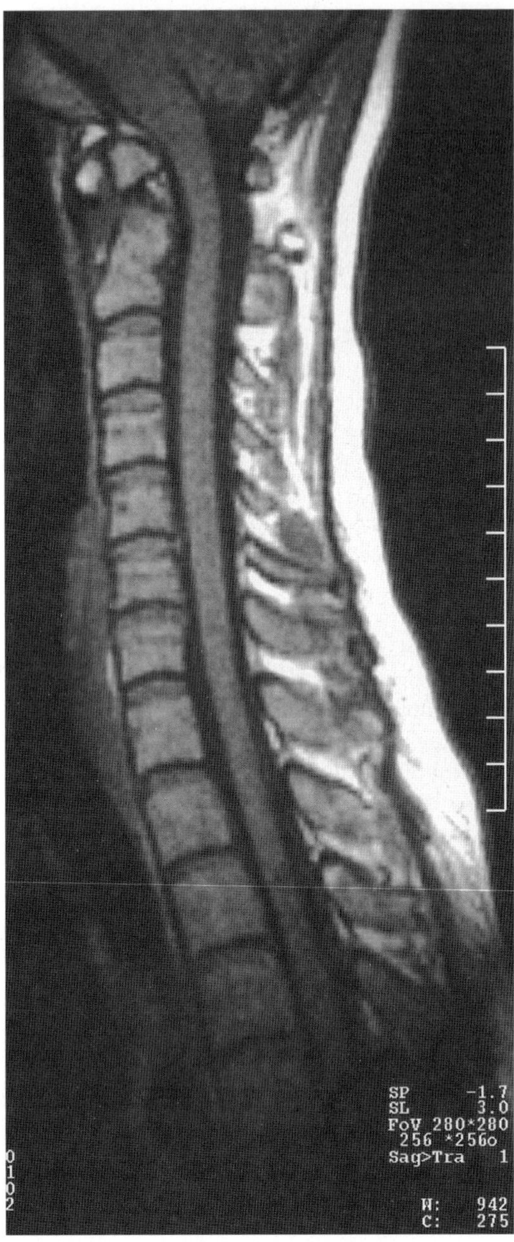

Fig. 2.24. Sagittal T1-weighted image of the cervical spine showing os odontoideum with marginal sclerosis of the two fragments and a gap of several millimeters between both fragments

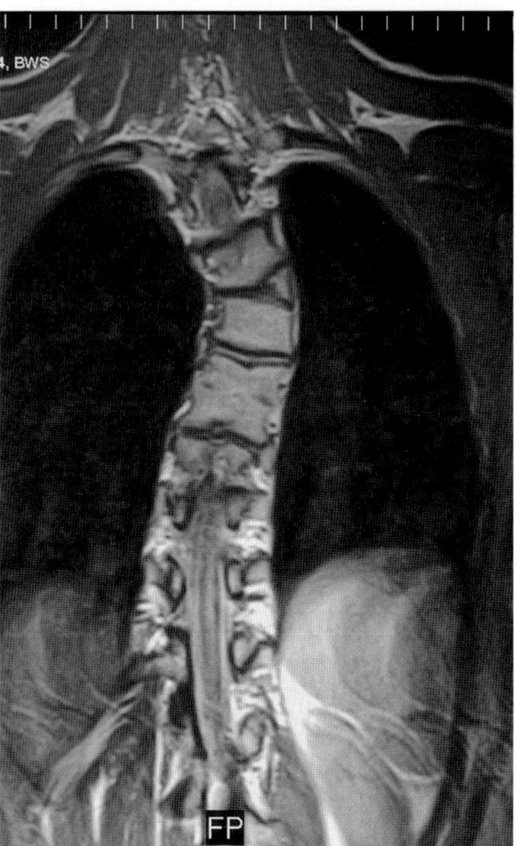

Fig. 2.25. Block vertebra. Coronal T2-weighted image showing fusion of T5-6 without an intervening disc. The height of the block does not correspond to that of the normal vertebrae. Two nerve roots are depicted on the left, corresponding to the T5 and T6 roots. Additional deformity due to a left hemivertebra at T3

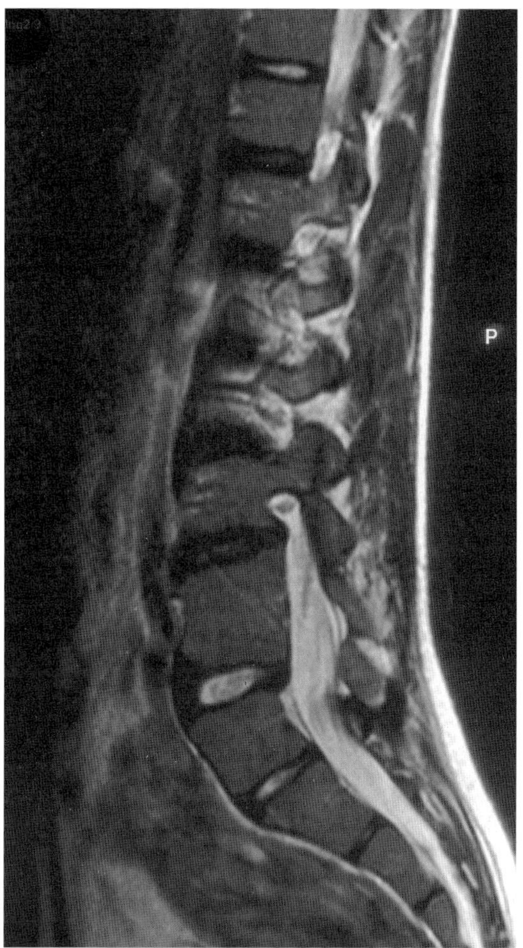

Fig. 2.26. Sagittal T2-weighted image of the lumbosacral junction showing a block vertebra at L4-5 with nearly complete absence of the intervening disc space. The lowest lumbar vertebra is abnormally large

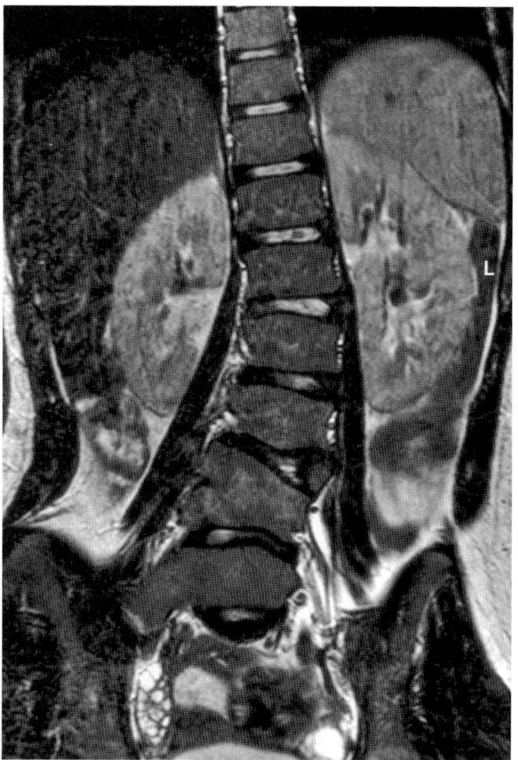

Fig. 2.27. Coronal T2-weighted image of the lumbar spine and lumbosacral junction showing incomplete right-sided vertebral fusion of L4-5 and a small left-sided wedge vertebra at L4. Accessory finding: cyst of the right ovary

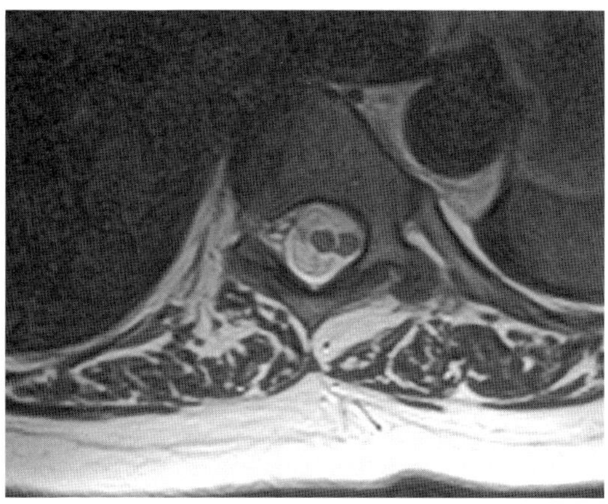

Fig. 2.28. Split cord malformation. Axial T2-weighted image through the T6 level showing the split cord in the spinal canal. The dural sac appears to be slightly distended

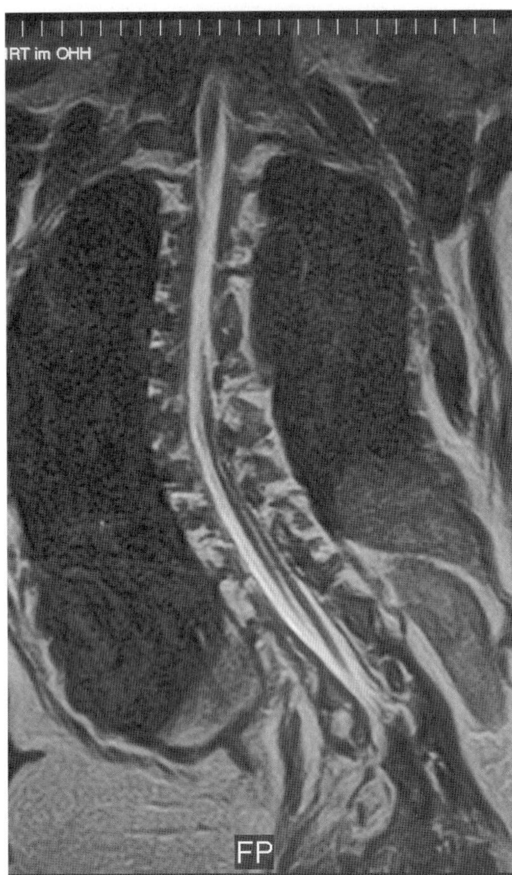

Fig. 2.29. Same patient. Coronal T2-weighted image. Only a faint bright line extending from T7 through T12 suggests splitting of the cord. Scoliosis with left concavity

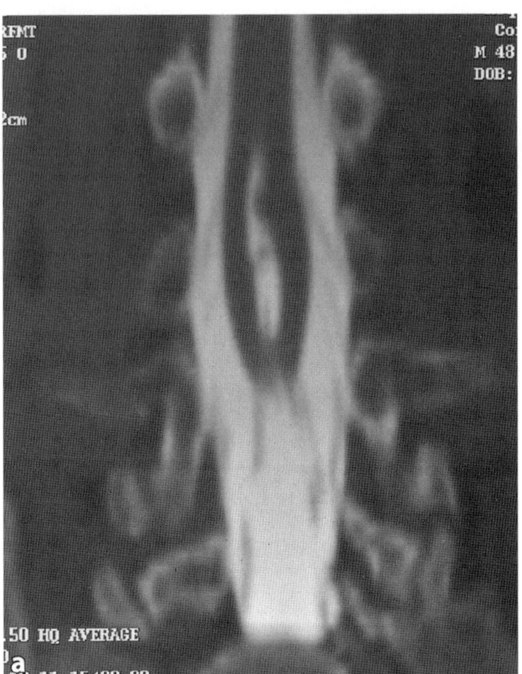

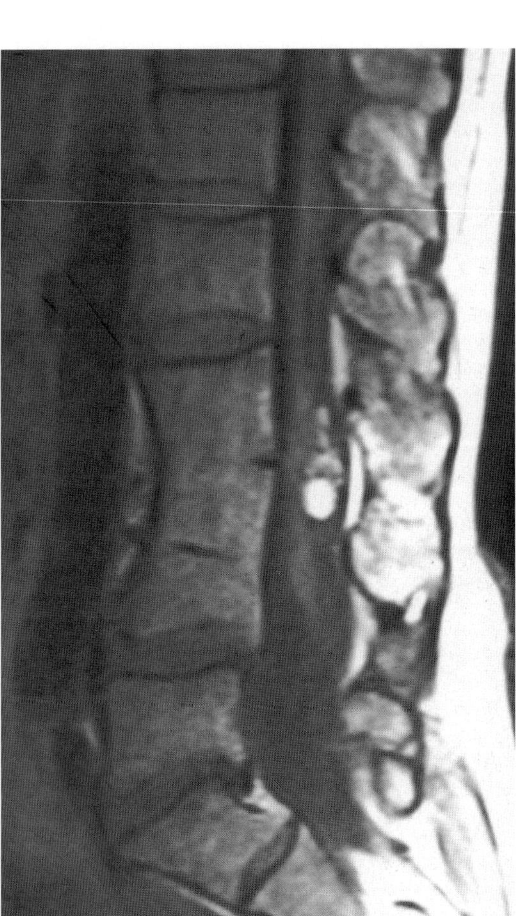

Fig. 2.30a, b. Sagittal T2- and T1-weighted images showing vertebral fusion from L2 through L4. Lipoma at the L3 level. Partial adhesion of the nerve roots to the posterior wall of the spinal canal

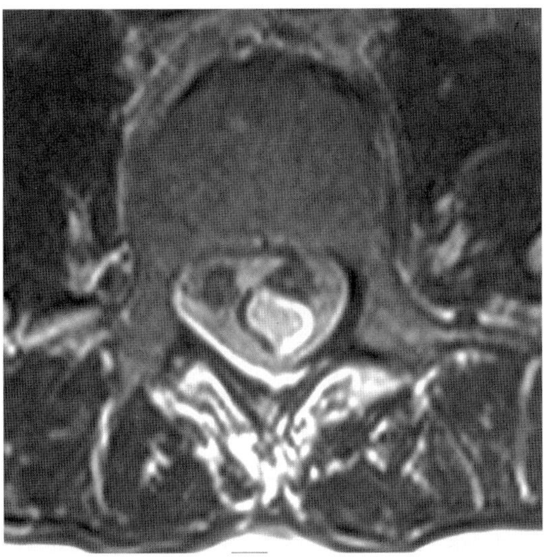

Fig. 2.31. Same patient. Axial T2-weighted image at the level of the lipoma

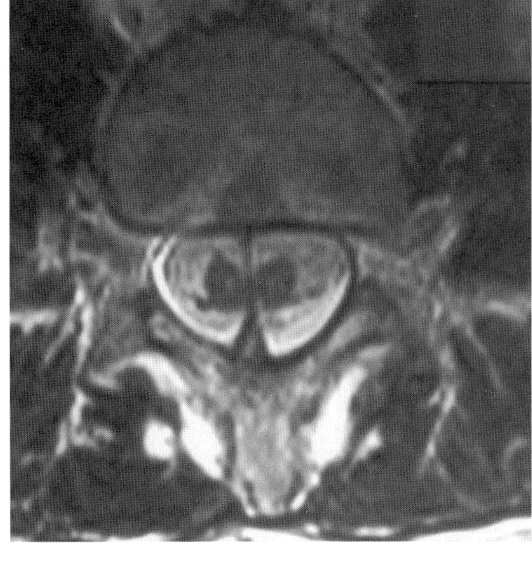

Fig. 2.32. T2-weighted image through the level of the bony spur

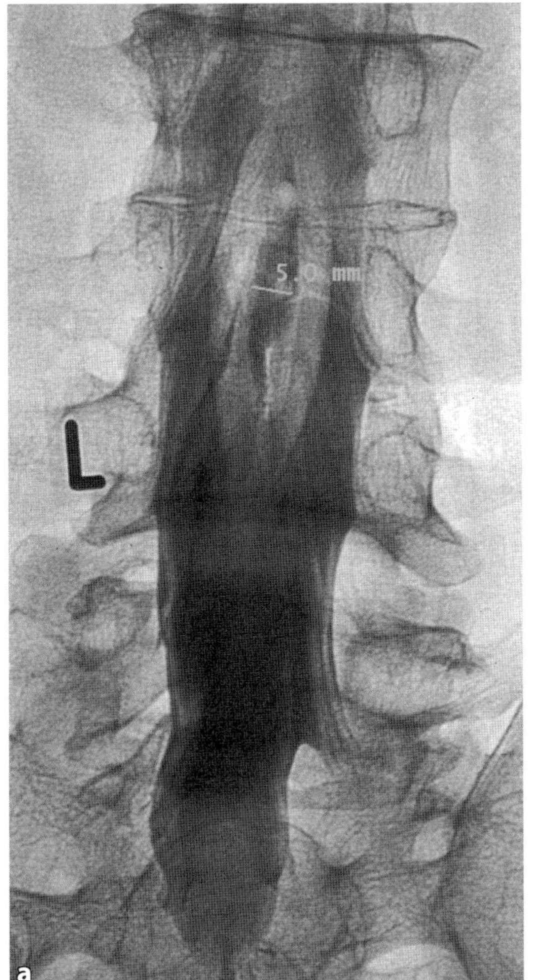

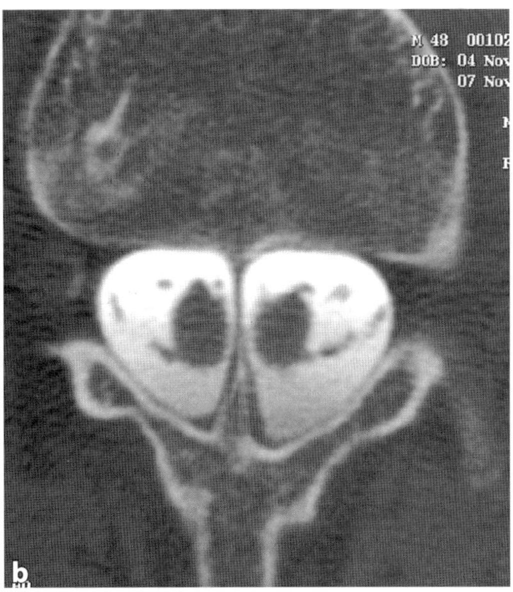

Fig. 2.33a, b. Conventional myelography and CT myelography of the lumbar region

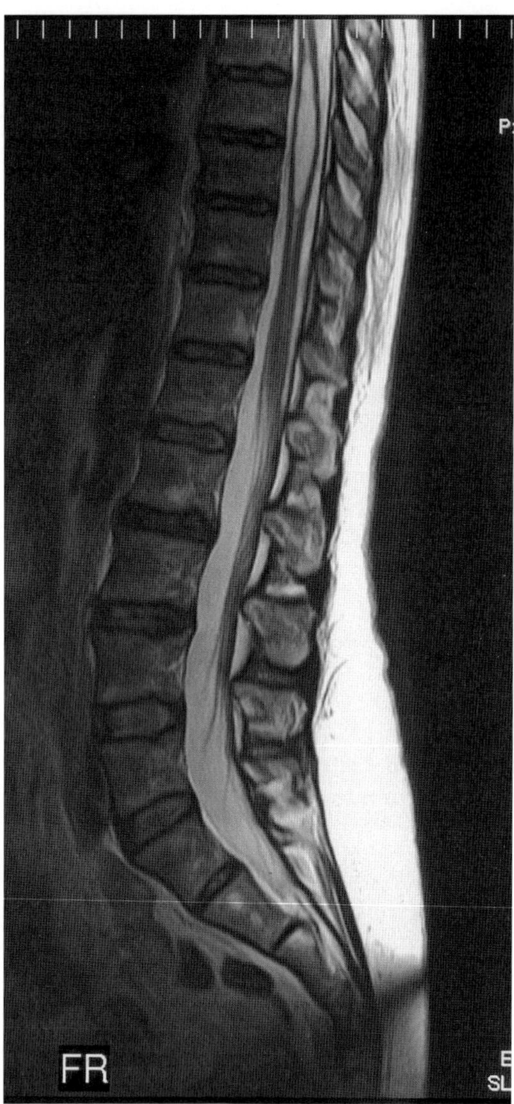

Fig. 2.34. Syringohydromyelia with cystic widening of the thoracic cord from T8 to T10. Sagittal T2-weighted image showing characteristic cystic signal intensity throughout the lesion with slight anterior and posterior displacement of the surrounding cord

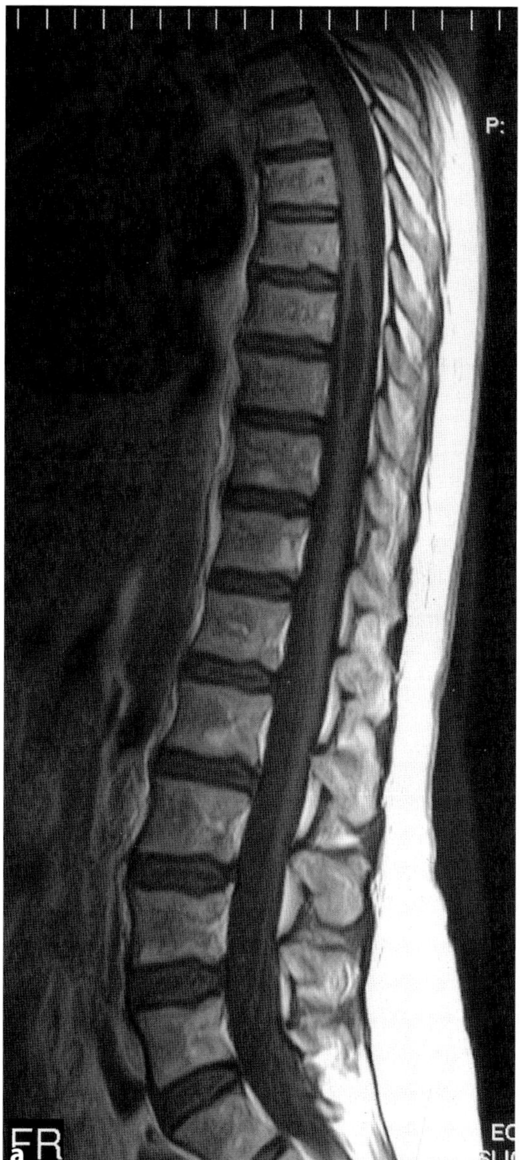

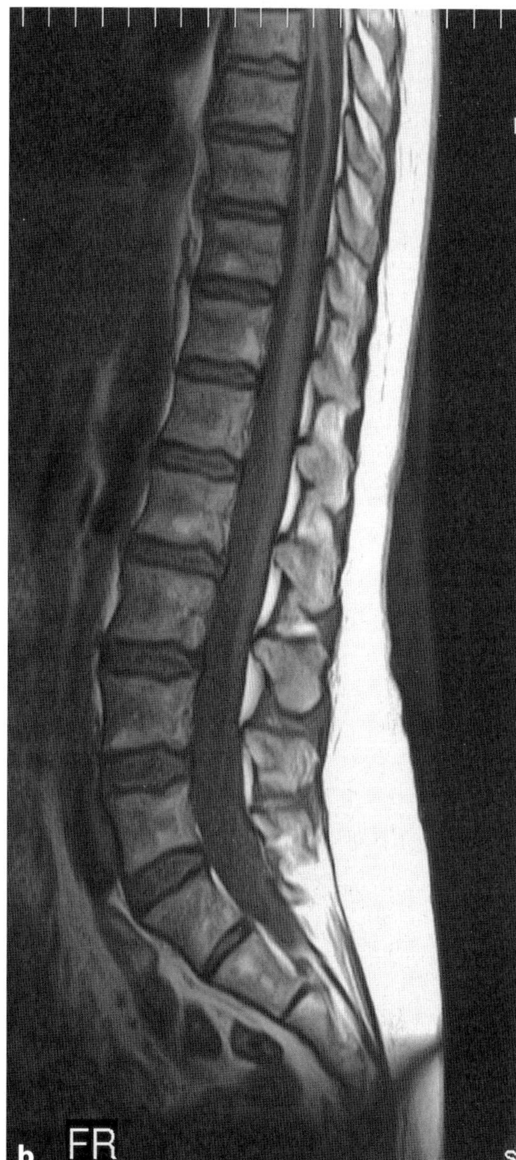

Fig. 2.35a, b. Same patient. Sagittal T1-weighted images before and after contrast administration. The intraspinal cystic lesion from T8 through T10 shows no contrast enhancement and there are no signs of irritation of the lower thoracic cord

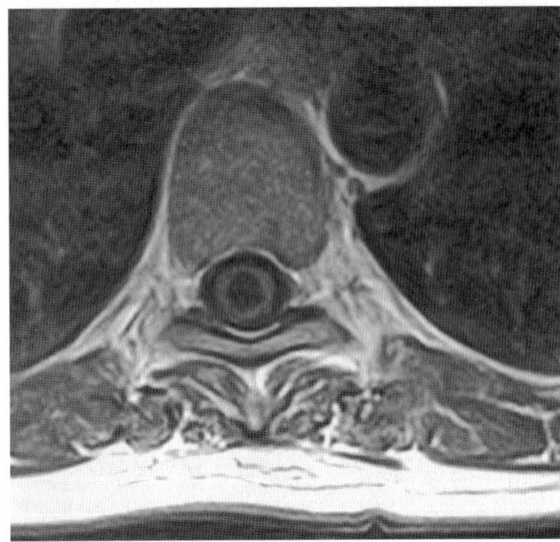

Fig. 2.36. Same patient. Axial T1-weighted image after contrast administration. Again, there is no enhancement of the intraspinal lesion. The surrounding cord is displaced and rarefied but shows no signs of irritation. Comment: On the basis of the available MR images, it is not possible to tell whether the lesion is hydromyelia or syringomyelia (dilatation of the central canal with increased fluid accumulation versus longitudinal fluid collection within the spinal cord but outside the central canal)

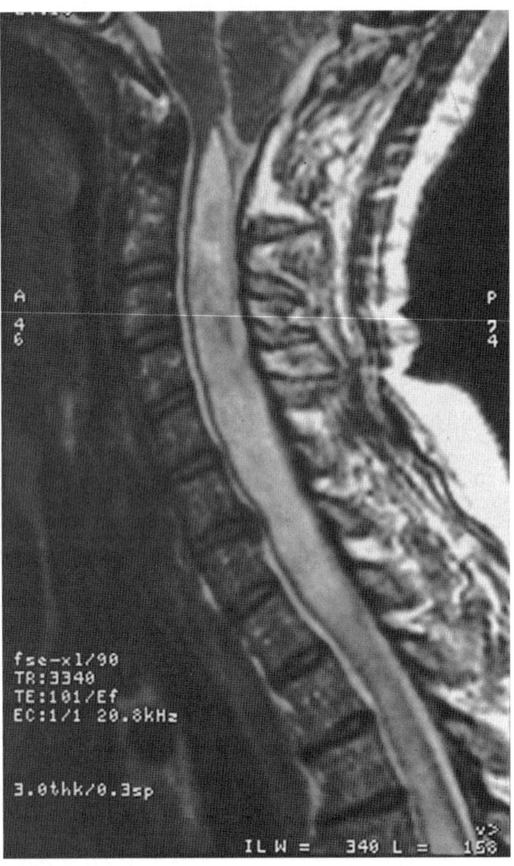

Fig. 2.37. Chiari type I malformation with syrinx cavity. Preoperative sagittal T2-weighted image showing low-lying cerebellar tonsils, sac-like syrinx cavity extending from C1 through T4 beyond the lower margin of the image. Spinal cord atrophy with tube-like appearance. CSF pulsation and flow artifacts in the upper portion of the syrinx from C2 through C4. Accessory finding: C6-7 disc herniation

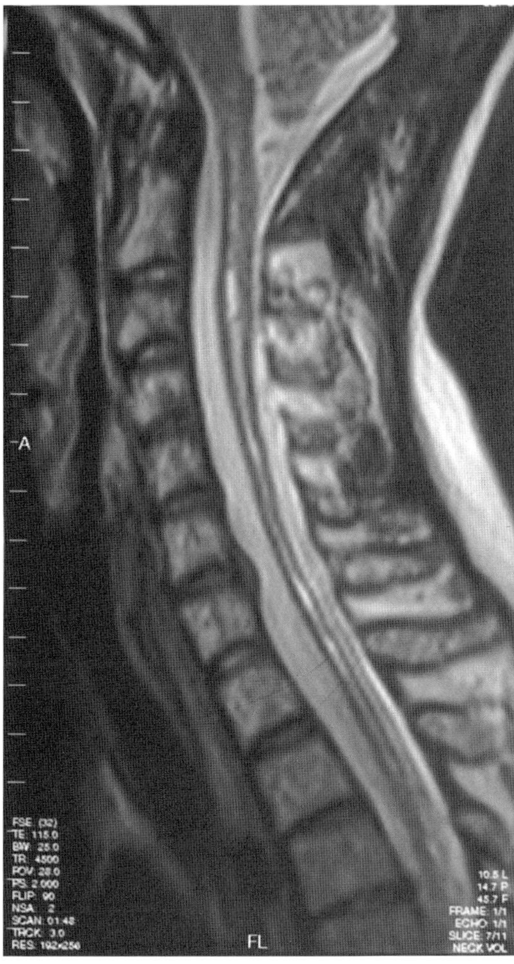

Fig. 2.38. Postoperative sagittal T2-weighted image showing collapse of the syrinx, surgically widened funnel at the level of the foramen magnum with unfolded, CSF-filled cisterna magna

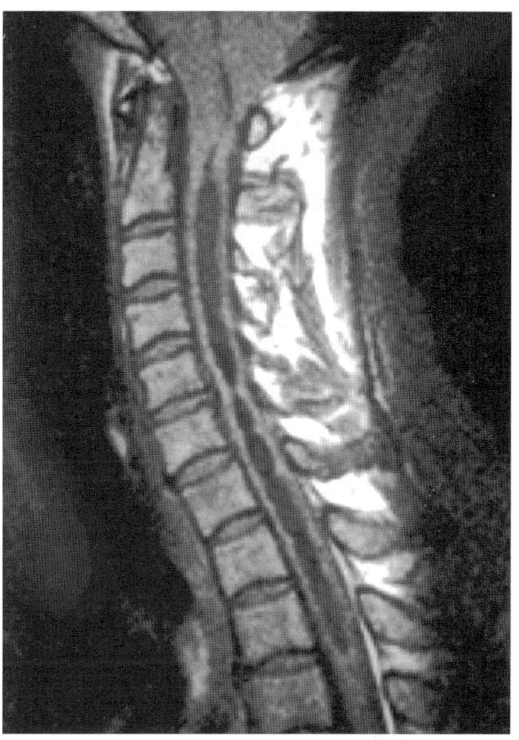

Fig. 2.39. Sagittal T1-weighted image before surgery showing syrinx cavity from C2 through T2-3, which creates a "string of pearls" appearance

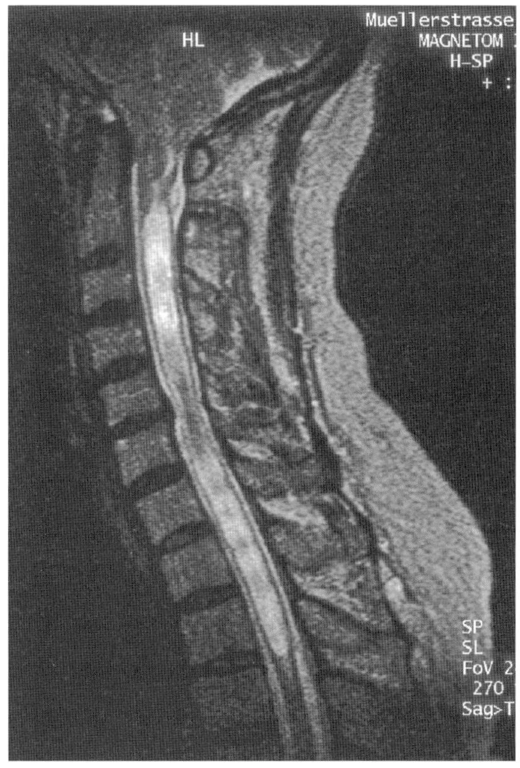

Fig. 2.40. Sagittal 2-weighted image before surgery

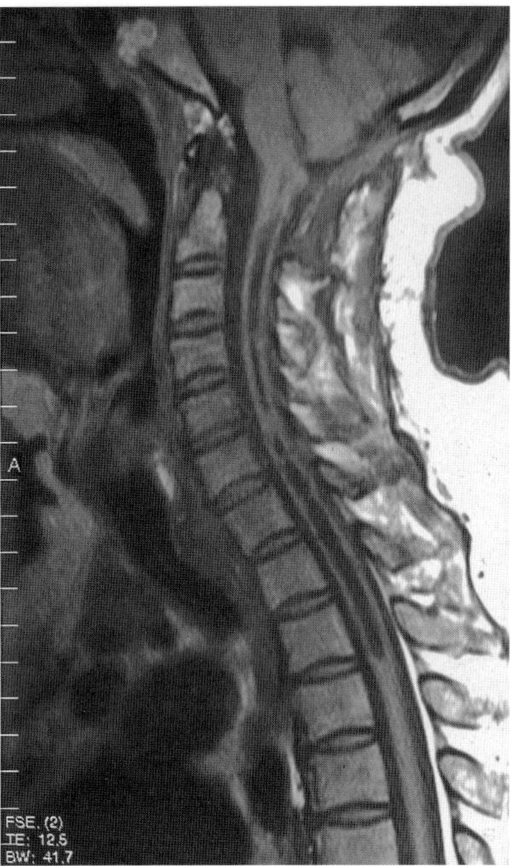

Fig. 2.41. Same patient. Sagittal T1-weighted image after surgery

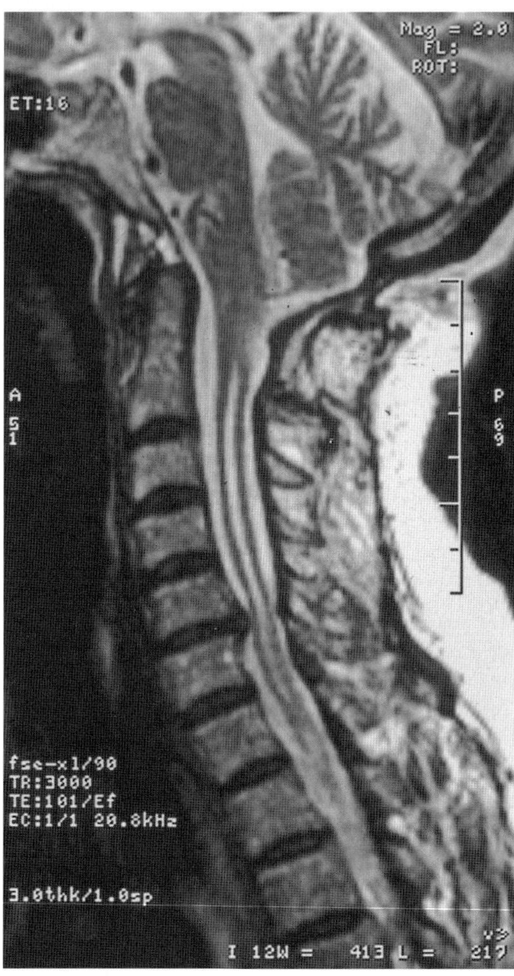

Fig. 2.42. Sagittal T2-weighted image. Follow-up three years postoperatively. Disc herniation at C5-6

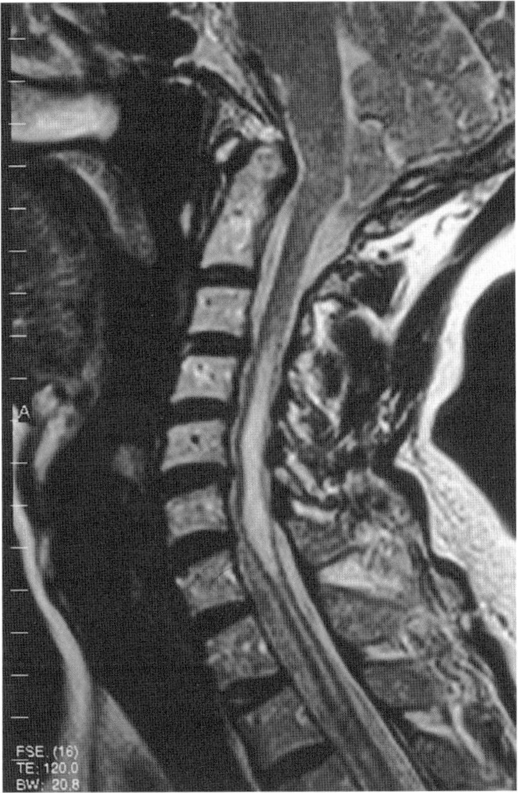

Fig. 2.43. Sagittal T2-weighted image. Syrinx extending from C3-4 through C7-T1 and narrowing of the spinal canal. Prominent additional narrowing through herniated discs at C5-6 and C3-4

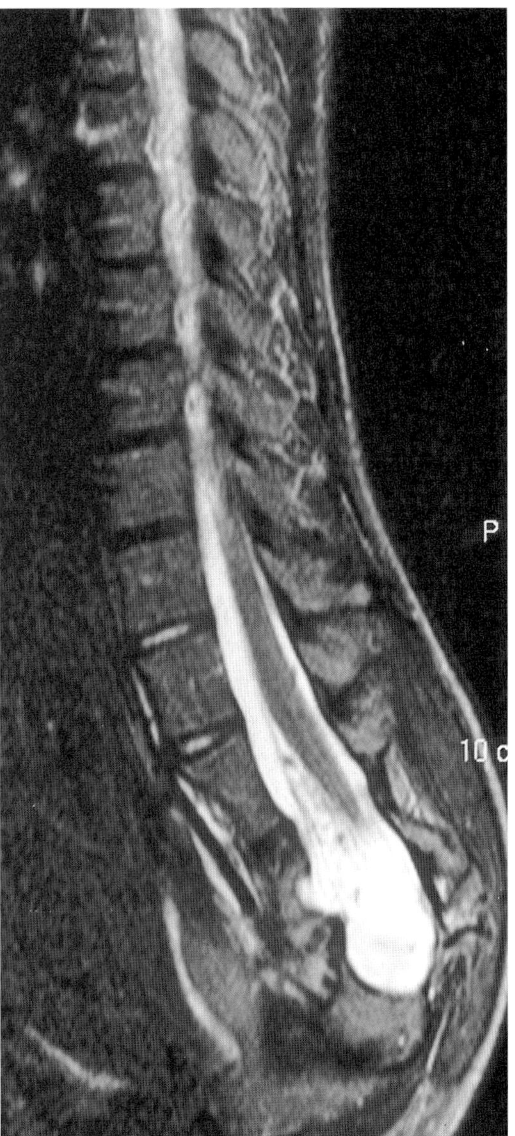

Fig. 2.45. Dysraphism. Sagittal T2-weighted image, overview

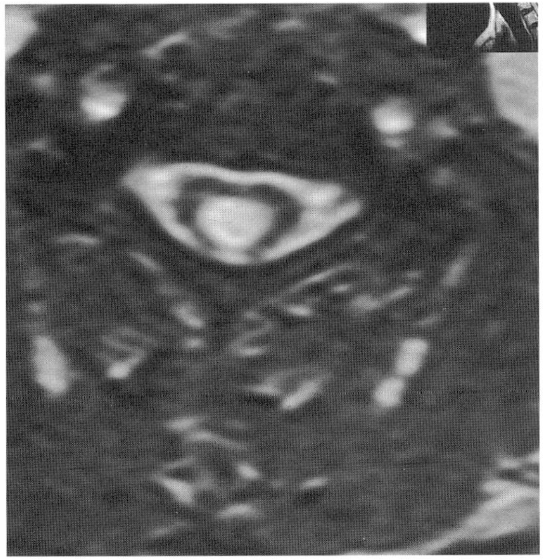

Fig. 2.44. Transverse T2*-weighted image. Large syrinx cavity with atrophy of the spinal cord

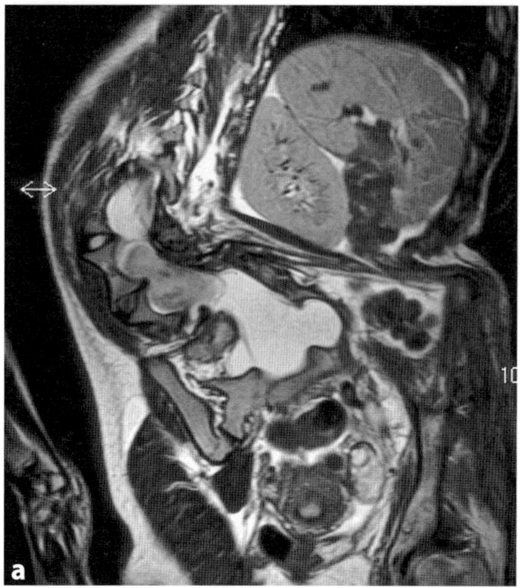

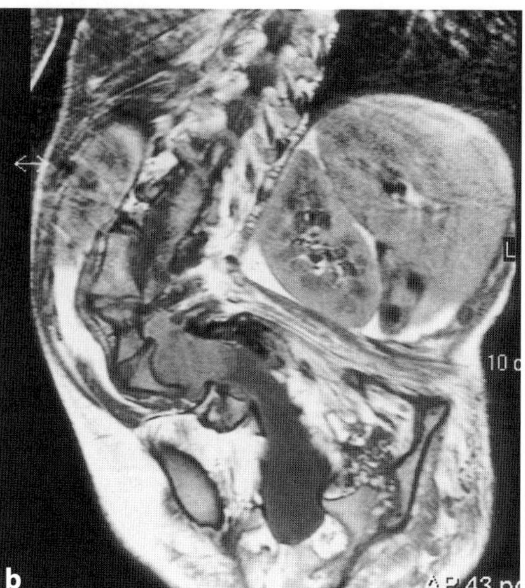

Fig. 2.46a, b. Coronal T2- and T1-weighted images

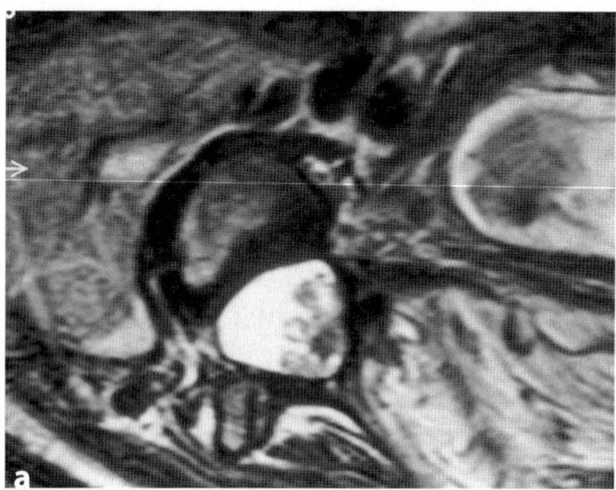

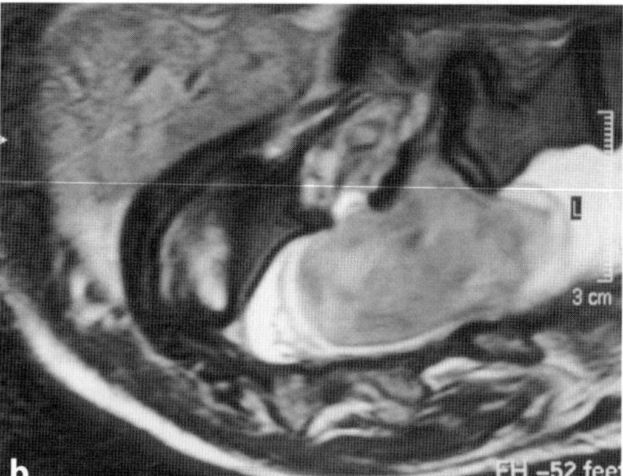

Fig. 2.47a, b. Transverse T2- and T1-weighted images

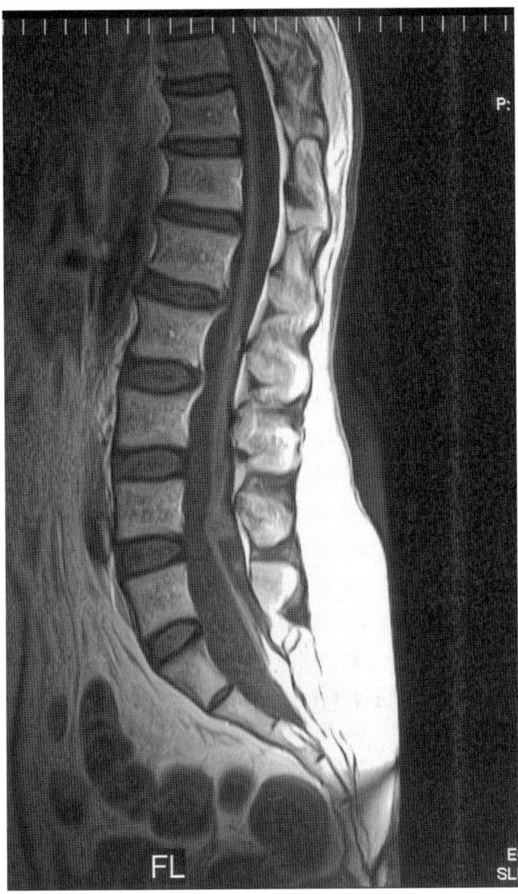

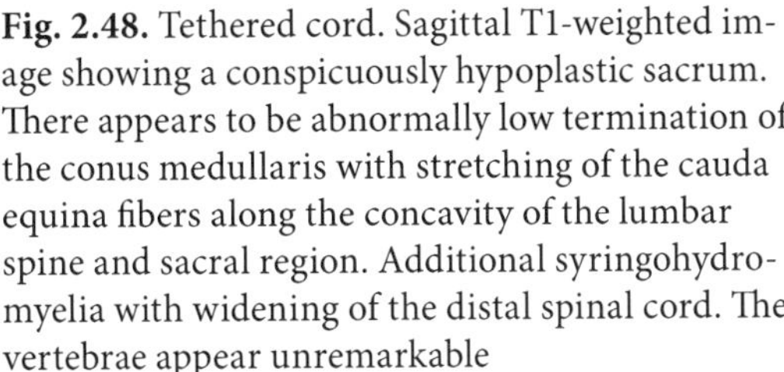
Fig. 2.48. Tethered cord. Sagittal T1-weighted image showing a conspicuously hypoplastic sacrum. There appears to be abnormally low termination of the conus medullaris with stretching of the cauda equina fibers along the concavity of the lumbar spine and sacral region. Additional syringohydromyelia with widening of the distal spinal cord. The vertebrae appear unremarkable

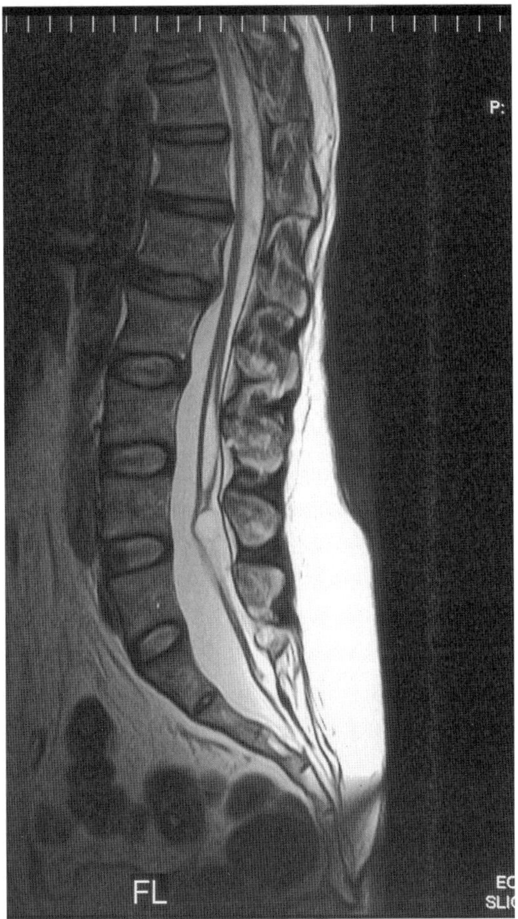

Fig. 2.49. Same patient. Sagittal T2-weighted image with more prominent depiction of the syringohydromyelia

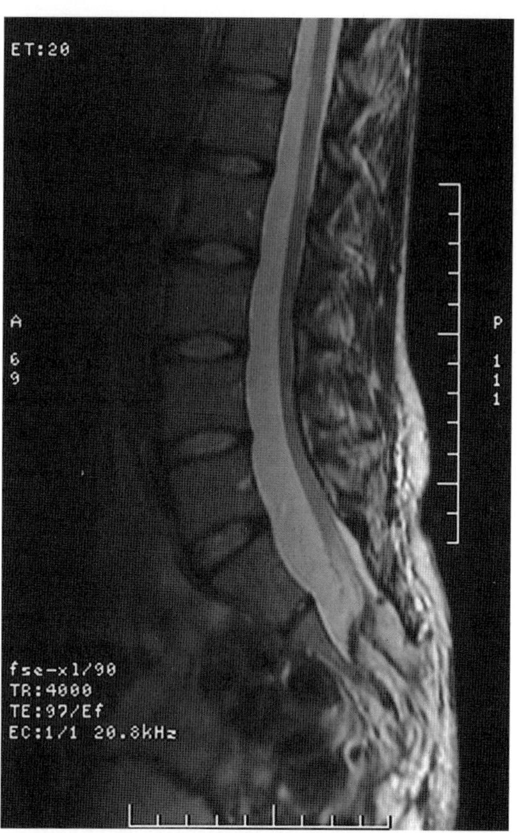

Fig. 2.50. Same patient. Sagittal T2-weighted image. Sacral tethering of the cord by lumbosacral lipoma with fusion defects of the sacral vertebral arches

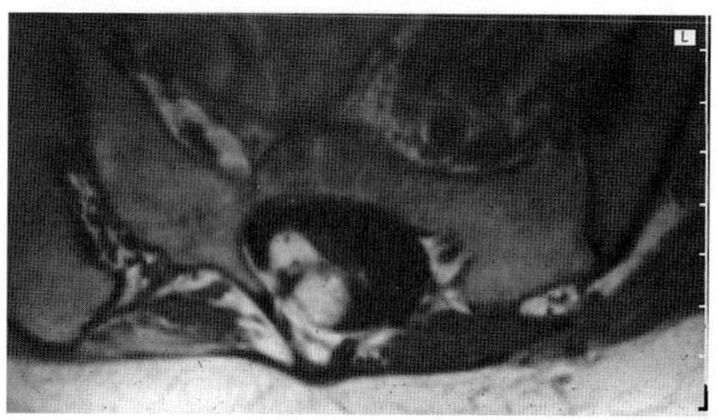

Fig. 2.51. Transverse T1-weighted image of the high-signal-intensity lipoma

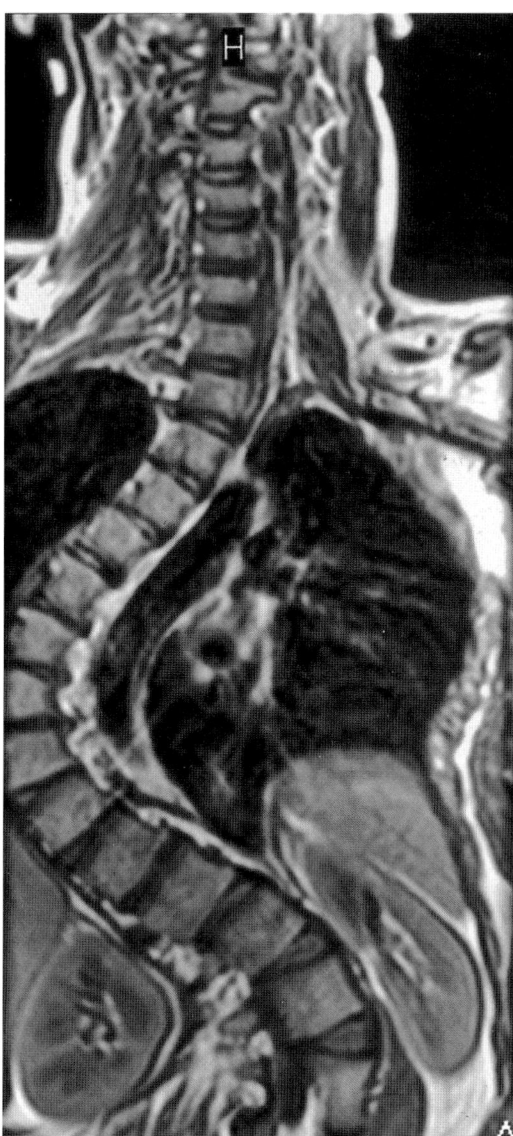

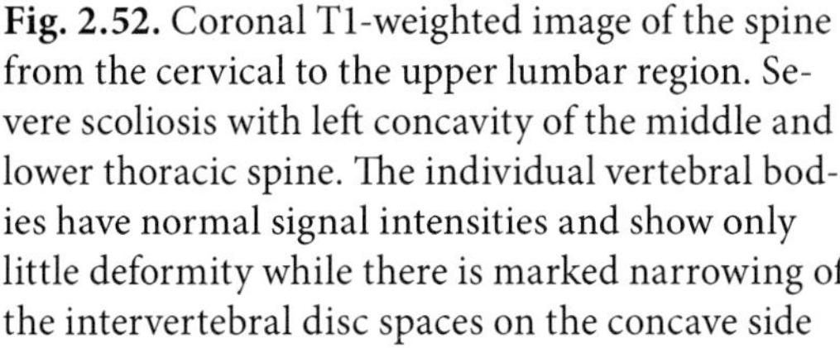
Fig. 2.52. Coronal T1-weighted image of the spine from the cervical to the upper lumbar region. Severe scoliosis with left concavity of the middle and lower thoracic spine. The individual vertebral bodies have normal signal intensities and show only little deformity while there is marked narrowing of the intervertebral disc spaces on the concave side

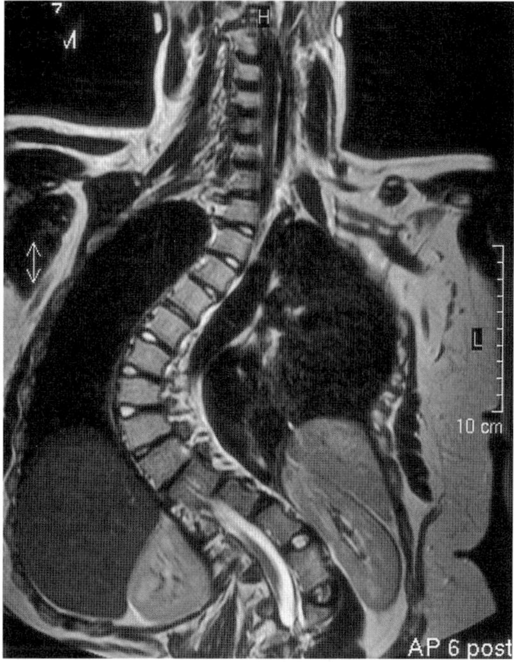

Fig. 2.53. Same patient. Coronal T1-weighted image passing through the spinal canal at the thoracolumbar junction. No major deformities of the individual thoracic vertebrae

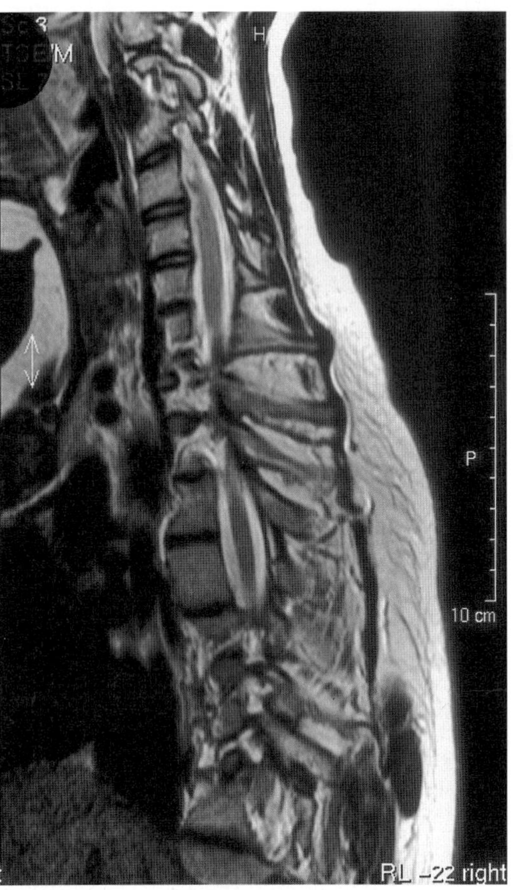

Fig. 2.54. Sagittal image through the spinal canal at the cervicothoracic junction. The spinal cord appears normal. Significant scoliosis often precludes visualization of the entire spinal cord on a single sagittal image, and several sagittal images are often required to evaluate the full length of the spine

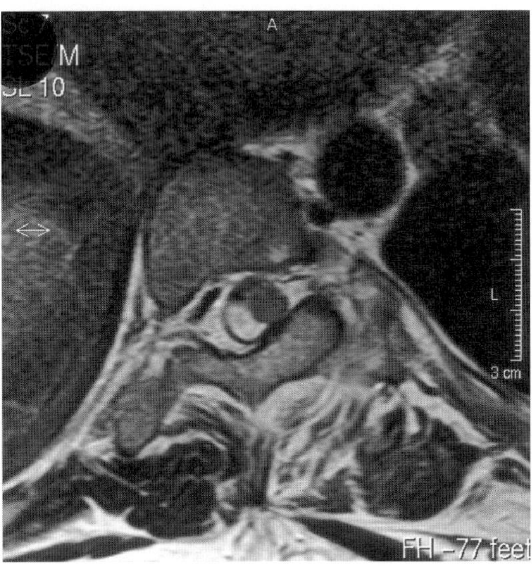

Fig. 2.55. Axial T2-weighted image. Typical appearance of the spinal cord on the concave side of a scoliotic curve. In the example, the concave side is on the left and the axial image passes obliquely through the vertebral body and spinal canal

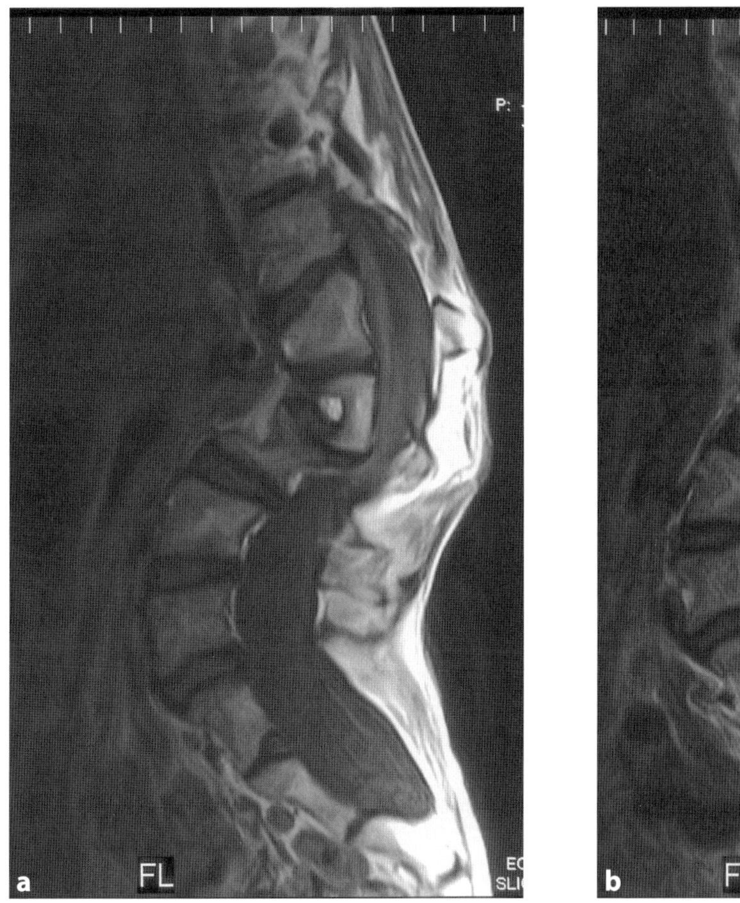

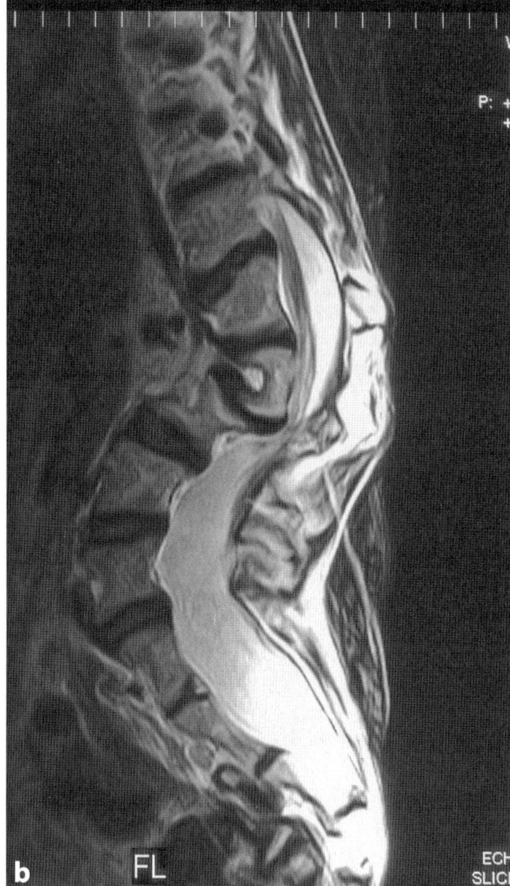

Fig. 2.56a, b. Sagittal T1- and T2-weighted images showing severe kyphoscoliosis with the apex at L2. Wedging of L2 is suggested. Spinal stenosis at the L2-3 level. Normal signal intensity of the vertebral bodies

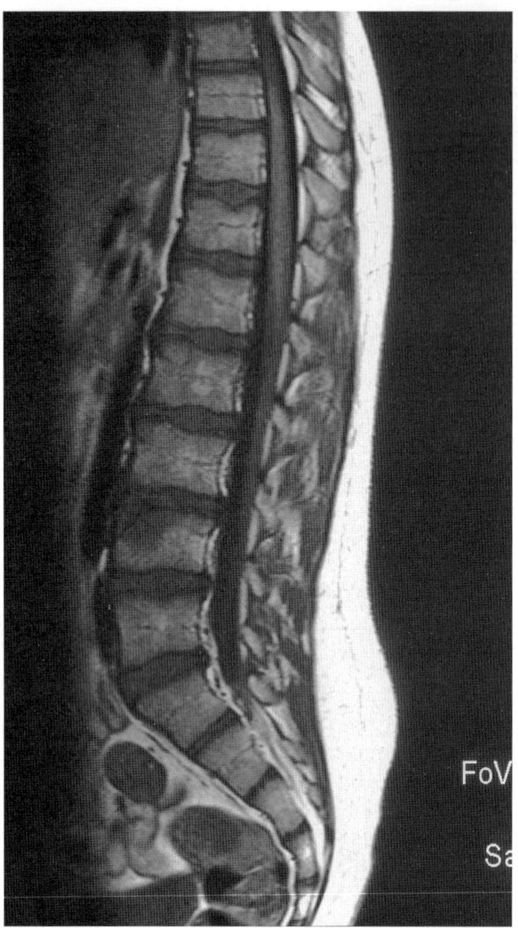

Fig. 2.57. Sagittal T1-weighted image of the lumbar region in a 14-year-old boy with low back pain. Irregular appearance of the superior and inferior endplates of T11 through L4 due to multiple Schmorl's nodes (herniation of disc tissue into adjacent vertebral body). Focal signal change and partial destruction of the upper anterior corner of L4 suggesting osteonecrosis as in Scheuermann's disease

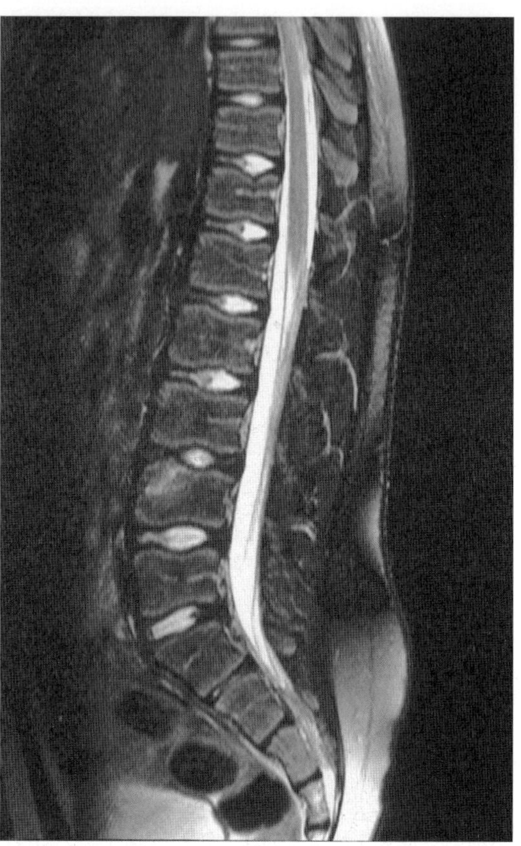

Fig. 2.58. Same patient. Sagittal T2-weighted gradient echo image of the lumbar region showing increased signal intensity of the focal osteonecrosis of L4

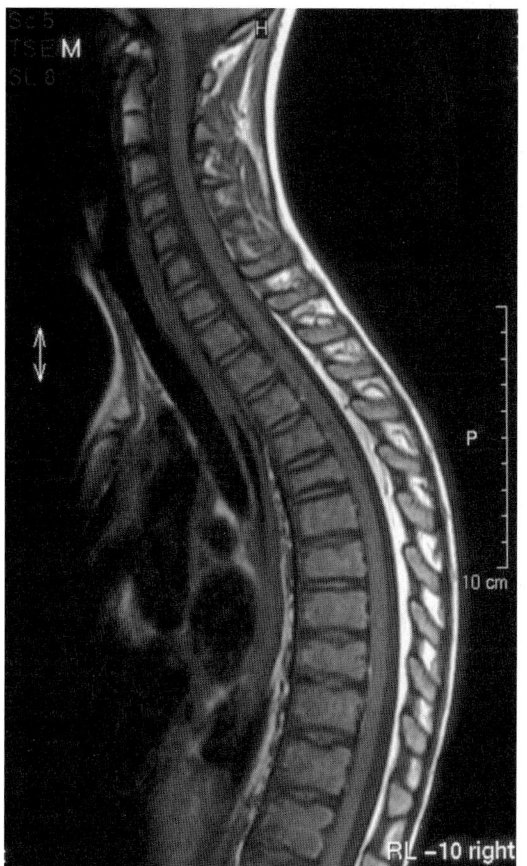

Fig. 2.59. Sagittal T1-weighted image of the cervical and thoracic region in a 15-year-old boy with kyphosis. Rounded upper and lower anterior edges with decreased signal intensity from T8 through T12. Wedging of T5 without signal changes that would suggest an acute event. Appearance consistent with older compression fracture with almost fully preserved posterior edge as in Scheuermann's disease. Irregular superior and inferior endplates of T7 through T12, consistent with small Schmorl's nodes

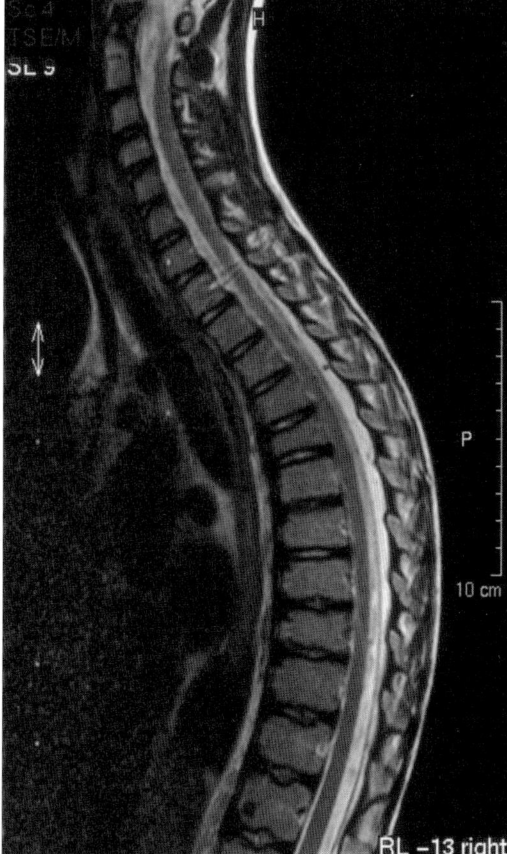

Fig. 2.60. Sagittal T2-weighted image of the cervicothoracic spine in the patient with Scheuermann's disease and kyphosis. Low-signal-intensity lesions of the anterior edges from T8 through T12. Wedging of T5

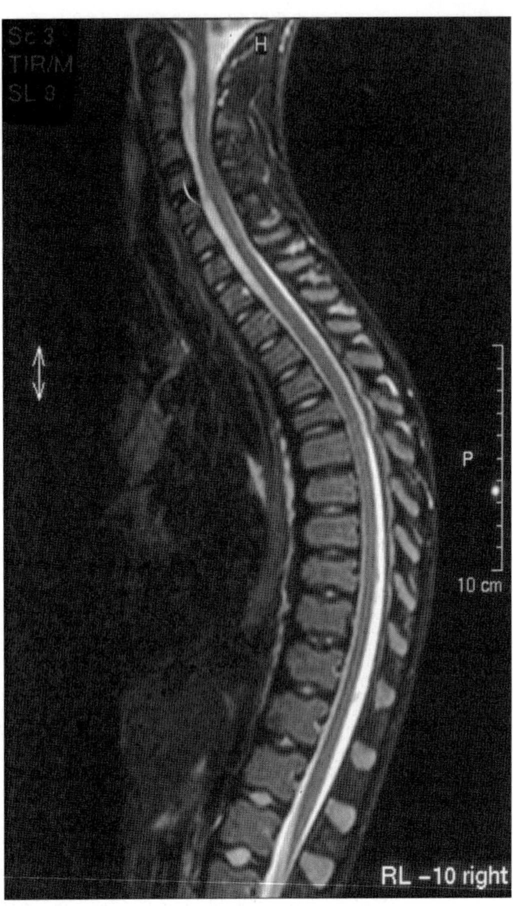

Fig. 2.61. Same patient as before. Sagittal T2-weighted image with fat saturation (STIR). Kyphosis due to T5 wedging. No edema; improved visualization of Schmorl's nodes from T7 through T12

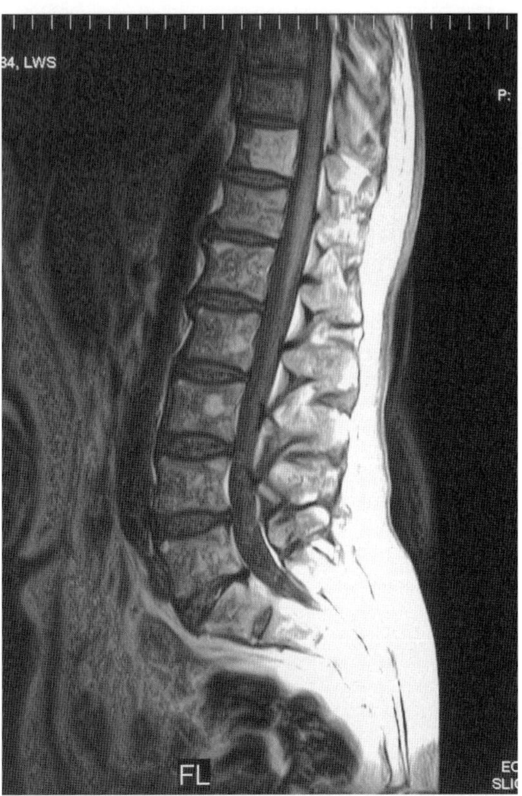

Fig. 2.62. 60-year-old patient with hemangioma. Sagittal T1-weighted image of the lower thoracic and lumbar regions showing increased signal intensity of the middle and posterior portions of T11. Normal size and shape of the vertebral body. Inhomogeneous appearance of the high-signal-intensity hemangioma through streaks of slightly lower signal

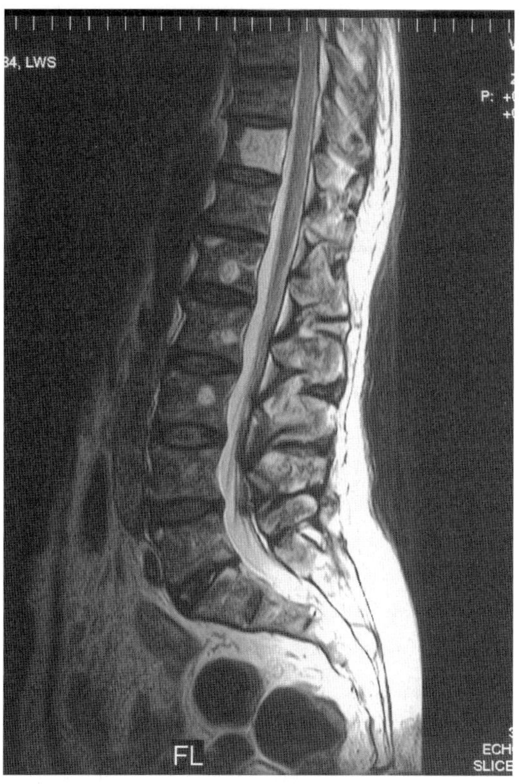

Fig. 2.63. Same patient as Fig. 2.62. Sagittal T2-weighted image showing T11 with the typical signal intensity of hemangioma. Also seen are additional smaller hemangiomas of L1 to L3

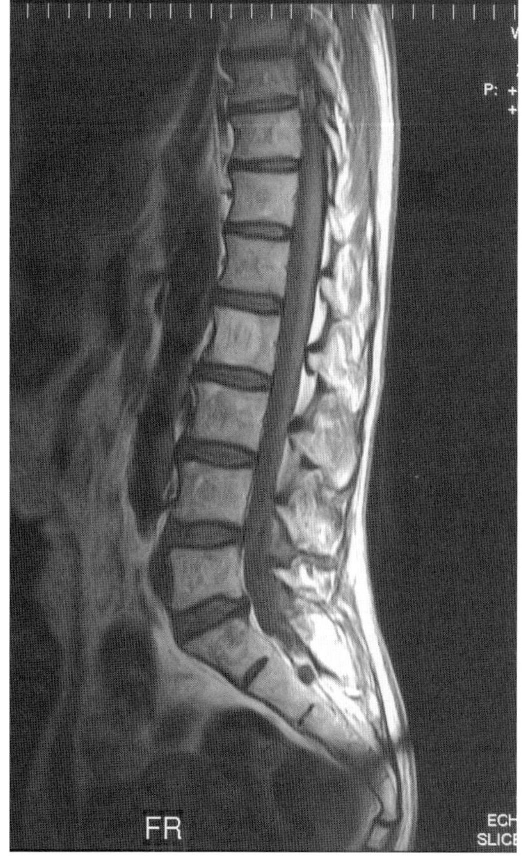

Fig. 2.64. Sagittal T1-weighted image of a hemangioma occupying the anterior and middle third of L2. Normal shape and size of the vertebral body

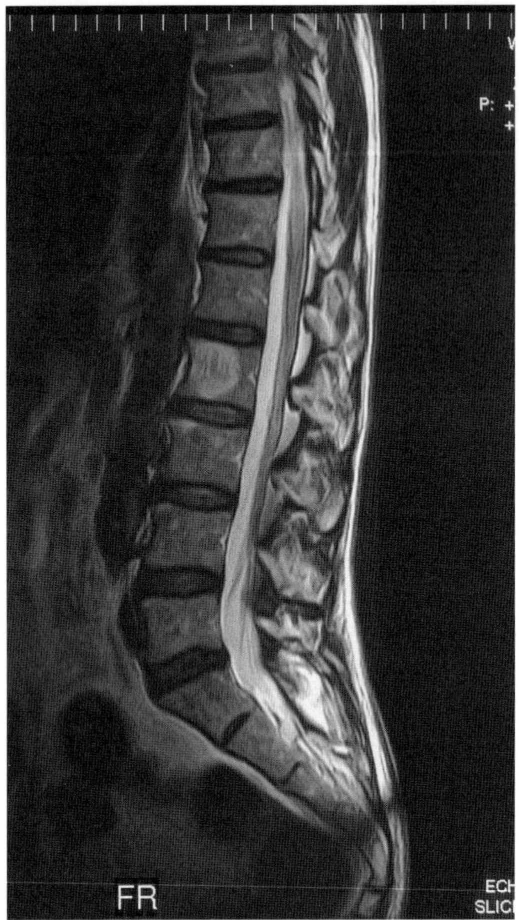

Fig. 2.65. Same patient. Typical appearance of the L2 hemangioma on sagittal T2-weighted image

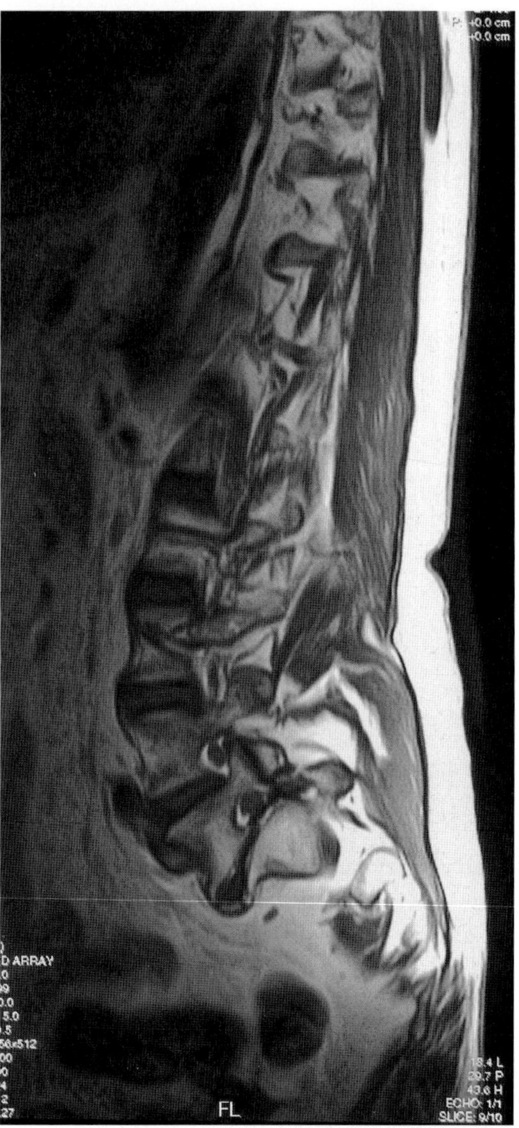

Fig. 2.66. Sagittal T1-weighted image in a patient with spondylolisthesis at L5-S1. Bony defect of the vertebral arch in the area of the pars interarticularis suggests spondylolysis. One-third anterior translation of L5 over S1, corresponding to grade 2 slippage according to the Meyerding classification

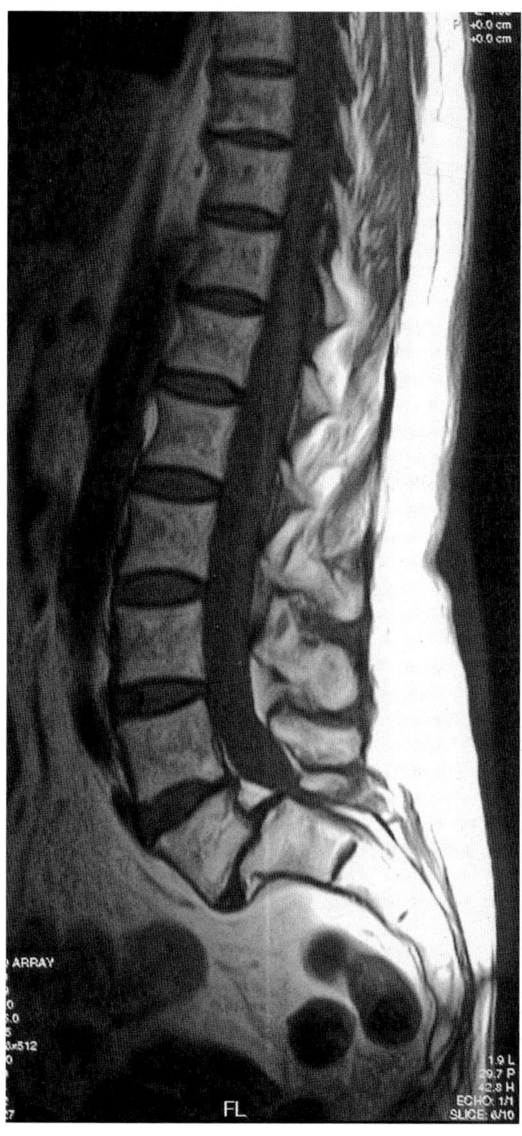

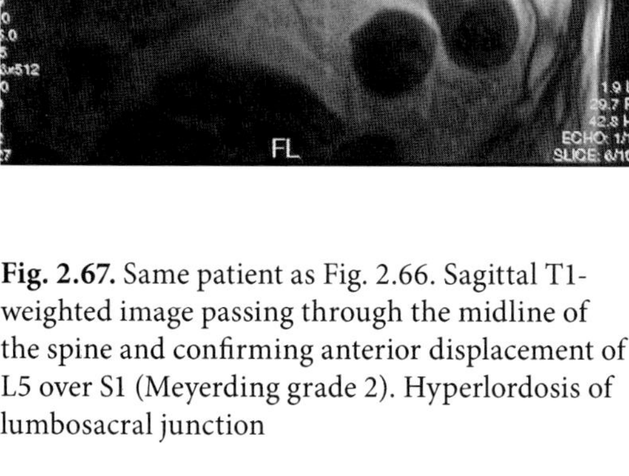

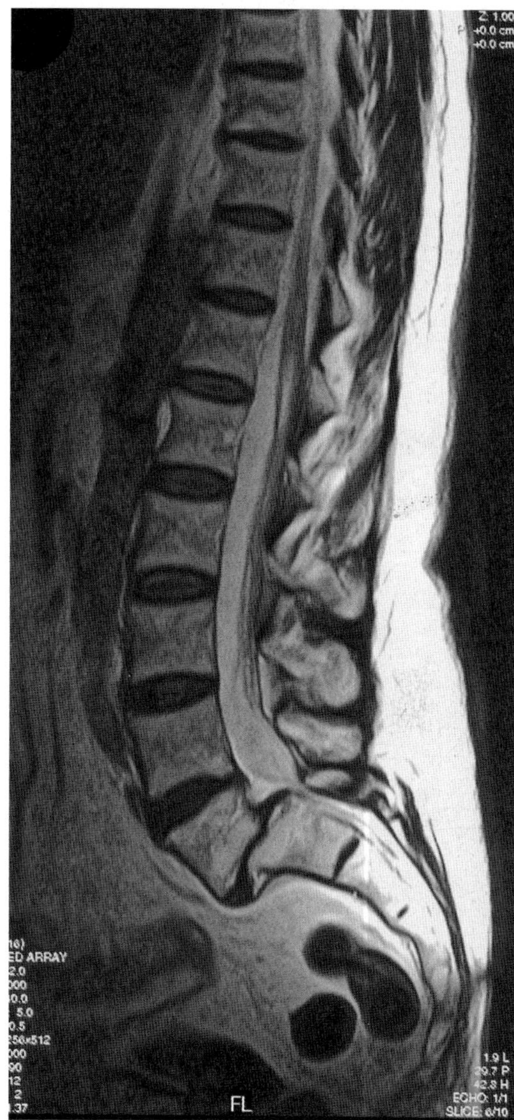

Fig. 2.67. Same patient as Fig. 2.66. Sagittal T1-weighted image passing through the midline of the spine and confirming anterior displacement of L5 over S1 (Meyerding grade 2). Hyperlordosis of lumbosacral junction

Fig. 2.68. Sagittal T2-weighted image of the patient with grade 2 spondylolisthesis due to spondylolysis

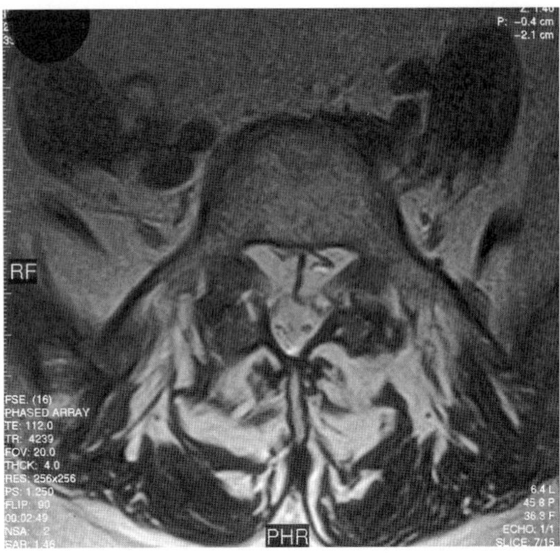

Fig. 2.69. Same patient. Axial T2-weighted image through the level of spondylolysis showing the defects as hyperostotic enlargement with contour irregularities of the vertebral arch

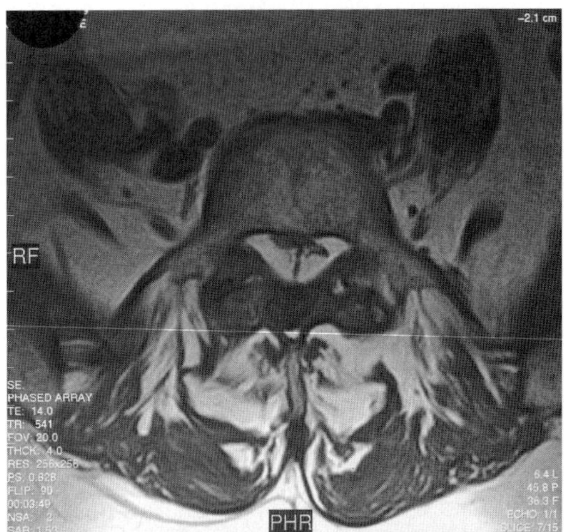

Fig. 2.70. Axial T1-weighted images of the bilateral spondylolysis

3 Trauma and Fractures

Pathoanatomy

Spinal injuries with damage to tissues may affect the intervertebral discs and ligaments or the bony structures either alone or in combination. Damage may involve the posterior elements (facet joints, vertebral arches, posterior ligaments) or the anterior elements (vertebral bodies, intervertebral discs, anterior and posterior longitudinal ligaments) or both.

In patients presenting with injuries to the anterior spinal elements, a crucial diagnostic question to be answered is whether the posterior surface of the affected vertebral body is intact.

Anatomically, injuries of the upper cervical spine have a special status: fractures of the occipital condyles, atlas, and dens axis as well as hanged man's fractures (traumatic spondylolisthesis of C2) and discoligamentous injuries with secondary instability – atlanto-occipital dislocation and atlantoaxial instability (translational and rotational).

Current classifications of injuries involving the spine from the mid-cervical to the lumbar region reflect the morphology and mechanisms of injury as well as prognostic implications. The most widely accepted classification is presented below.

Classification of spinal injuries from the mid-cervical to lumbar region (based on Magerl et al. 1994)

Type A: Vertebral body compression
- A1 Impaction fracture
- A2 Split fracture
- A3 Burst fracture

Type B: Distraction injury of anterior and posterior elements
- B1 Posterior ligament disruption
- B2 Posterior disruption includes arch
- B Anterior disruption through disc

Type C: Anterior and posterior elements with rotation
- C1 Type A with rotation
- C2 Type B with rotation
- C3 Rotation and shear

Osteoporotic fractures are low-trauma fractures that occur secondary to a low bone mass and microarchitectural deterioration of bone tissue. Vertebral fractures in osteoporosis have characteristic features (fish vertebra, wedge vertebra), typically with preservation of the superior endplate.

Pathomechanism

Spinal injuries are caused by different kinds of forces comprising flexion, distraction, axial compression, extension, rotation, and shearing mechanisms. The underlying mechanism is reflected in the type of injury and is taken into account in current classifications of spinal injuries.

Traffic accidents represent about 40% of all cervical and 30% of thoracolumbar injuries, sports injuries 20% of cervical and 10% of thoracolumbar injuries, and falls from great heights about 20% of cervical injuries and about 40% of thoracolumbar injuries. The remaining 10% to 20% of cases are accounted for by various other causes. Osteoporotic fractures are different in that they characteristically occur after minimal trauma.

The ankylosed spine is very susceptible to fracture due to progressive loss of mobility and secondary osteoporosis. As a consequence, the spine is less able to absorb impacts and fractures can be caused by minimal trauma, in particular shear forces. Such fractures predominantly occur at the vulnerable junctions, mostly the lower cervical region. Spinal injuries involving the anterior elements in patients with ankylosing spondylitis typically affect the intact intervertebral disc with concomitant fracture of syndesmophytes.

3.1 Dens Fractures

MR Technique

Patients with suspected dens fracture are examined with T1- and T2-weighted sequences in sagittal, axial, and coronal planes, often supplemented by T2-weighted imaging with fat saturation (STIR technique). Acquisition of a proton density-weighted sequence may be useful to identify fresh hemorrhage in the subdural space and surrounding soft tissue.

MR Findings

Three types of dens fractures are distinguished according to the anatomic level of the fracture (tip of dens, base of dens, body of C2) in the scheme of Anderson and D'Alonzo. The extent to which dens fractures can be evaluated on coronal and sagittal images depends on the course of the fracture line and the degree of fracture displacement. Concomitant narrowing of the spinal canal is best appreciated on axial and sagittal images. Axial images are also most suitable for identifying associated damage to the transverse ligament, which is important in assessing stability. The ligament is seen as a low-signal-intensity structure posterior to the dens on both T1 and T2.

Fresh fractures are often accompanied by small bone marrow edema, which is best seen on T2-weighted images in combination with a STIR technique. Irritation of surrounding soft tissue is also most impressively visualized with fat saturation. Fresh bleeding can produce a variety of signal intensities. Hemorrhage in the subdural space is best seen on sagittal and axial images in most cases. T2-weighted images depict acute hemorrhage as a slightly hyperintense lesion but usually with a signal intensity lower than that of CSF. On T1-weighted images, acute hemorrhage is nearly isointense with muscle. Here, it may be useful to acquire an additional proton density-weighted sequence. Some days after the acute event, T1-weighted images usually identify bleeding by its high signal intensity (Figs. 3.1–3.7).

MR Pitfalls

It is sometimes difficult to reliably distinguish between old and fresh fractures. In general, older fragments can be identified by the presence of marginal sclerosis, while edema is not present immediately after an acute fracture. Depiction of a bony structure with homogeneous marrow signal and marginal sclerosis is also consistent with congenital os odontoideum. However, with this anomaly, the surrounding soft tissue structures usually appear unremarkable. Diagnostic problems may also arise in individuals with aplasia or hypoplasia of the dens.

3.2 Axis Fractures

MR Technique

Patients with suspected fracture of the axis are typically imaged using axial T1- and T2-weighted sequences and T2-weighted sequences with fat saturation (STIR). Coronal images are superior only in cases with more severe fracture dislocation. Images in sagittal orientation enable good assessment of fractures involving the anterior portion of the C2 vertebra.

MR Findings

Fractures of the C2 neural arch are associated with disruption of the posterior tension band. The most common type is hanged man's fracture, or traumatic spondylolisthesis, which is defined as a fracture through the pedicles of the axis with or without vertebral translation. The fracture is best identified on sagittal and axial images, which will show discontinuity of the anterior portion of the arch. Depending on the extent of subluxation, there may be concomitant injury to the C2-3 disc. Involvement of the disc is suggested by abnormal signal intensities, possibly with depiction of hemorrhage in the disc space.

Hanged man's fractures are classified according to Effendi. The main role of MRI is to identify and evaluate concomitant C2-3 disc injury. The spinal cord and width of the spinal canal are best evaluated on axial and sagittal images.

A so-called teardrop fracture is a vertebral fracture with avulsion of a triangular-shaped fragment from the anteroinferior corner of the vertebral body by the anterior longitudinal ligament. This type of fracture is identified on sagittal images by signal alterations and depiction of the characteristically shaped fragment, from which this fracture derives its name (Figs. 3.8–3.12).

3.3 Spinal Contusion

MR Technique

Imaging in two planes using T2- and T1-weighted sequences; T2-weighted images with fat suppression to identify bone marrow edema (bone bruise); gradient echo sequences to detect bleeding (Fig. 3.13).

MR Pitfalls

Excellent visualization even of small traumatic bone lesions; however, microfractures of cancellous bone may mimic more extensive traumatic lesions.

Small bone fragments (in the spinal canal) are more difficult to identify than with CT.

3.4 Atlas Fractures

MR Findings

Atlas fractures are less conspicuous and may be difficult to detect on MR images due to the small size of the bony structures involved. MRI serves to evaluate the ligamentous structures (transverse ligaments) and the topographic relationship of the dens axis to the spinal cord. The different types of Jefferson fractures and unilateral fractures of the arch or lateral mass are classified as stable or unstable fractures, depending on the course of the fracture line and concomitant injury to the transverse ligament.

MRI shows interruption of the affected part on T1- and T2-weighted images (typically axial images). Evaluation of the cervical cord is important to exclude concomitant injury or potentially deleterious bleeding.

3.5 Stable Vertebral Fractures

MR Technique

MRI is predominantly performed using T1- and T2-weighted sagittal and axial images, supplemented by T2-weighted imaging with fat saturation as needed. Sagittal T2-weighted images are most useful for evaluating spinal anatomy in younger patients with a low fat content of the vertebral bodies.

Acute trauma is associated with extensive edematous changes of the bony structures. The edematous changes gradually resolve but may be detectable for up to six months after the event.

MR Findings

Vertebral fracture is identified by deformity of the vertebral body and a reduced height. Specific injury patterns vary with the type of force that caused it (compression, hyperflexion, hyperextension, shearing, and rotation). Images must be carefully scrutinized for involvement of the three weight-bearing columns (anterior, middle, and posterior portion of vertebral body). Evaluation of the posterior column is most important, since it may be damaged even without a conspicuous height reduction. An intact posterior margin and normal height of the posterior portion indicate a stable vertebral fracture (Figs. 3.14–3.19).

MR Pitfalls

A vertebral fracture is sometimes difficult to differentiate from tumorous or inflammatory destruction. In these cases, the patient's history, determination of inflammatory parameters, and careful evaluation of the localization and extent of the destructive changes may suggest the correct diagnosis. Malignant tumors often affect the pedicles and posterior third of the vertebra. The signal alterations seen in spondylodiscitis typically affect the vertebral bodies on both sides of the disc.

3.6 Unstable Vertebral Fractures

MR Technique

Sagittal and coronal images serve to assess vertebral body height. Axial images are most suitable for evaluating spinal canal width. As with stable fractures, images are acquired with T1- and T2-weighting (T2 with fat saturation).

MR Findings

The defining feature of unstable vertebral fractures is involvement of the posterior column, which is suggested by the demonstration of cortical interruption or a reduced height.

Occasionally, only discreet indentations with only minimal loss of height may be present. In such cases, signal alterations extending to the posterior cortical layer suggest instability.

Additional displacement of the vertebral bodies relative to each other suggests rupture of anterior and/or posterior ligaments and is often associated with edema or bleeding (Figs. 3.20–3.26).

MR Pitfalls

A fresh fracture at a previous fracture site (e.g. "sintering" of osteoporotic fractures) can be missed on MR images because there may be a marked loss of height of the affected vertebral body but only minimal edema.

3.7 Fractures of Transverse and Spinous Processes

MR Technique

Fractures of the transverse and spinous processes are typically caused by hyperextension or hyperflexion injuries.

These fractures are best evaluated on images perpendicular to the fracture line. Displaced bone fragments of a transverse or spinous process can be identified in all three planes. Images obtained during the acute phase will demonstrate edema and/or bleeding around the fracture.

MR Findings

Displaced fragments of the spinous or transverse processes are best seen on sagittal and axial images while fragments of the transverse processes may also be located on coronal images. Acute avulsion of a vertebral process is accompanied by edema around the fracture and in surrounding soft tissue. Often, a fat-saturated T2 sequence is needed to reliably demonstrate edema. Occasionally, the ligaments/muscles attaching around the fracture site display signal alterations indicating edema/hemorrhage (Figs. 3.27–3.34).

3.8 Disc Injuries

MR Technique

Disc injury is evaluated on sagittal, axial, and coronal T1- and T2-weighted images, supplemented by T2-weighted images with fat saturation as needed.

MR Findings

Traumatic injury to the intervertebral disc is associated with damage to the ligamentous supportive structures of the spine and often causes instability of the affected spinal segment, which may have to be confirmed by additional flexion and extension radiographs.

Traumatic disc injury may cause rupture of the annulus fibrosus with release of gelatinous disc material. MRI will show if disc material extends beyond the normal disc space. Posterior protrusion may cause marked narrowing of the spinal canal or obstruction of the neural foramina. The changes are best seen on sagittal and axial images (Figs. 3.35–3.37).

3.9 Osteoporotic Fractures

MR Technique

Suspected fractures in patients with osteoporosis are evaluated on T1- and T2-weighted sagittal, axial, and coronal images. T2-weighted STIR images are acquired to detect a fresh fracture.

MR Findings

Osteoporotic spinal bone changes are seen as a loss of trabecular structure on sagittal and axial images. Other vertebral bodies may be reduced in height due to old fractures, which can be distinguished from an acute vertebral fracture by an unchanged signal intensity on STIR images. An acute osteoporotic fracture alters the appearance of the vertebral body. The changes may be confined to the anterior and middle columns, but may occasionally also extend to the posterior portion. Edema is seen as an increase in signal intensity on T2-weighted images, most impressively on STIR images. The bone matrix is difficult to evaluate on MRI. Additional radiographs help corroborate the tentative MRI diagnosis of osteoporosis/osteopenia (Figs. 3.38–3.46).

MR Pitfalls

Vertebral compression fractures due to metastasis and porotic fractures may be similar in appearance. Osteoporotic fractures have no destructive component and typically spare the pedicles.

Osteoporotic fractures, which have low signal intensity on unenhanced images, show some enhancement on postcontrast T1-weighted images, resulting in near isointensity with the surrounding marrow. Tumorous vertebral fractures typically show slightly more pronounced enhancement, but it is nevertheless next to impossible to distinguish these two types of fractures on the basis of their signal enhancement.

3.10 Posttraumatic Syrinx

MR Technique

Sagittal T1- and T2-weighted images and axial images; contrast-enhanced T1-weighted sequence to exclude tumorous syrinx. Coronal images may be helpful in individual cases.

MR Findings

Longitudinal lesion with fluid signal in the spinal cord (Figs. 3.47–3.55).

MR Pitfalls

Pulsation or motion artifacts may mimic a syrinx, in particular on T2-weighted images. Comparison of the appearance on axial images is necessary.

3.11 Spinal Cord Injuries

See Figs. 3.56 to 3.58.

3.12 Ligament Injuries

MR Findings

Ligaments have low or absent signal on T1- and T2-weighted images. Traumatic injury to a ligament may be indicated by a focal disruption or rarefaction of the normal ligamentous structure. Acute ligamentous injury is associated with marginal edematous swelling, which is identified on T2-weighted images by an increase in signal intensity. Hemorrhage will be depicted as a focal area of increased signal intensity on T2-weighted images and shortly afterwards also on T1-weighted images.

Isolated ligament injuries may be difficult to evaluate by MRI. They can be demonstrated by flexion and extension radiographs. Small bony avulsions may be missed on MR images, while larger avulsed bone fragments attached to the ligament are depicted with bone signal. Bleeding or reactive edema is often apparent at the site of avulsion. These structures may help evaluate the extent of bone damage on CT scans (Fig. 3.59–3.61).

3.13 Fractures in Ankylosing Spondylitis

MR Technique

Patients with ankylosing spondylitis and suspected spinal fracture are examined using sagittal and axial T1- and T2-weighted images. These may be supplemented by coronal images and a T2-weighted sequence with fat saturation (STIR technique).

MR Findings

Spinal fracture in ankylosing spondylitis is suggested by a horizontal fracture line through a vertebra/intervertebral space with involvement of the vertebral arch structures. In addition, MRI shows the typical changes of the disc spaces associated with the underlying disease. The fractures tend to heal poorly due to excessive motion at the affected level as a result of stiffening of adjacent motion segments. As with acute fractures in general, edema of surrounding anatomy may be present as well as irritation of soft tissue and hemorrhage (Figs. 3.62–3.64).

3.14 Clinical Significance of MRI in Spinal Injuries

Adequate therapeutic management of spinal trauma crucially relies on the comprehensive evaluation of the extent of damage to the bony structures, in particular the posterior column of affected vertebral bodies, the discoligamentous structures, and the paravertebral soft tissue. While not being the primary imaging modality in the initial evaluation of patients with spinal injuries, MRI can provide important additional information supplementing the clinical, radiographic, and CT findings. CT is superior to MRI in delineating the presence and extent of bony injuries, and the advent of spiral CT scanners has fundamentally altered the management of patients with acute spinal injuries. Nevertheless, MRI is invaluable for evaluating damage to discoligamentous structures occurring alone or in conjunction with other injuries. Moreover, MRI is also indispensable for assessing spinal canal involvement and impingement on the cord in patients with neurologic deficits.

About 70% of all osteoligamentous injuries of the cervical spine and about 20% of all thoracolumbar fractures treated in a hospital are associated with neurologic deficits. Spinal injuries may be accompanied by severe neurologic deficits even when no major compression of neural structures is apparent – e.g. because spontaneous (partial) repositioning has occurred. Moreover, patients may develop severe neurologic deficits secondary to spinal trauma when fractures or other injuries that could explain the deficits are absent. This may be the case after transient hyperextension of the spinal cord or spinal vessels.

In patients with osteoporotic vertebral fractures, especially if these are multiple, MRI can help distinguish between acute and chronic fractures.

Fractures associated with ankylosing spondylitis are often missed at initial diagnosis because they are difficult to see on radiographs (severe osteoporosis, overlying structures in the lower cervical region, injury patterns involving the intervertebral disc and syndesmophytes) and because they are often caused by minor trauma. Here, MRI is an indispensable supplementary diagnostic tool.

Spinal fractures in patients with ankylosing spondylitis should be stabilized surgically even if no fracture dislocation is apparent. Surgery is indicated because the underlying disease with stiffness of adjacent motion segments exposes the fracture level to excessive motion, especially in the cervical region, thereby increasing the risk of dislocation. Moreover, the unfavorable biomechanical situation also precludes spontaneous healing or beneficial effects of conservative measures in most patients. Instead, these patients are at risk of persistent secondary discoligamentous destruction (Andersson 2 lesion) with chronic instability.

3.15 Nerve Root Avulsion

Pathoanatomy and Pathophysiology

The ventral and dorsal nerve roots unite to form the segmental spinal nerves directly distal to the spinal ganglia in the intervertebral foramina. A nerve root may rupture due to traction forces acting on the distal plexus in spinal trauma. On their intraspinal course, the nerve roots are protected by the dura and, in the cervical region, there is some additional protection from the fibrous portions of the deep cervical fascia, providing attachment for the nerves along their extraforaminal course. The fascia provides stronger protection for the C5 and C6 nerves, which explains why avulsion more commonly affects the lower cervical nerve roots. The preferred rupture site is at the lateral margin of the foramen (postganglionic injury). Avulsion of dorsal and ventral nerve roots occurs directly after the nerve roots have emerged from the cord. The arachnoid membrane ensheathing the nerve root also ruptures and herniates into the intervertebral foramen, giving rise to a characteristic pseudomeningocele.

MR Findings

MRI depicts the characteristic pseudomeningocele, while the nerve root is no longer discernible (Figs. 3.65 and 3.66).

MR Pitfalls

The demonstration of a pseudomeningocele is virtually regarded as diagnostic of nerve root avulsion. Nevertheless, it is known that a pseudomeningocele may be present without nerve root avulsion. Definitive demonstration of an intrathecal nerve root avulsion is also difficult by MRI.

Clinical Significance

There have been various attempts to reimplant avulsed nerve roots into the cord but all attempts have thus far shown that direct repair is not possible. The surgical option available in nerve root avulsion is nerve transfer (neurotization).

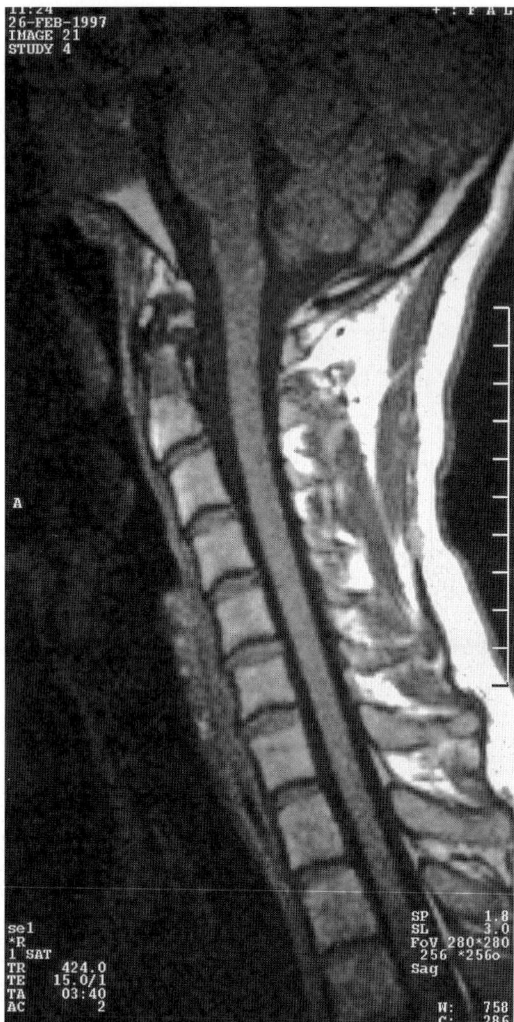

Fig. 3.1. Sagittal T1-weighted image of a 34-year-old patient after a motorcycle accident. Transverse fracture through the tip of the dens with posterior displacement of the fragment. No displacement or indentation of the cervical cord. Discreet areas of low signal intensity around the fracture suggest marrow edema of the dens

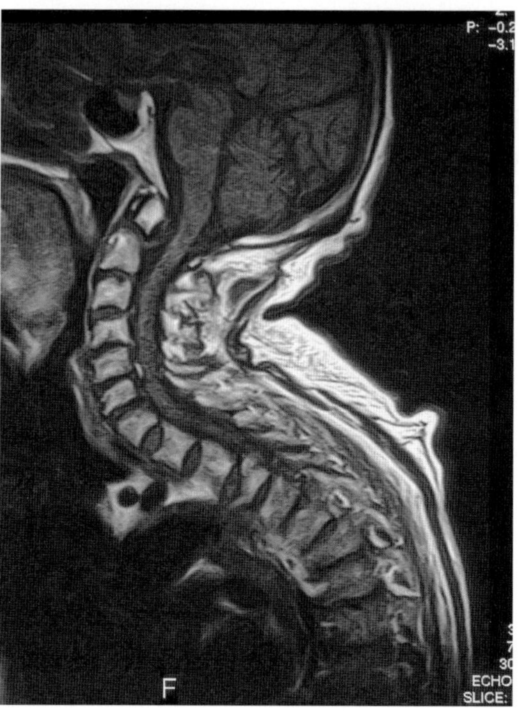

Fig. 3.2. Sagittal T1-weighted image of a 78-year-old patient after a fall. Image showing a transverse fracture through the middle portion of the dens and moderate posterior displacement of the dens fragment with only minimal displacement of the cord at the fracture level. Also seen is severe degeneration of the cervical spine with protrusions and narrowing of the spinal canal. This image does not show any signal alterations of the cord at the fracture level. Note that T1-weighted images are not very sensitive to such changes and a normal appearance on T1 therefore does not exclude injury to the spinal cord or malacia

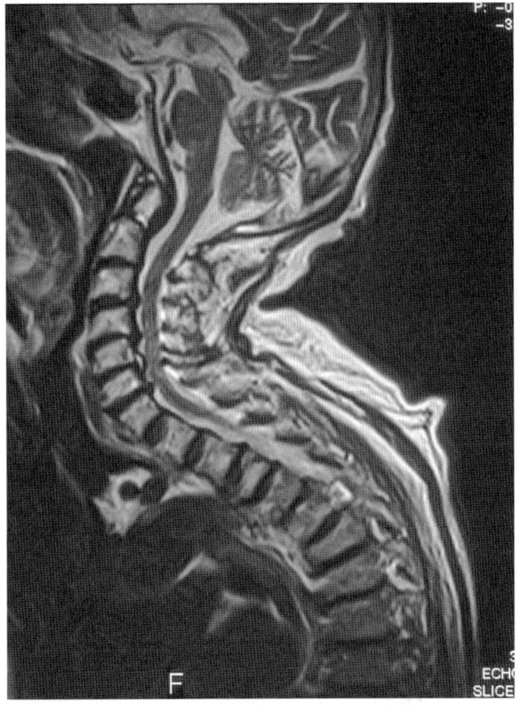

Fig. 3.3. Same patient as Fig. 3.2. Sagittal T2-weighted image of the dens fracture. Indentation of the subdural space at the C2 level is now somewhat more conspicuous than on the T1-weighted image. No significant hematoma or other lesion is seen around the fracture. This appearance suggests an older fracture. No signs of injury/malacia of the spinal cord

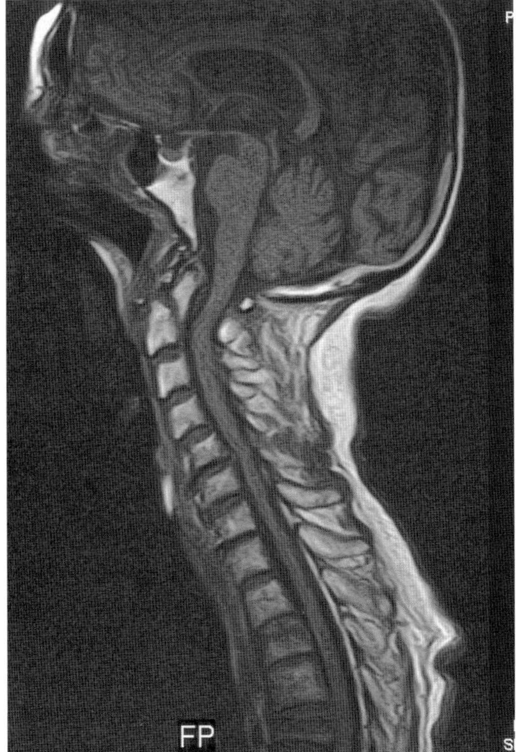

Fig. 3.4. Sagittal T1-weighted image of a 90-year-old patient who fell from her bed. Dislocated dens fracture through the middle portion of the dens with posterior tilting of the fragment. Irregular appearance of the fracture margins but normal signal intensity. No signs of hematoma

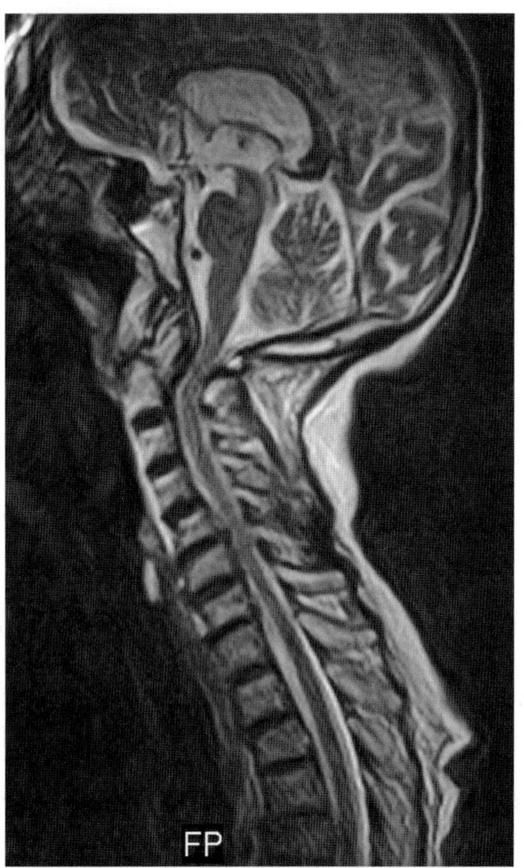

Fig. 3.5. Same patient as Fig. 3.4. Sagittal T2-weighted image showing the oblique fracture through the middle portion of the dens with posterior displacement of the fragment and stenosis of the spinal canal at the C1-2 level. The fragments have a slightly higher signal intensity than the adjacent vertebrae

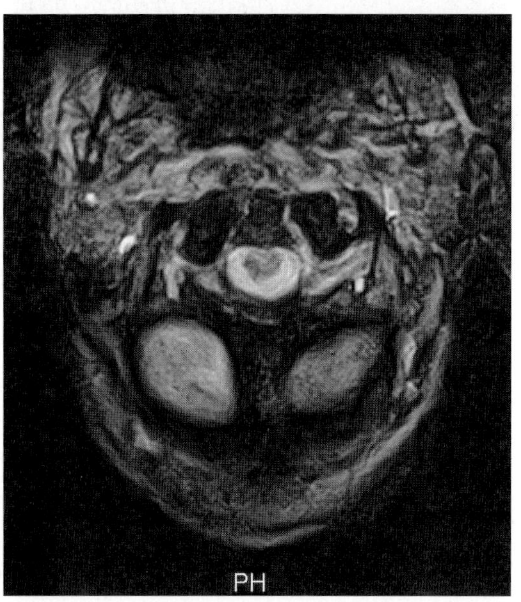

Fig. 3.6. Axial T2-weighted image of the same patient. The narrowing of the anterior subdural space at the fracture level seen on the sagittal images is less prominent in the axial plane. There is slight posterior displacement of the spinal cord. Mild hyperintensities in the anterior aspect of the spinal cord without significant expansion

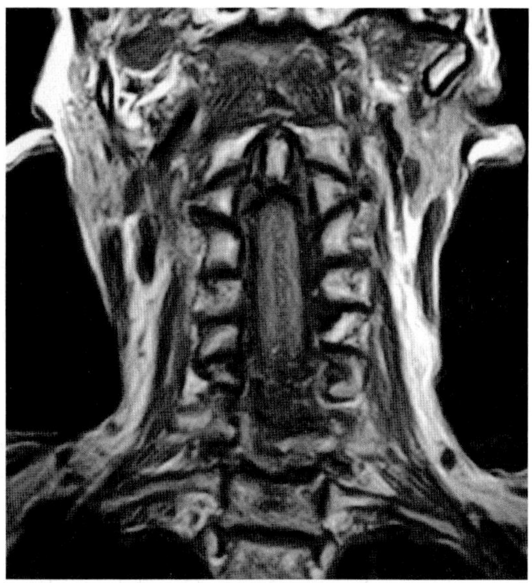

Fig. 3.7. Same patient. Coronal T1-weighted image showing protrusion of the dens fragment into the spinal canal at the C1-2 level

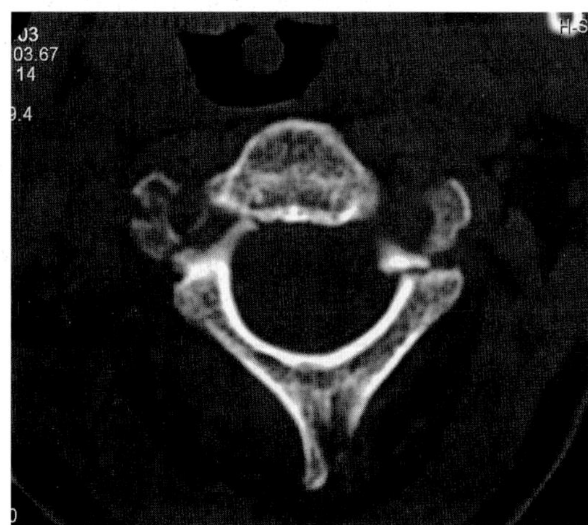

Fig. 3.8. Axial CT scan of a 40-year-old patient with bilateral fracture of the arch of the axis. The fracture line on the right is directly adjacent to the neural foramen. The fracture on the left is posterior to the foramen and there is slight displacement of the anterior part of the axis

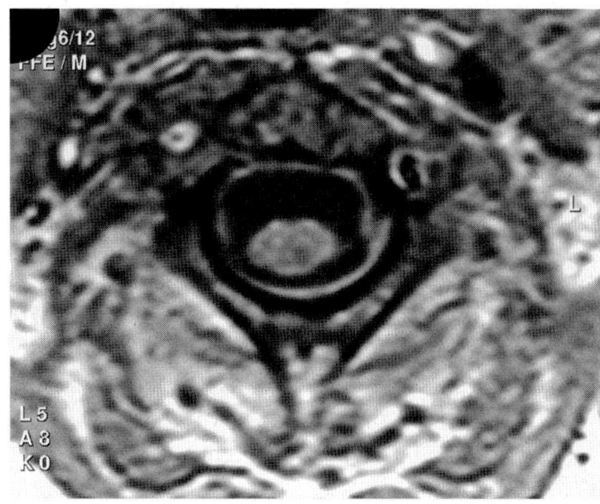

Fig. 3.9. Corresponding axial T1-weighted image of the bilateral arch fracture at C2 already demonstrated by CT. The fractures are indicated by discontinuities

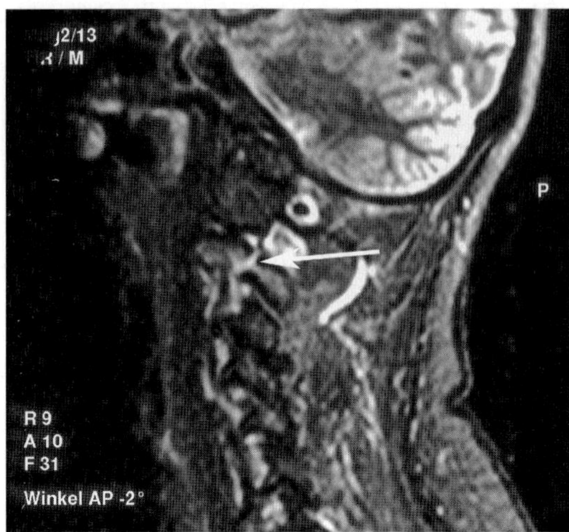

Fig. 3.10. Same patient. Sagittal T2-weighted image with fat saturation showing a band of increased signal intensity in the area of the right pedicle of C2 *(arrow)*

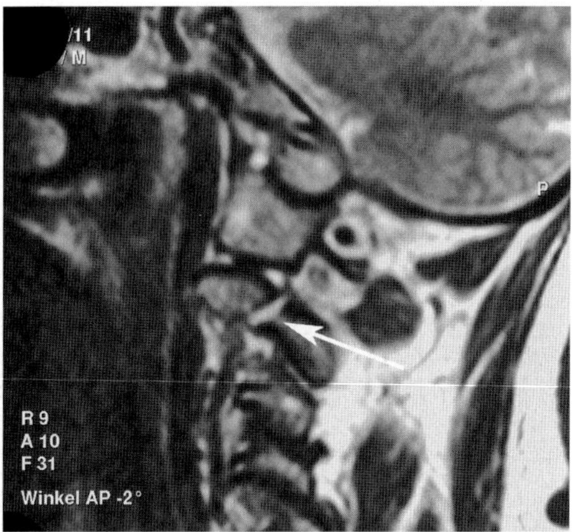

Fig. 3.11. Sagittal T2-weighted image of the axis fracture *(arrow)*

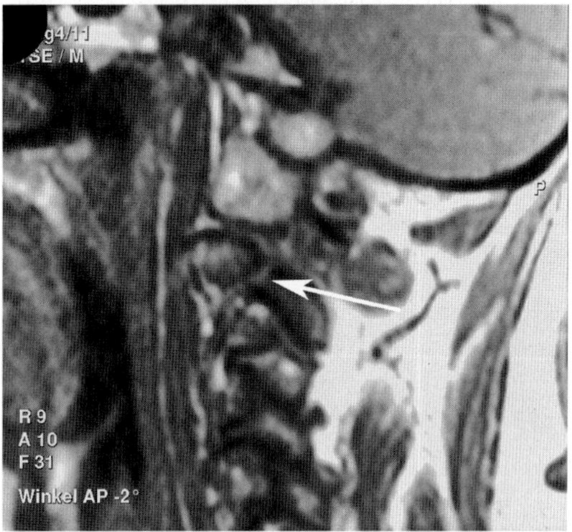

Fig. 3.12. Sagittal T1-weighted image showing the C2 arch fracture on the right without surrounding edema or hematoma *(arrow)*

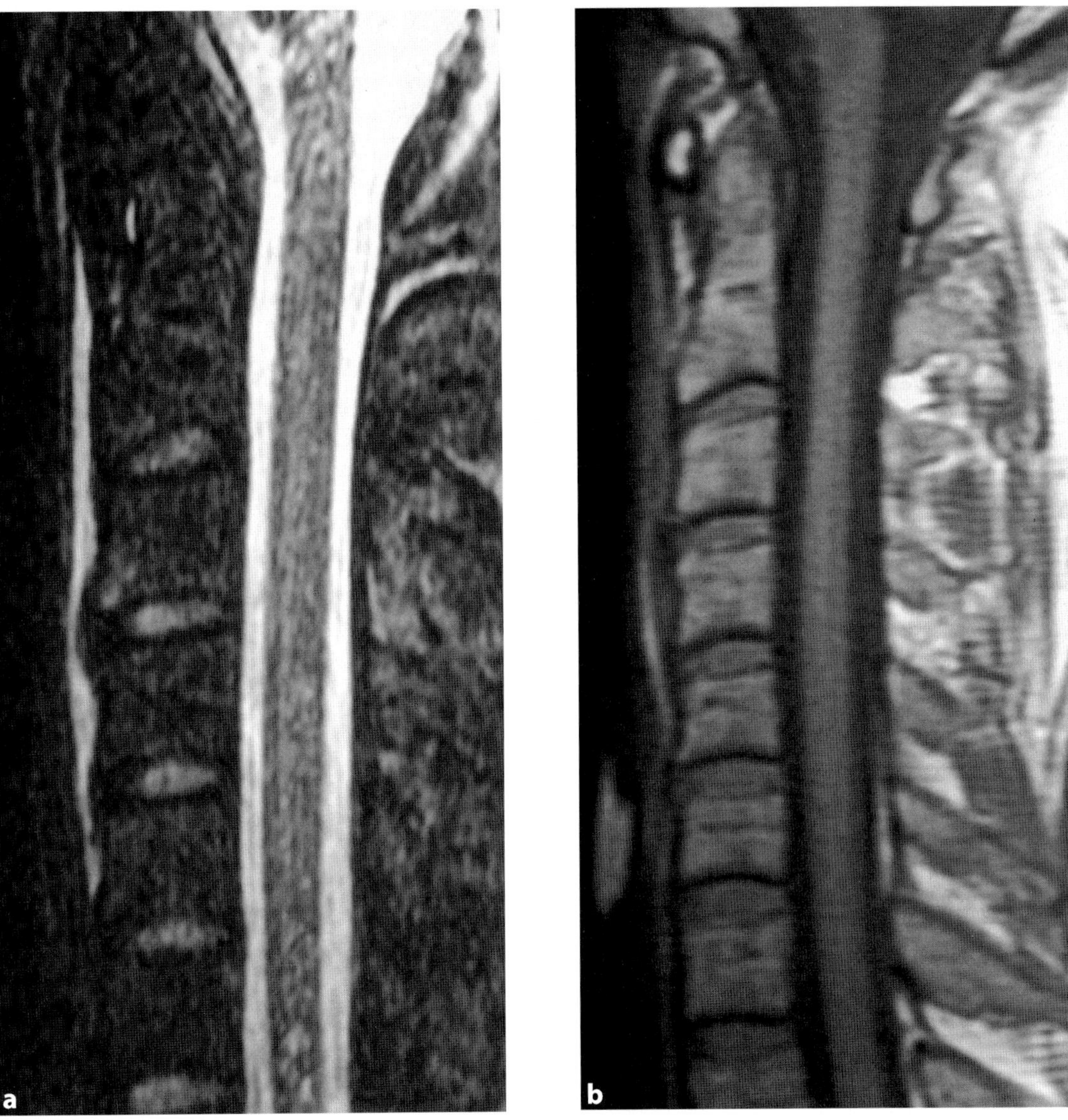

Fig. 3.13a, b. Spinal contusion. Fat-suppressed sagittal T2- and T1-weighted images showing bone bruises of the anterior edges of C3 and C4 with prevertebral hematoma/edema and bone marrow edema

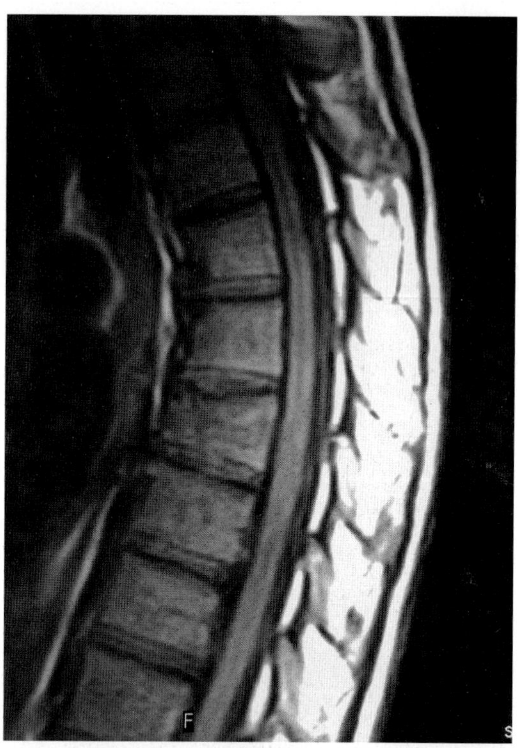

Fig. 3.14. Sagittal T1-weighted image of the mid-thoracic spine in a patient with postural kyphosis. The image demonstrates an irregular superior endplate of the T9 vertebra and blurring of this area. Mild signal reduction of the marrow below the T9 endplate. Stable posterior edge

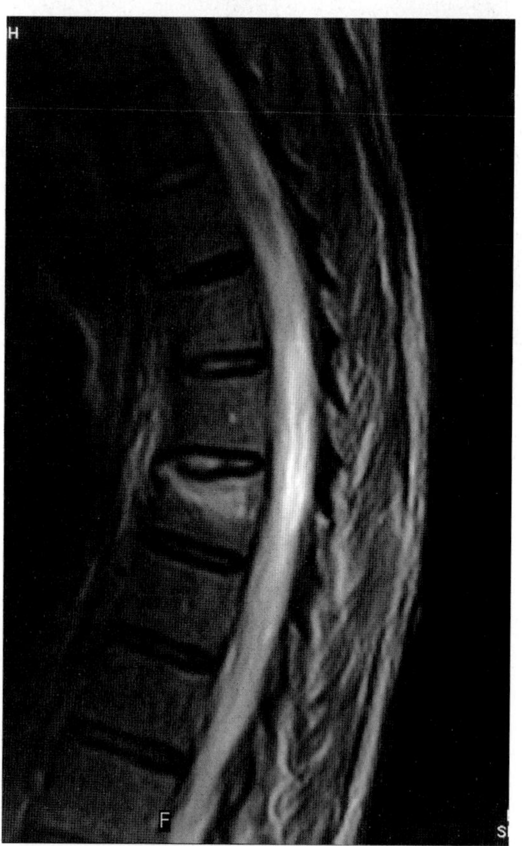

Fig. 3.15. Same patient as Fig. 3.14. Sagittal T2-weighted image with fat saturation of the mid-thoracic spine. Large bone marrow edema of the T9 vertebra below the irregular superior endplate. The findings are consistent with a more recent impression fracture involving the anterior and middle portions but sparing the posterior portion

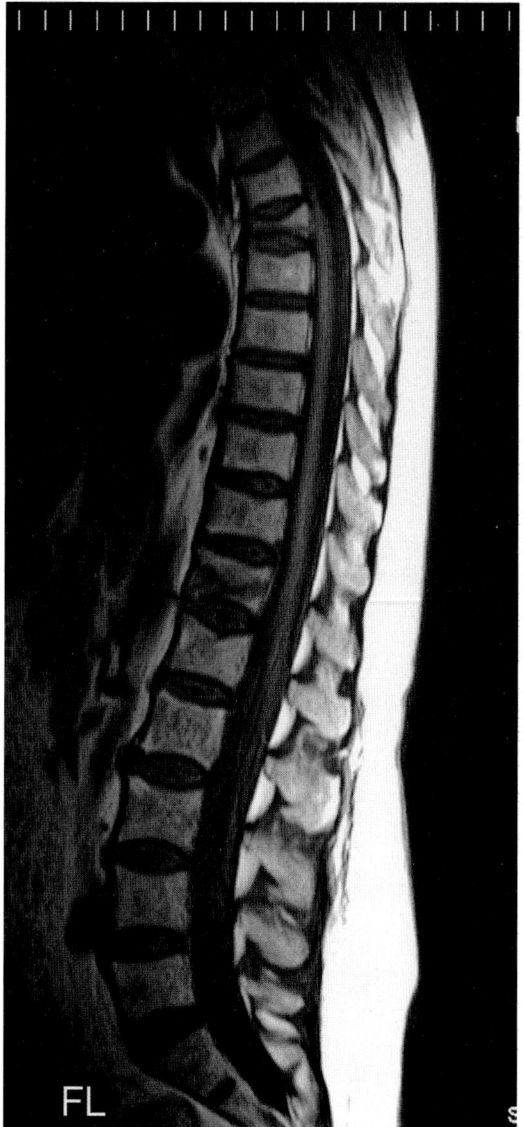

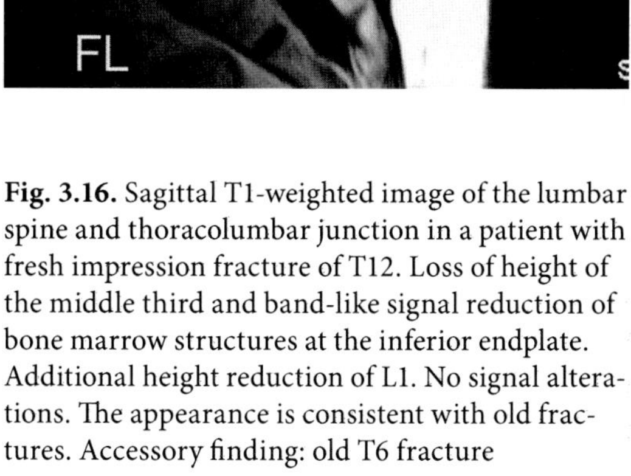
Fig. 3.16. Sagittal T1-weighted image of the lumbar spine and thoracolumbar junction in a patient with fresh impression fracture of T12. Loss of height of the middle third and band-like signal reduction of bone marrow structures at the inferior endplate. Additional height reduction of L1. No signal alterations. The appearance is consistent with old fractures. Accessory finding: old T6 fracture

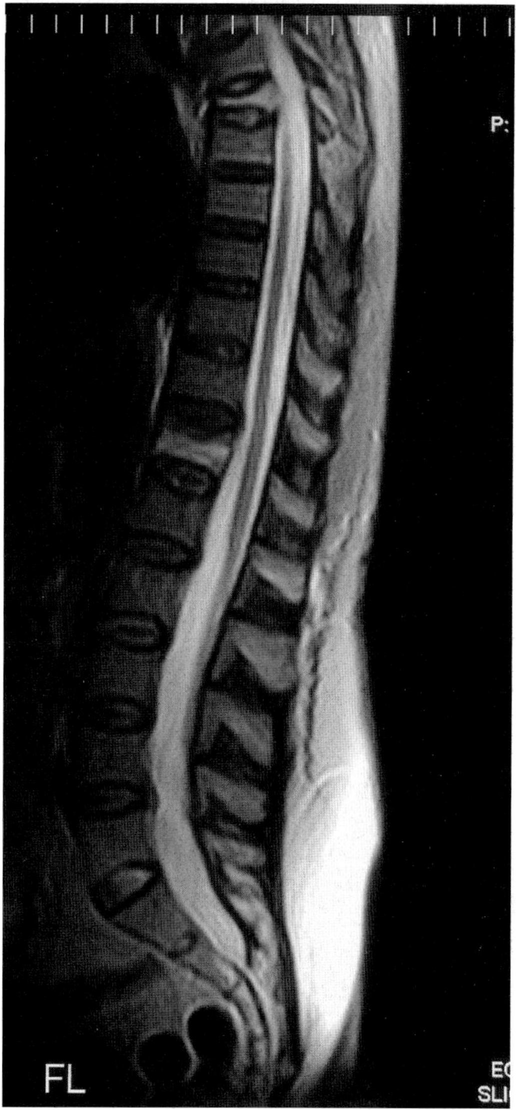

Fig. 3.17. Sagittal T2-weighted image of the thoracolumbar region. There is a band of increased signal intensity in the lower portions of the vertebral body which represents bone marrow edema extending to the posterior margin. The height of the posterior column is not reduced. The findings suggest a stable T12 compression fracture as the loss of height is confined to the anterior and middle columns

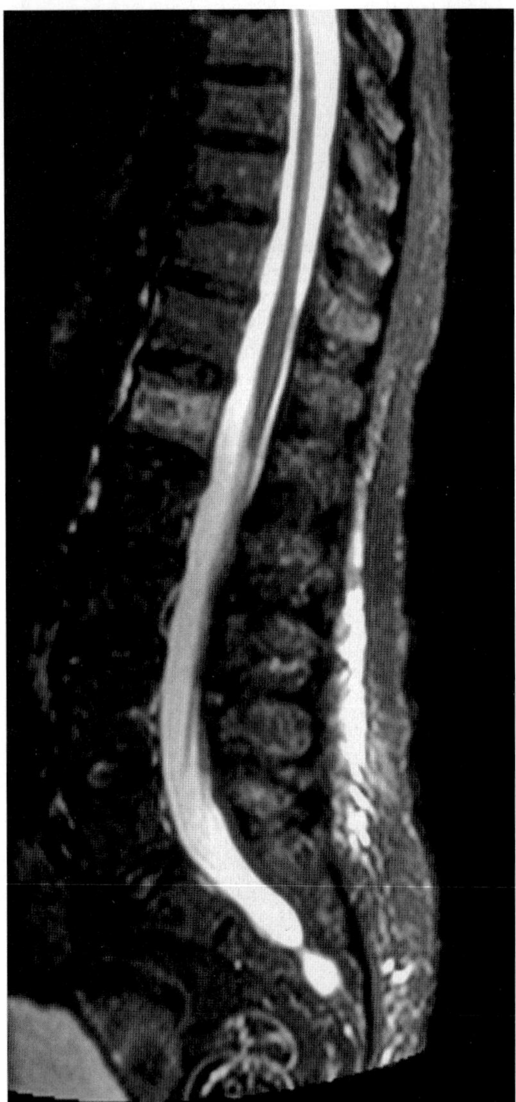

Fig. 3.18. Sagittal T2-weighted image with fat saturation of the lumbar region including the thoracolumbar junction in a patient after trauma. Area of high signal intensity in the L1 vertebral body with intact posterior margin and only minimal loss of height of anterior column. In this patient with trauma, the appearance is consistent with large bone marrow edema but only discreet fracture of the anterior column without any signs of instability

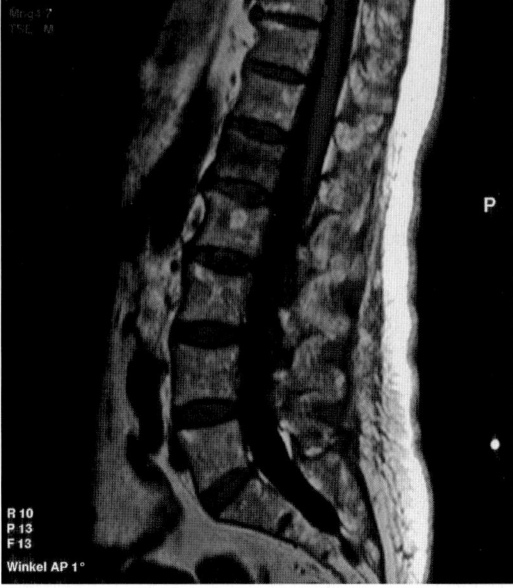

Fig. 3.19. Sagittal T1-weighted image of the stable L1 fracture showing only mild signal reduction of the vertebral body which is nearly normal in shape and size with an intact posterior margin

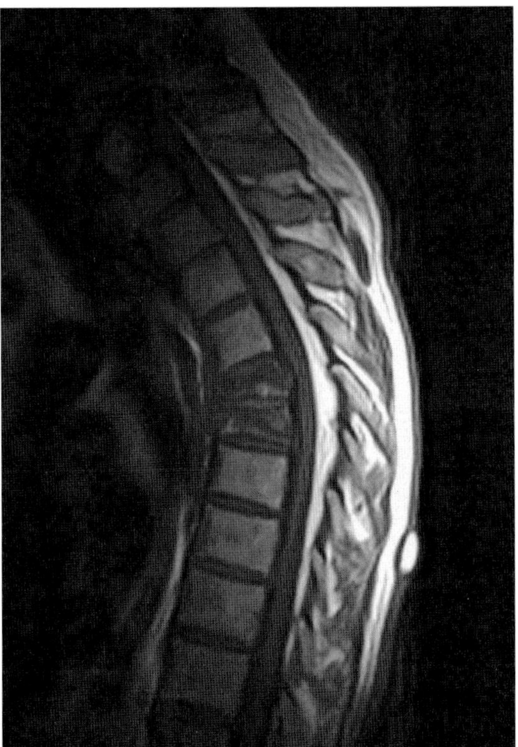

Fig. 3.20. Sagittal T2-weighted image of the thoracic region in a 43-year-old patient after a fall. The painful region is indicated by a fat capsule attached to the skin. The image demonstrates reduced signal intensity and deformity of the T7 and T8 vertebral bodies above the capsule. In addition, there is slight indentation and displacement of the thoracic cord without signs of a mass or hematoma in the area around the fractured vertebrae

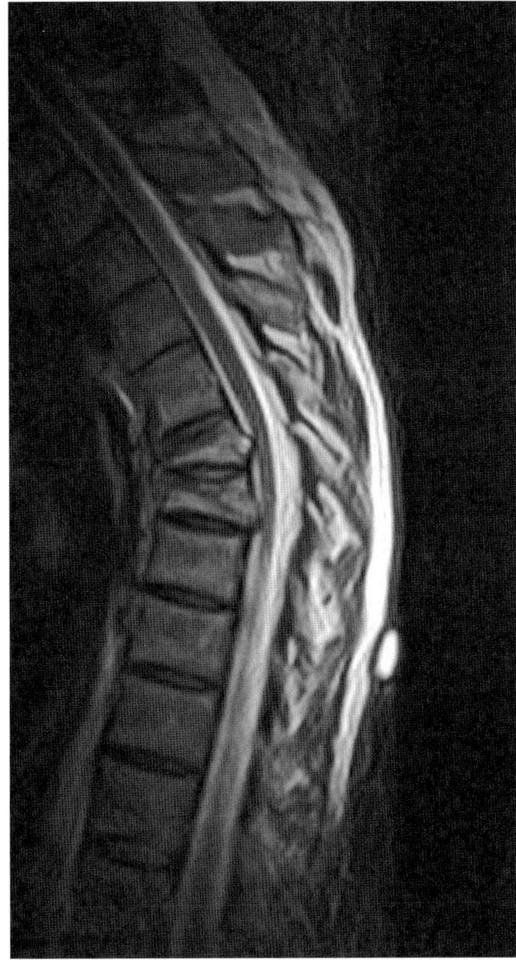

Fig. 3.21. Same patient. Sagittal T2-weighted image of the thoracic region showing the height reduction of all three columns of the T7 and T8 vertebral bodies. In addition, there is dislocation of bone structures from the middle third of T7 and lower third of T8 which are contiguous with the thoracic cord. Suggestion of a slight signal increase in the spinal cord at this level, consistent with edema. The T7 and T8 fractures are unstable because all three columns are involved

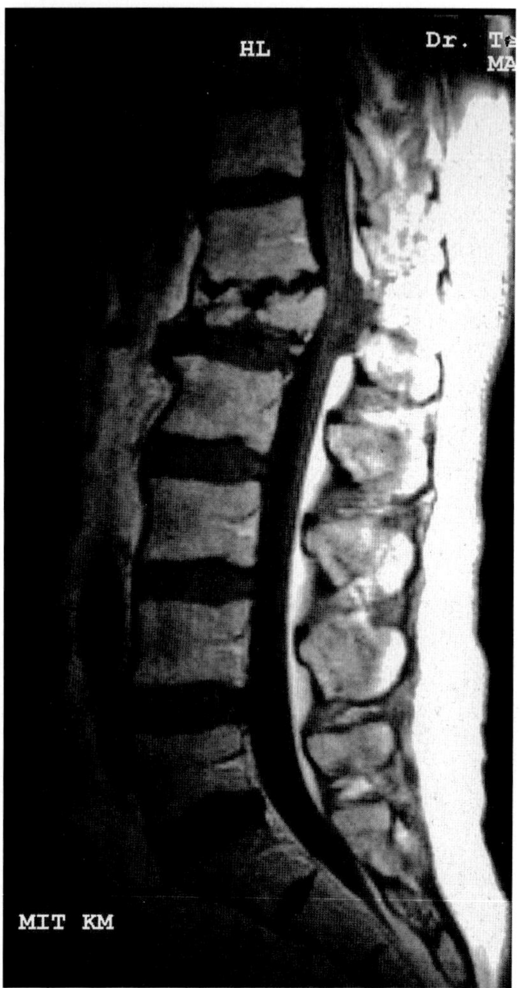

Fig. 3.22. Sagittal T1-weighted image of a 55-year-old patient obtained five months after a traffic accident. There is a pronounced loss of height of the entire L1 vertebral body with marked irregularities of the L1 superior endplate and T12 inferior endplate. The posterior margin of L1 protrudes into the spinal canal and displaces the conus medullaris/cauda equina. The unchanged signal intensity of the L1 vertebral body suggests an older fracture

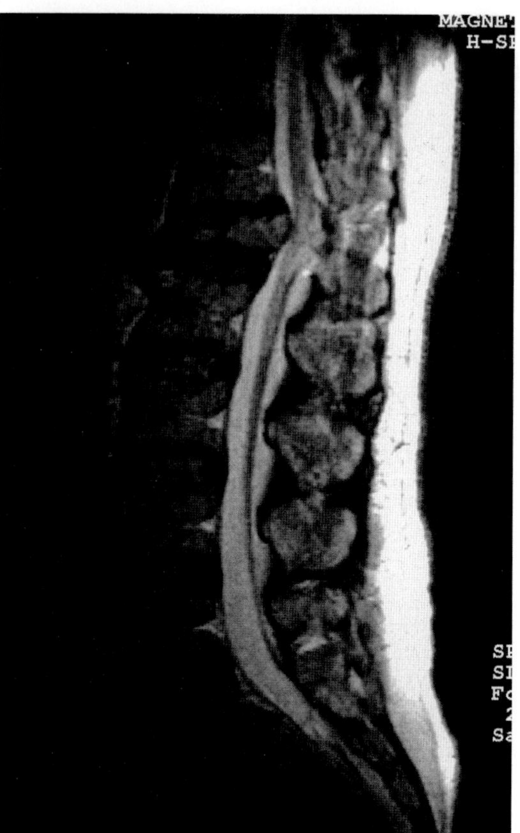

Fig. 3.23. Same patient. Sagittal T2-weighted image. The posterior portion of L1 indents the spinal canal with narrowing and displacement of the conus/cauda equina. The unaltered vertebral signal intensity is consistent with an older fracture sustained about five months previously

Fig. 3.24. Sagittal T2-weighted image of the cervical spine and cervicothoracic junction showing an impression fracture of the anterior and middle columns of C7. Increased fluid in the former C6-7 interspace is suggested by an increased signal intensity. There is mild posterior displacement of C7 over C6 with narrowing of the spinal canal and slight cord displacement at this level. This appearance suggests an unstable fracture although the anterior margin is intact

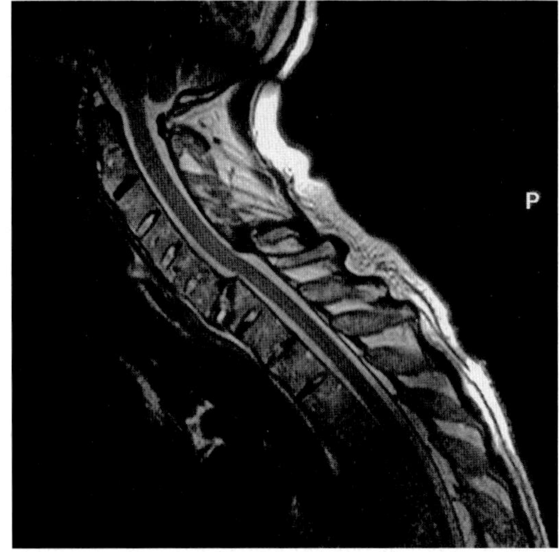

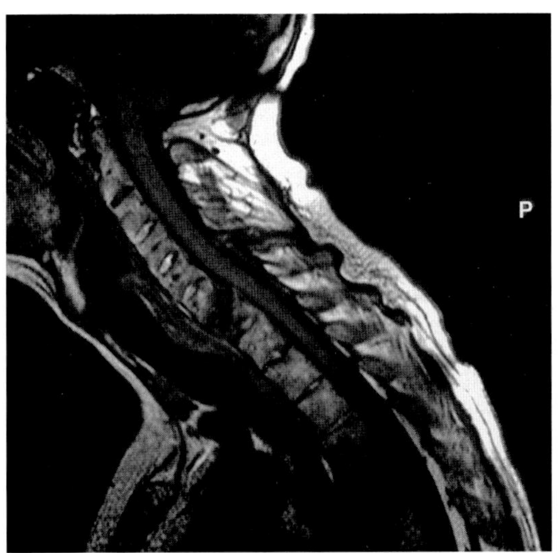

Fig. 3.25. Same patient. Sagittal T1-weighted image of the unstable C7 fracture with low signal intensity indicating increased fluid in the upper portion of C7 and the C6-7 interspace. There is involvement of posterior structures but no evidence of hemorrhage

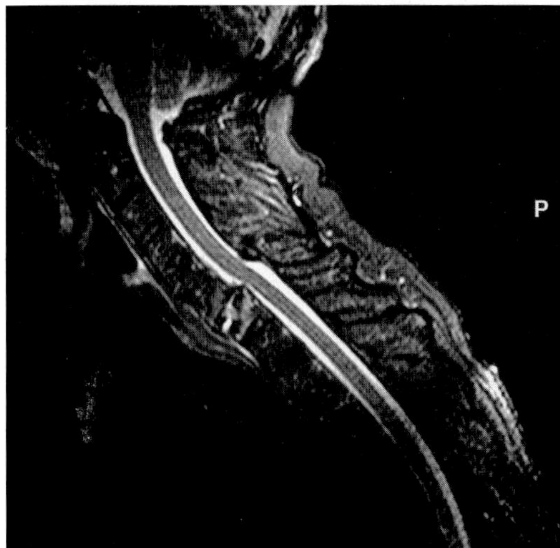

Fig. 3.26. Sagittal T2-weighted image with fat saturation showing high signal intensity of C7 consistent with an acute impression fracture. There is involvement of the anterior and middle columns while the posterior edge is intact. Nevertheless, displacement of C6 over C7 and involvement of posterior vertebral structures suggest an unstable fracture

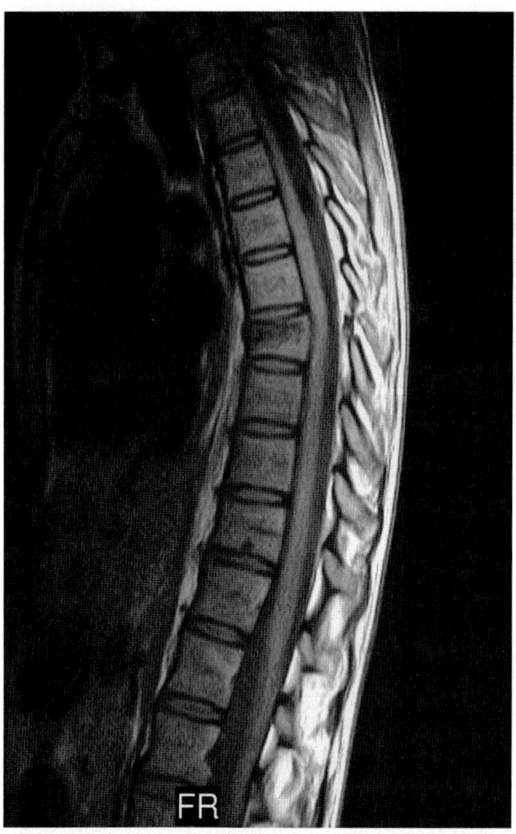

Fig. 3.27. Sagittal T1-weighted image of the thoracic region in a 27-year-old patient after a traffic accident. Loss of height of the middle and anterior columns of T8 with reduced signal intensity at superior endplate. Mild abnormal convexity of the posterior edge of T8. The appearance suggests an acute vertebral fracture. The fracture of the transverse process is not visualized on the sagittal image

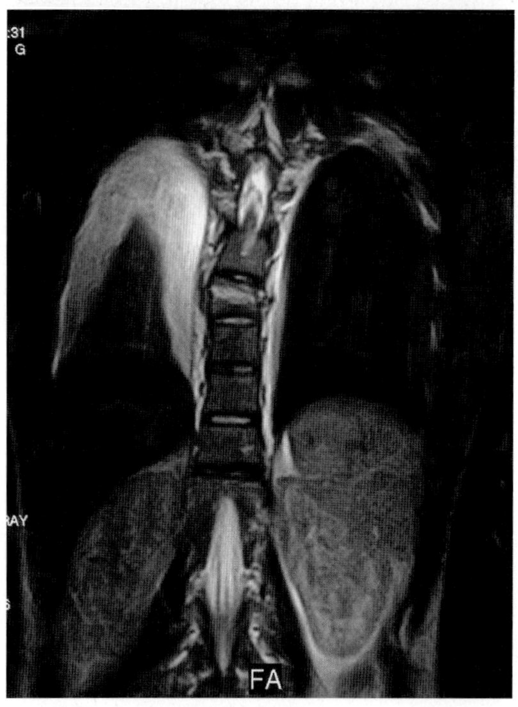

Fig. 3.28. Same patient. Coronal T2-weighted image of the T8 fracture. Vertebral compression is more prominent on the left. There are band-like hyperintensities of the bone marrow in the fracture area. Slight postural scoliosis with left concavity and pleural effusion on the right

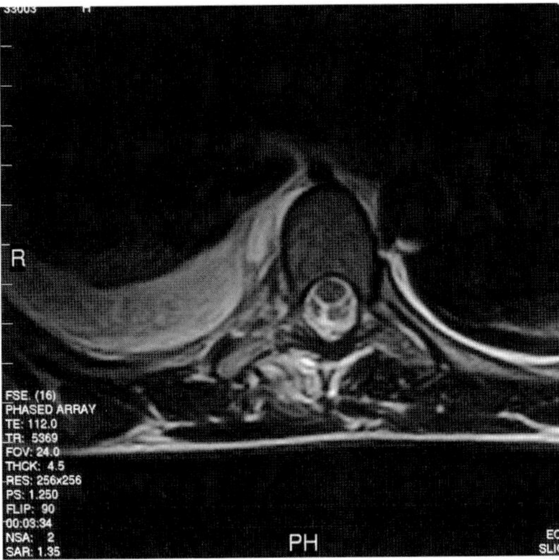

Fig. 3.29. Same patient. Axial T2-weighted image. Discontinuity of the right transverse process with surrounding edema and signal alterations of soft tissue structures. Pleural effusion on the right

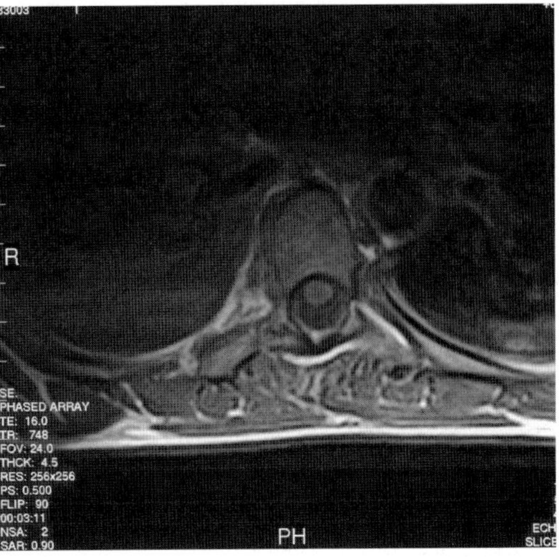

Fig. 3.30. Same patient. Axial T1-weighted image showing the fracture of the transverse process on the right. Surrounding edema is only suggested indirectly by blurring of soft tissue septa

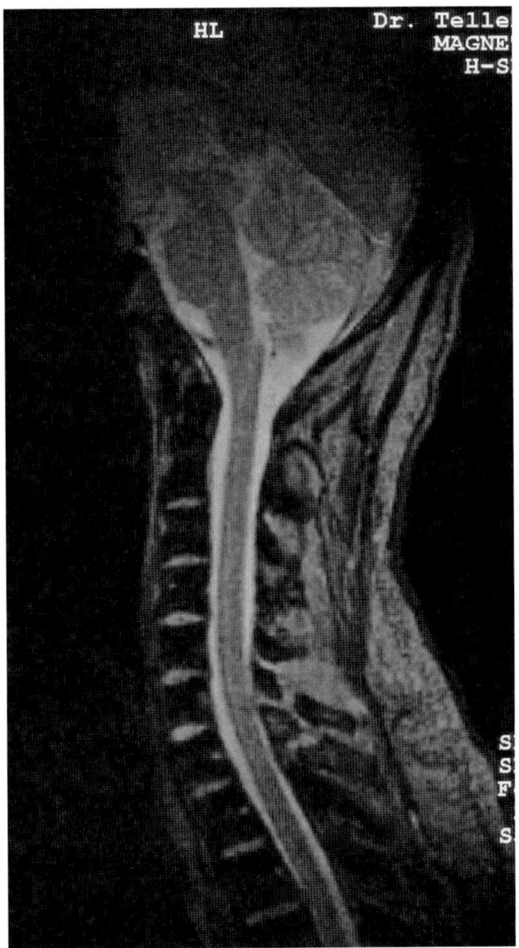

Fig. 3.31. Multiple spinous process fracture. 48-year-old patient presenting with posterior cervical pain after falling from a ladder. Sagittal T2-weighted image with fat saturation of the cervical region. Perpendicular disruption of the C6 and C7 spinous processes with slight posterior displacement and mild edema and hemorrhage of surrounding structures

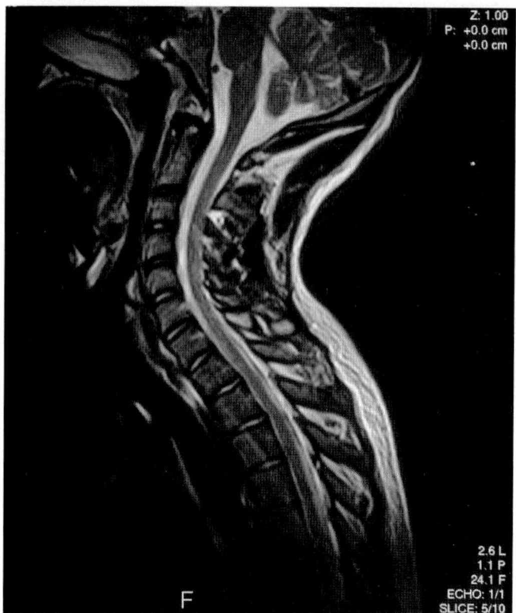

Fig. 3.32. Sagittal T2-weighted image of the cervical and upper thoracic regions in a 22-year-old patient after a rear-end collision. Mild hyperlordosis of the cervicothoracic junction. Nearly perpendicular discontinuity of the C6 spinous process and increased signal intensity without significant edema or other changes in surrounding structures

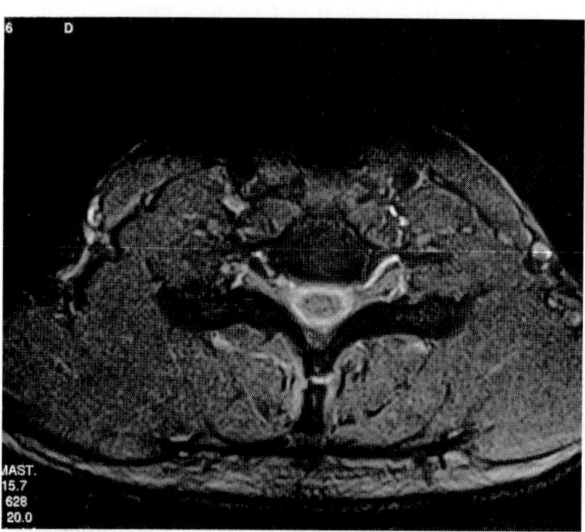

Fig. 3.33. Axial T2-weighted image of the cervical region at the C6 level. The fracture is identified by a band of increased signal intensity through the C6 spinous process

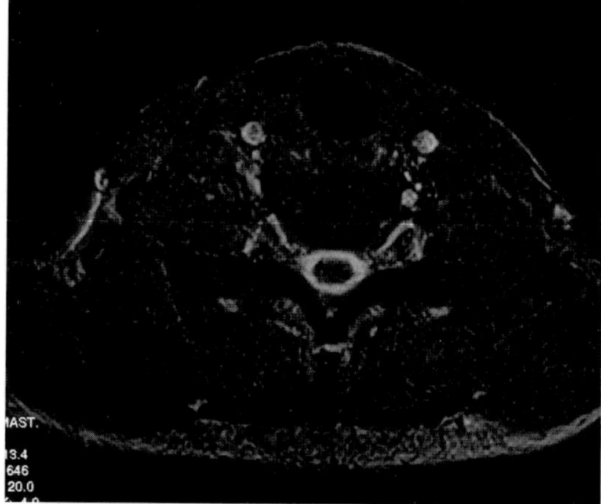

Fig. 3.34. Axial T2-weighted image with fat saturation. Slightly improved visualization of the fracture line and focal fluid collection at the level of the C6 spinous process

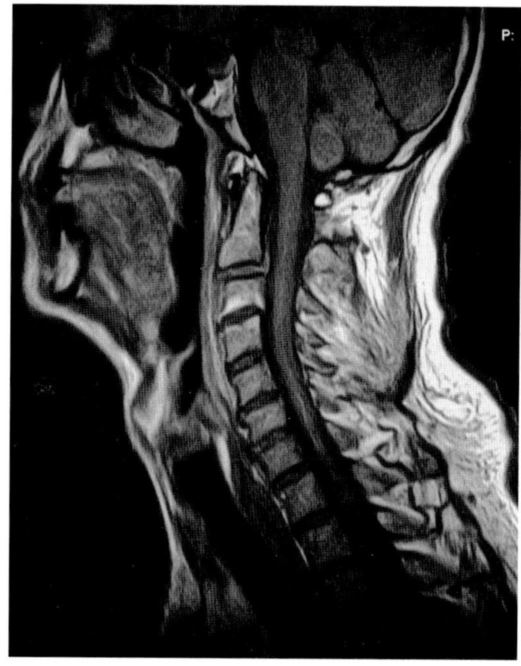

Fig. 3.35. Sagittal T1-weighted image of the cervical region in a 77-year-old patient after a fall. Degenerative changes of the intervertebral disc spaces with signs of chronic osteochondrosis at C3-4 and fat signal in the lower portions of the C3 vertebra. The C2-3 disc is conspicuously hyperintense and there is posterior herniation with portions of the herniated disc extending upward behind C2. In addition, a slightly inhomogeneous mass of high signal intensity extends prevertebrally from C1 through C5, consistent with diffuse hematoma. The overall appearance suggests disc injury with intradiscal hemorrhage

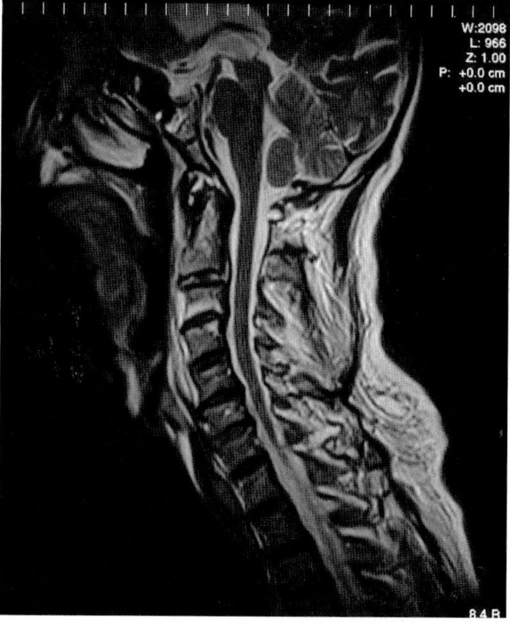

Fig. 3.36. Sagittal T2-weighted image. Abnormal high signal intensity of the C2-3 disc with intact bony structures

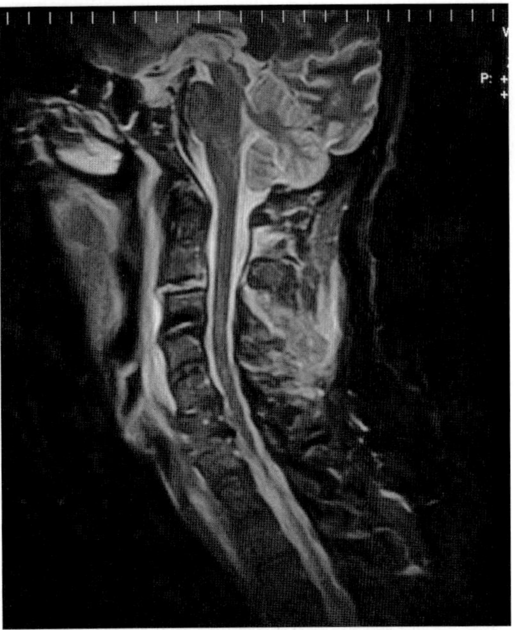

Fig. 3.37. Sagittal T2-weighted image with fat saturation of the cervical region. Abnormal hyperintensity of the C2-3 disc with edema and possible hemorrhage. The appearance is consistent with more recent disc injury. In addition, there is soft tissue edema posterior to C3 through C5

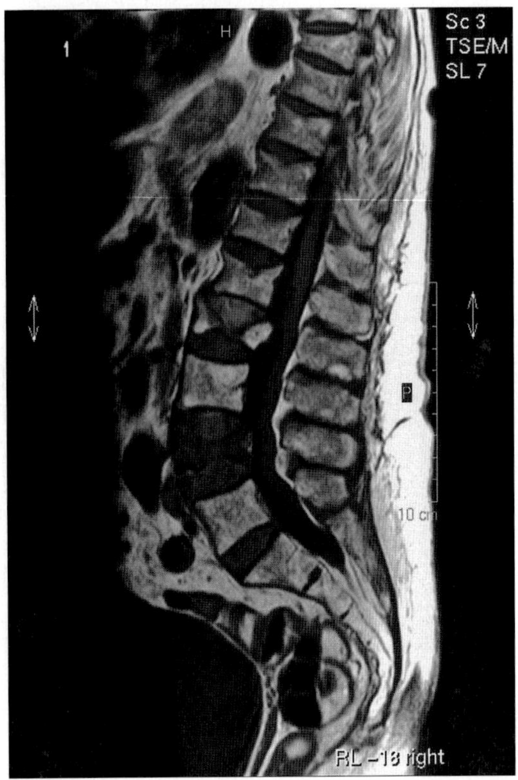

Fig. 3.38. 76-year-old patient; lumbar pain without trauma that could explain the symptoms. Sagittal T1-weighted image of the lumbar region including the lower thoracic spine. There is abnormal signal intensity of the L4 vertebral body with a marked loss of height and deformity of both endplates. In addition, there is deformity of L2 with displacement of the posterior margin toward the spinal canal. The signal intensity is normal. Impression fractures of the superior endplates of L1, T11, and T12. Wedging of T8. The reduced signal intensity of the L4 vertebral body suggests an acute fracture. No signs of a malignant process

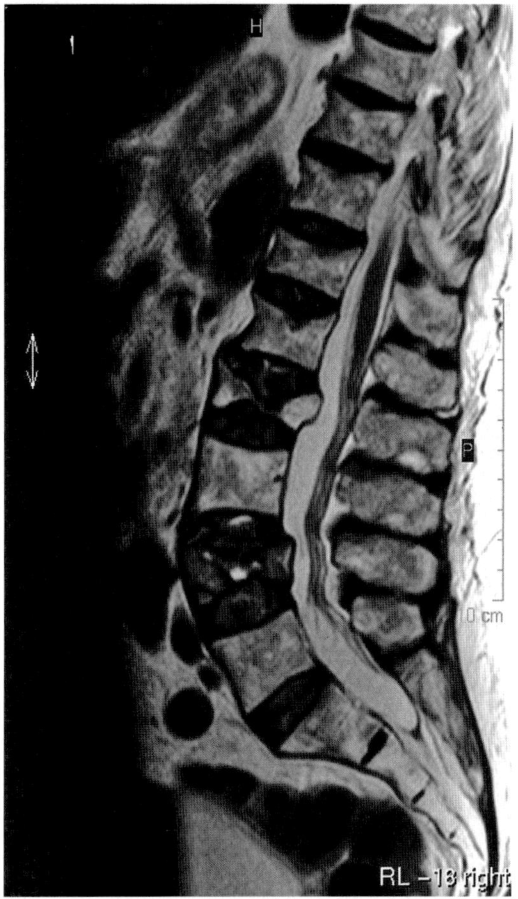

Fig. 3.39. Same patient. Sagittal T2-weighted image showing small central fluid collection of high signal intensity in the acutely fractured L4 vertebral body. Older compression fracture of L2. Inhomogeneous bone marrow signal of the remaining vertebral bodies, consistent with osteoporosis

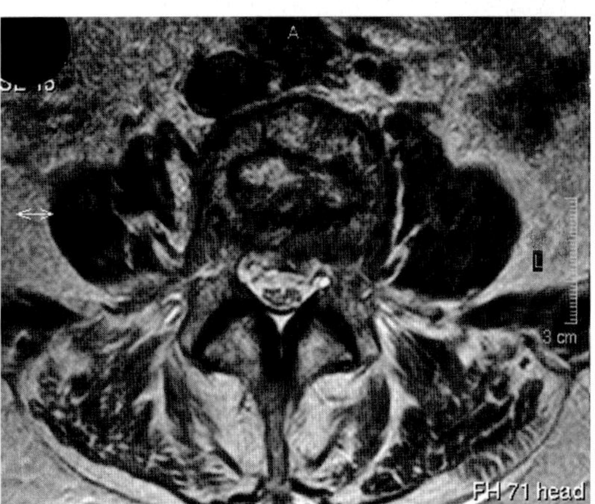

Fig. 3.40. Same patient. Axial T2-weighted image through the L4 vertebra showing inhomogeneous appearance and several fracture lines. Only mild perifocal edema or hematoma

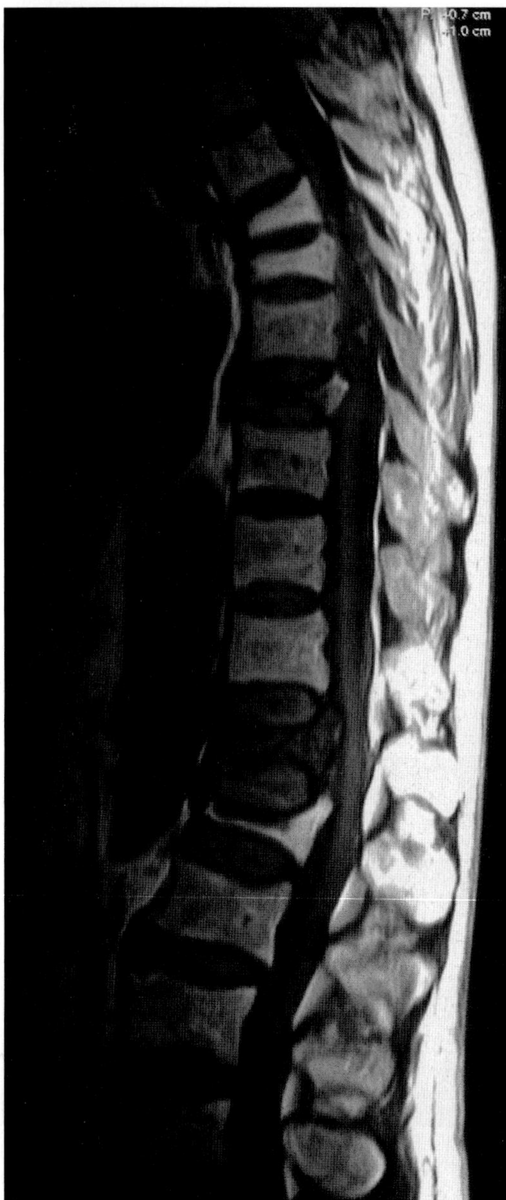

Fig. 3.41. 80-year-old patient with thoracic spine pain. Sagittal T1-weighted image of thoracolumbar regions. The signal intensity of the T8 and T12 vertebral bodies is reduced. The T5, T6, and L1 vertebrae show deformities while their signal intensities are nearly normal, consistent with older fractures. The more recent fractures of T12 and T8 are associated with displacement of the posterior margins toward the spinal canal

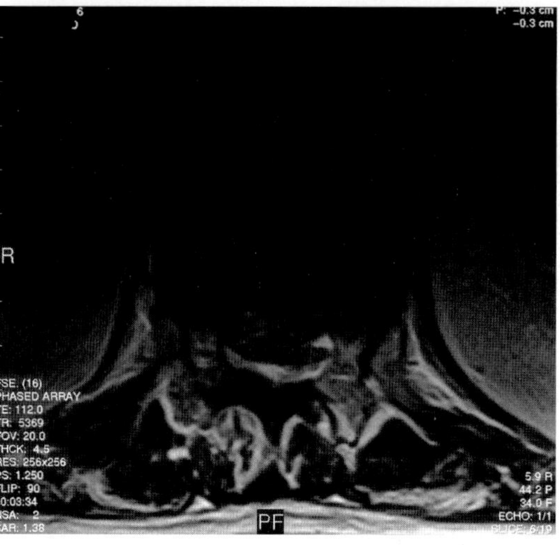

Fig. 3.42. Same patient. Axial T2-weighted image through the T8 vertebra. Marked indentation of the dural sac with spinal stenosis at the level of the fracture; no evidence of bony destruction. Slightly inhomogeneous appearance of the bone marrow, consistent with osteoporosis

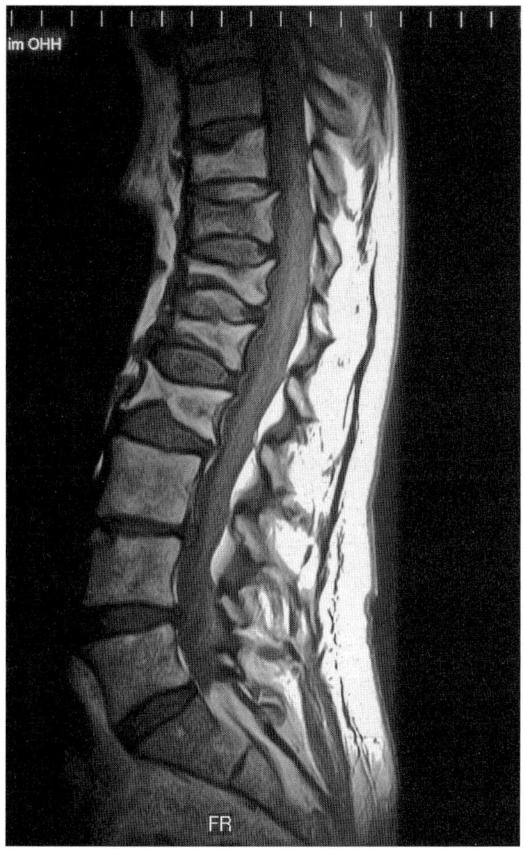

Fig. 3.43. 72-year-old patient with known osteoporosis. Sagittal T1-weighted image showing wedge and fish deformities of the vertebral bodies from T10 through L2. A band of low signal intensity in the T11 vertebra suggests a more recent fracture

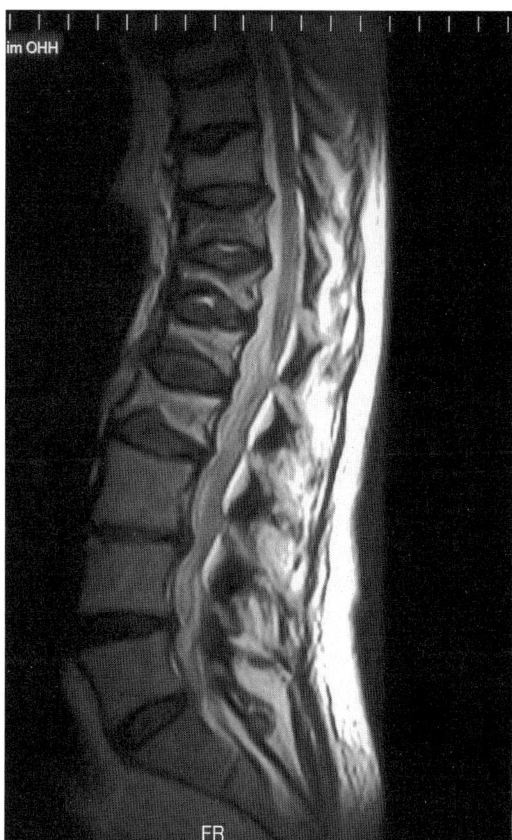

Fig. 3.44. Sagittal T2-weighted image of the same patient showing multiple porotic fractures and sintering from T10 through L2

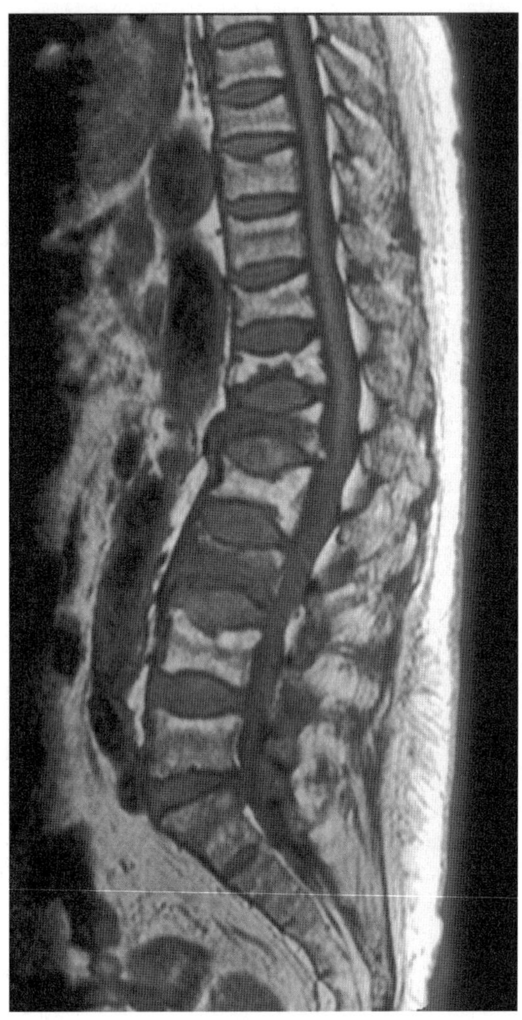

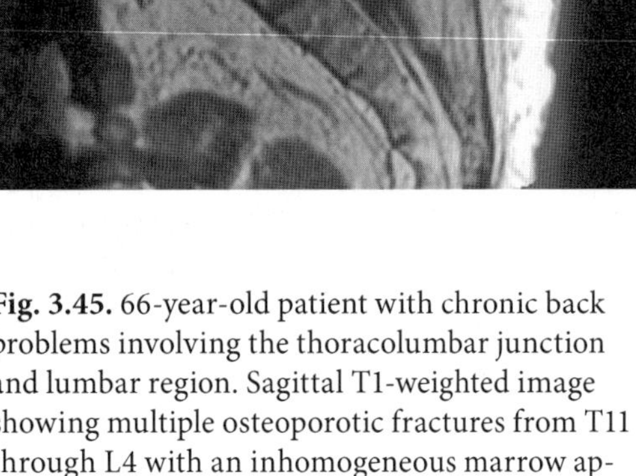

Fig. 3.45. 66-year-old patient with chronic back problems involving the thoracolumbar junction and lumbar region. Sagittal T1-weighted image showing multiple osteoporotic fractures from T11 through L4 with an inhomogeneous marrow appearance. Areas/bands of reduced signal intensity in L1 and L3 on T1-weighted image suggest acute fractures of these vertebral bodies

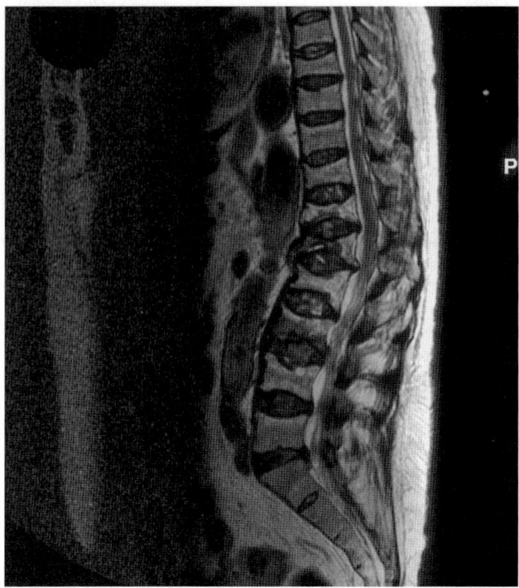

Fig. 3.46. Sagittal T2-weighted image. Slight narrowing of the spinal canal at the L3-4 level. No signs of posterior displacement of the fractured vertebral bodies

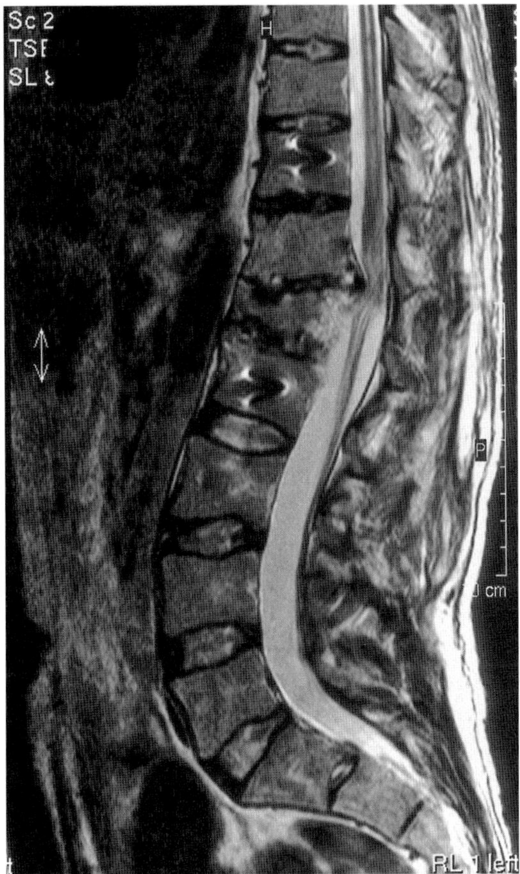

Fig. 3.47. Sagittal T2-weighted image of the lumbar spine and thoracolumbar junction obtained in a 40-year-old man following osteosynthesis of an L1 fracture. There is marked deformity of the L1 vertebra and susceptibility artifacts obscure the T11 and L2 vertebrae. Posterior protrusion of the T12-L1 intervertebral disc with spinal narrowing. Posttraumatic syrinx is suggested by a band of increased signal intensity in the lower spinal cord

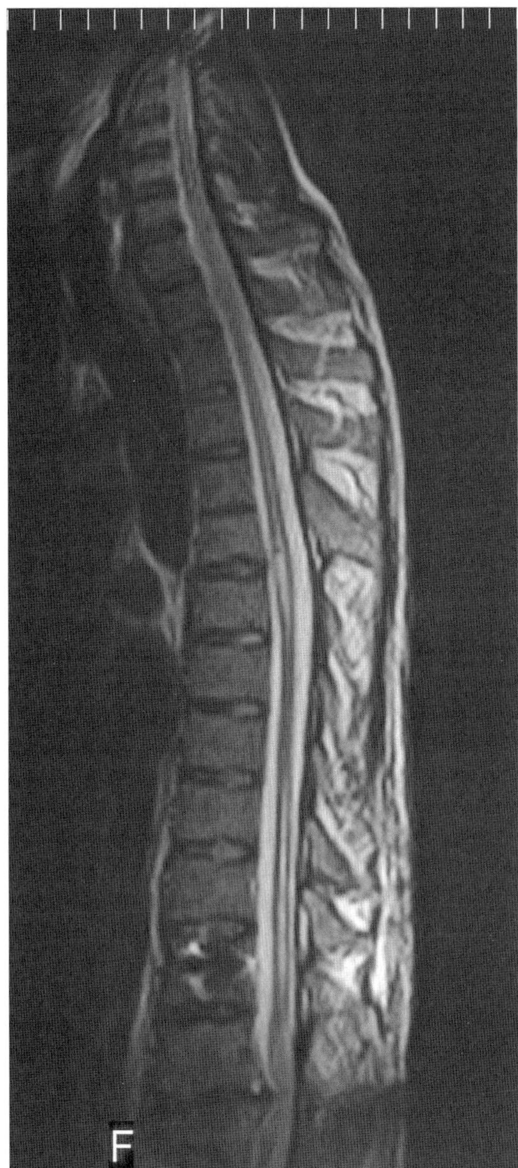

Fig. 3.48. Sagittal T2-weighted image of the thoracic region showing a band of increased signal intensity in the center of the spinal cord extending from the cervical spine to the thoracolumbar junction and suggesting (posttraumatic) syrinx. No evidence of tumor

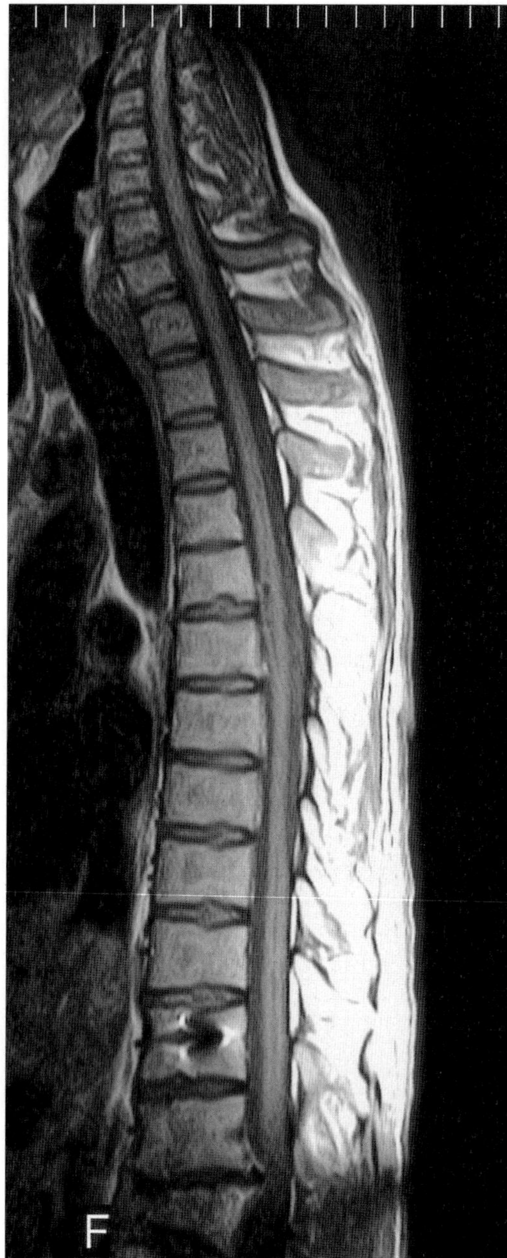

Fig. 3.49. Same patient. Sagittal T1-weighted image with only discreet signs of the syrinx in the thoracic and lumbar spinal cord

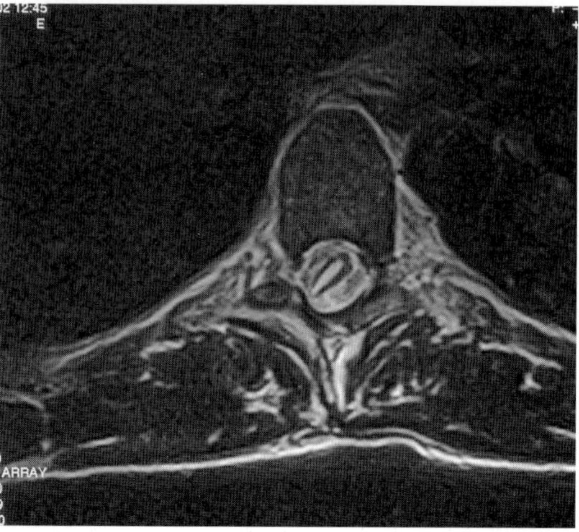

Fig. 3.50. Axial T2-weighted image showing the posttraumatic syrinx described in the preceding figures at the T8 level. Atrophy of the spinal cord with a saber-sheath-like cystic fluid collection

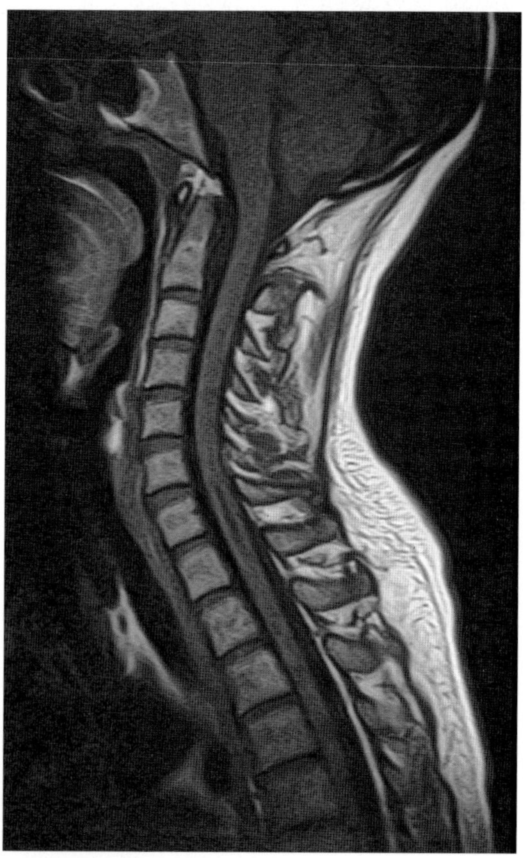

Fig. 3.51. Sagittal T1-weighted image of the cervical and cervicothoracic junction in a 38-year-old patient. The image shows oval cystic widening of the spinal cord from C6 through T1. The increase in spinal cord volume is minimal and the surrounding soft tissue and bone structures appear unremarkable

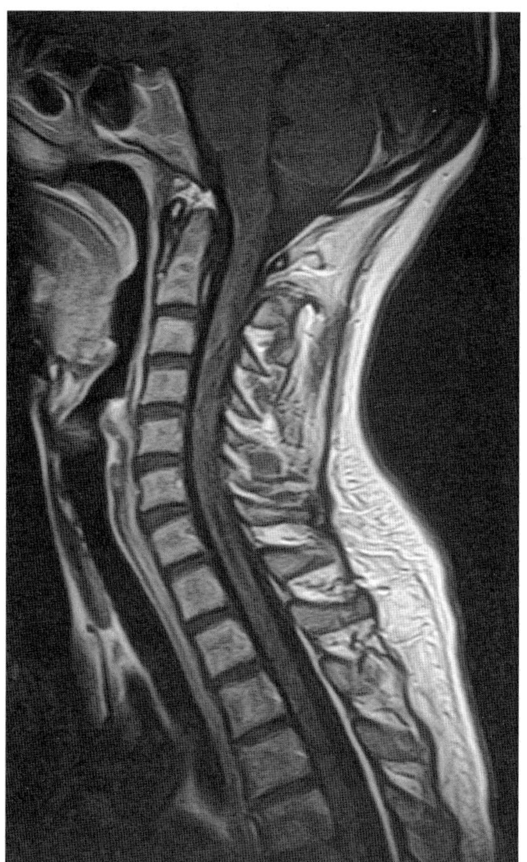

Fig. 3.52. Sagittal T1-weighted image of the same patient after contrast administration. There is no enhancing focal lesion in the spinal cord. The post-traumatic syrinx is slightly more conspicuous

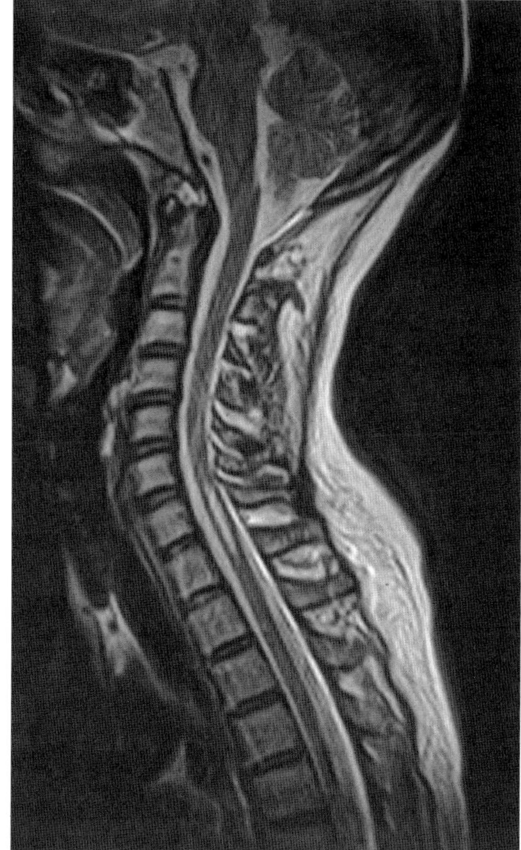

Fig. 3.53. Sagittal T2-weighted image of the markedly hyperintense syrinx extending from C6 to T1

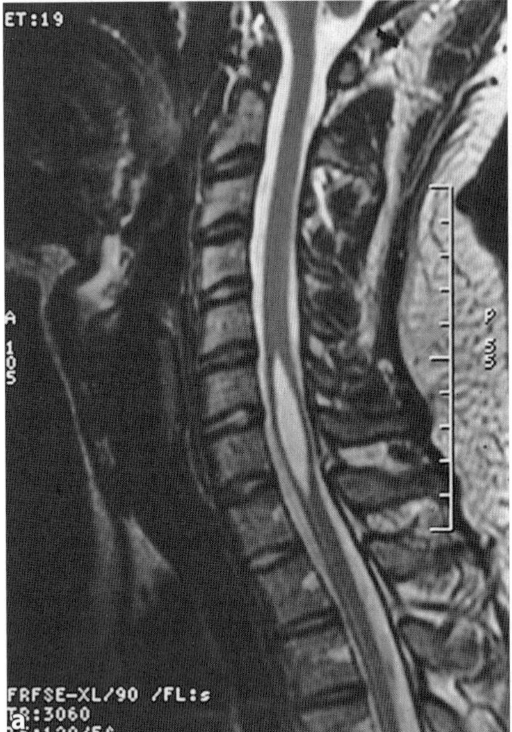

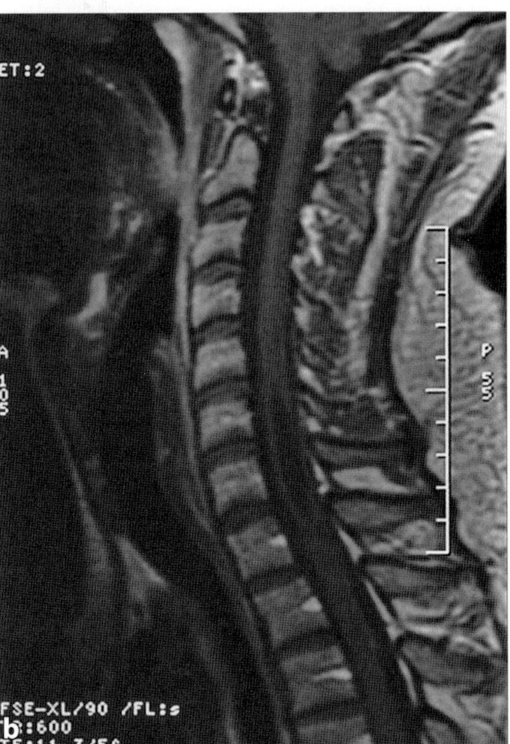

Fig. 3.54a, b. T2- and T1-weighted sagittal images: syrinx in the cervical spinal cord extending from C5-6 to C7-T1 (status post contusion)

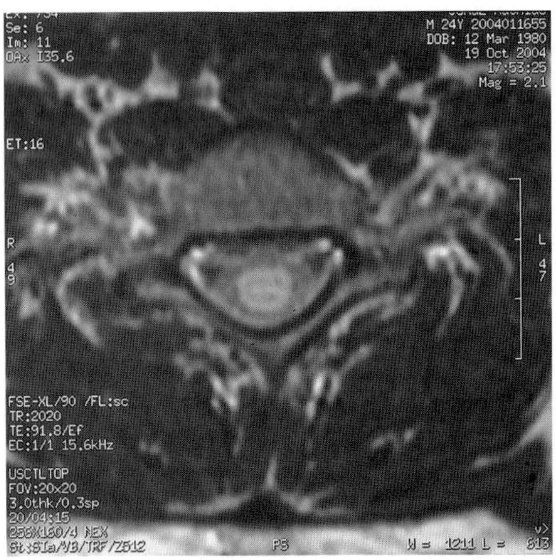

Fig. 3.55. Transverse T2-weighted image of the syrinx demonstrating the mass effect with enlargement of the spinal cord diameter and compression of the subarachnoid CSF space

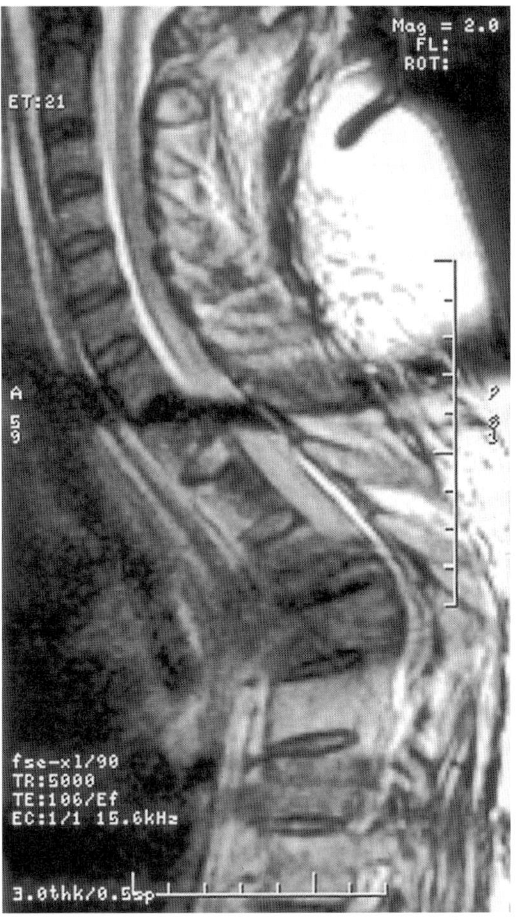

Fig. 3.56. Gunshot injury of the spinal cord at T1. Sagittal T2-weighted image showing longitudinal edematous widening of the cervicothoracic cord below C5-6. There is distortion due to the projectile

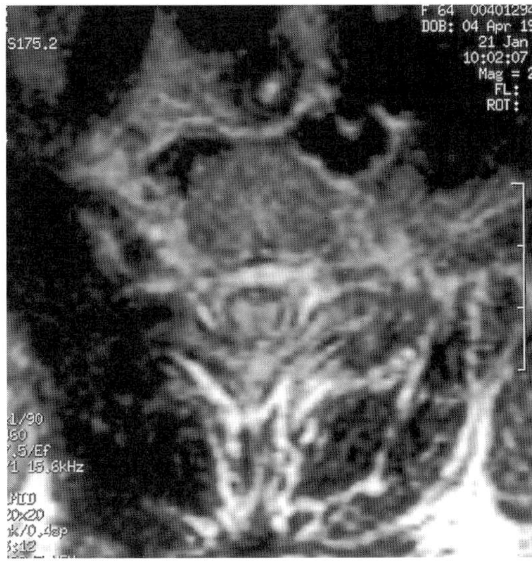

Fig. 3.57. Transverse T2-weighted image

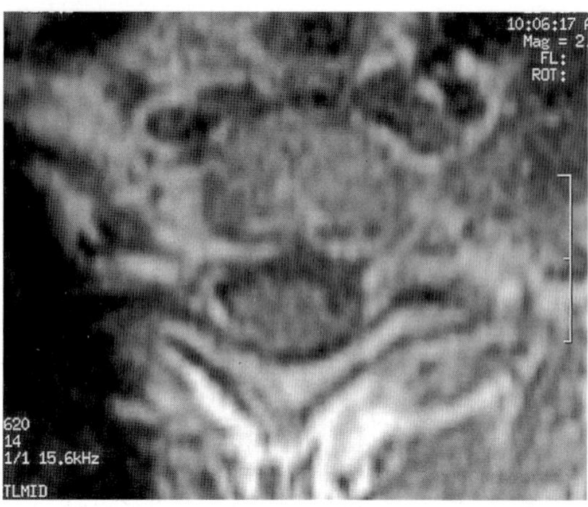

Fig. 3.58. Transverse T1-weighted image showing extensive paravertebral bleeding on the left and signal voids due to artifacts. Traumatized and edematous spinal cord

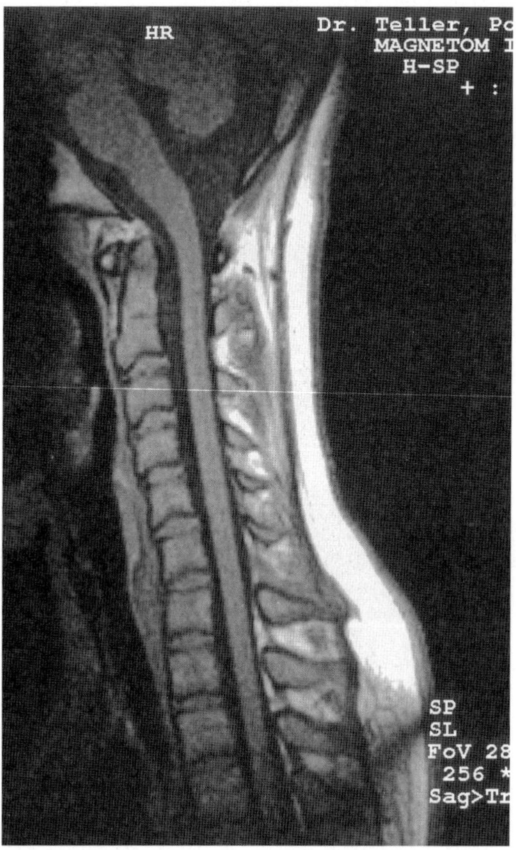

Fig. 3.59. 15-year-old patient with posterior symptoms at the cervicothoracic junction after a traffic accident. Sagittal T1-weighted image with age-appropriate bone marrow signal. Upright cervical spine and suggestion of kyphosis with the apex at C6-7. Suggestion of a mass isointense to muscle at the tip of the C7 spinous process

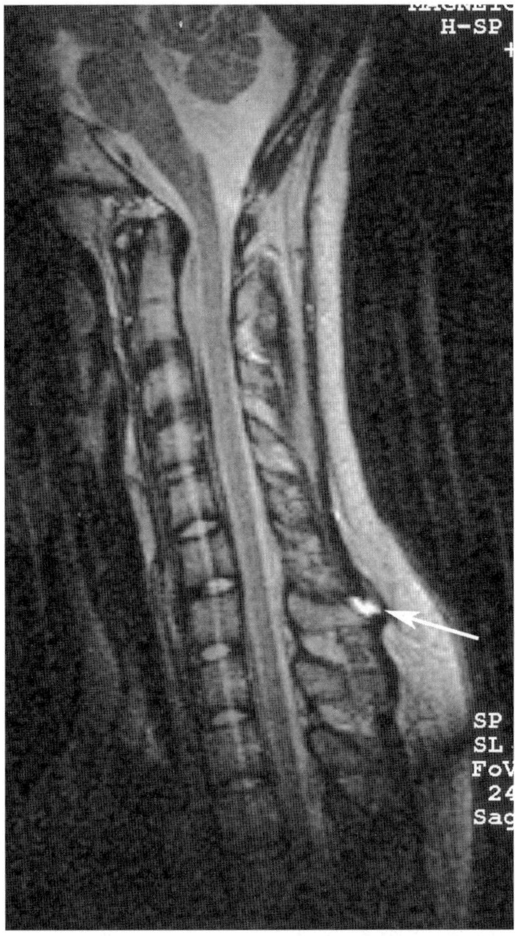

Fig. 3.60. Same patient. Sagittal T2-weighted image slightly degraded by motion artifacts showing a sharply marginated focal mass of high signal intensity in the area of the nuchal ligament directly at the tip of the C7 spinous process *(arrow)*. The appearance suggests rupture of the ligament. There is no irritation of surrounding soft tissue structures and no abnormal bone signal

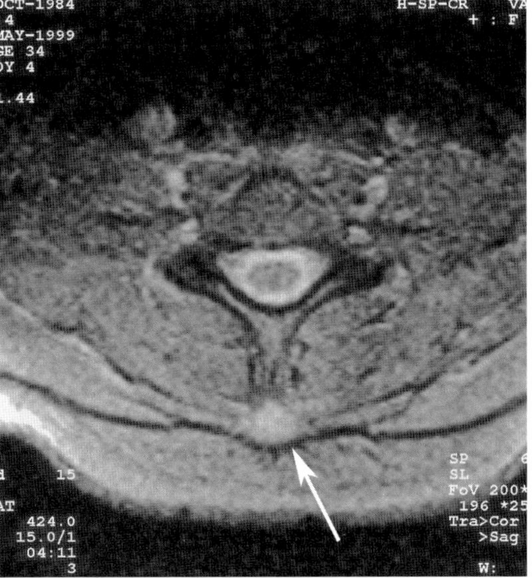

Fig. 3.61. Axial T2-weighted image through the level of the C7 spinous process showing the focal, slightly blurred lesion at the C7 spinal process *(arrow)* indicating the site of ligament rupture

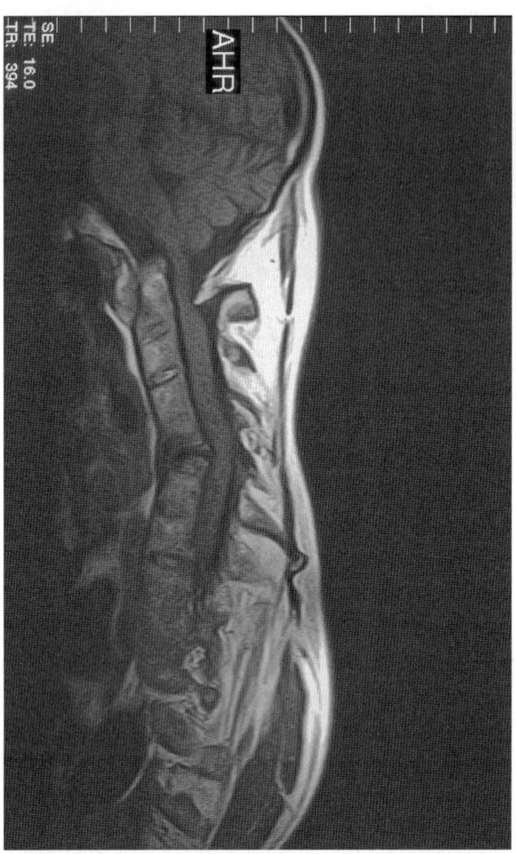

Fig. 3.62. 56-year-old patient with known ankylosing spondylitis. Sagittal T1-weighted image showing the typical spinal changes associated with ankylosing spondylitis and basilar impression. There is a fracture at the C5-6 level with abnormal signal and kyphotic curvature but no irritation of surrounding soft tissue structures

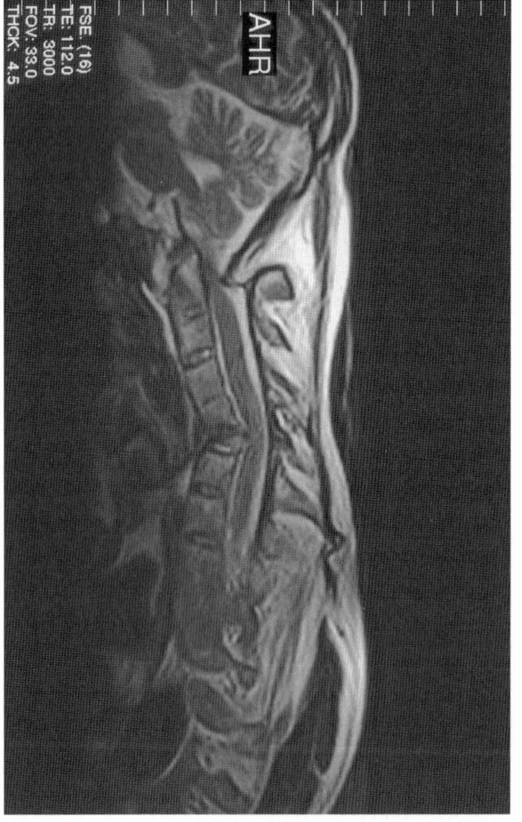

Fig. 3.63. Sagittal T2-weighted image of the cervical region showing the kyphotic curvature at C5-6 and posterior displacement of the spinal cord. The signal intensities are normal. Basilar impression with spinal narrowing at the craniocervical junction

Fig. 3.64. Coronal T1-weighted image showing the fracture at the C5-6 level with right concave scoliosis

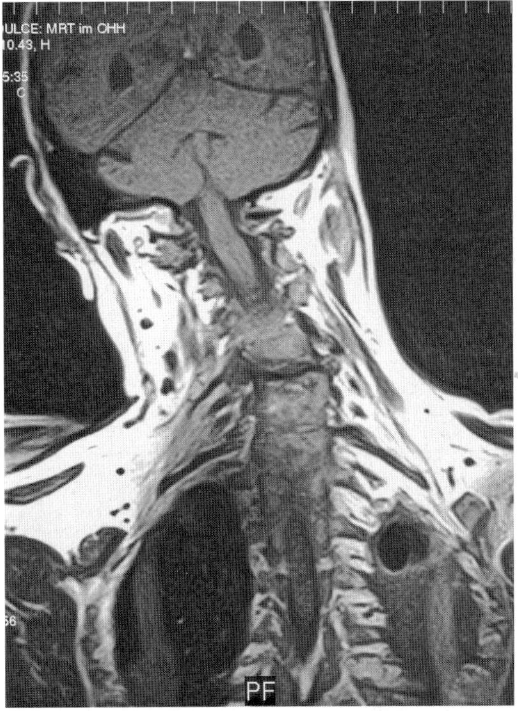

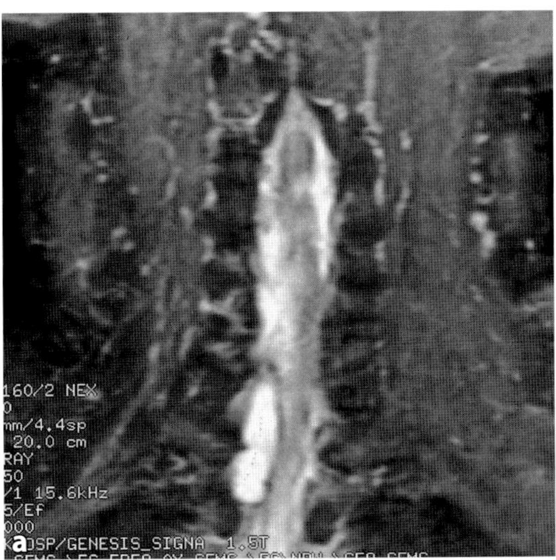

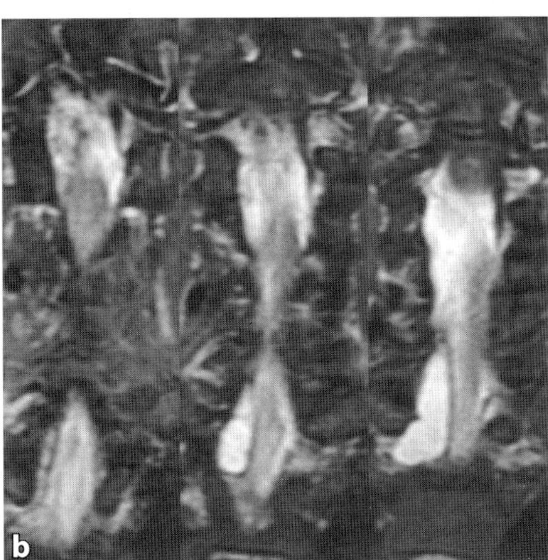

Fig. 3.65a, b. Coronal fat-suppressed T2-weighted images

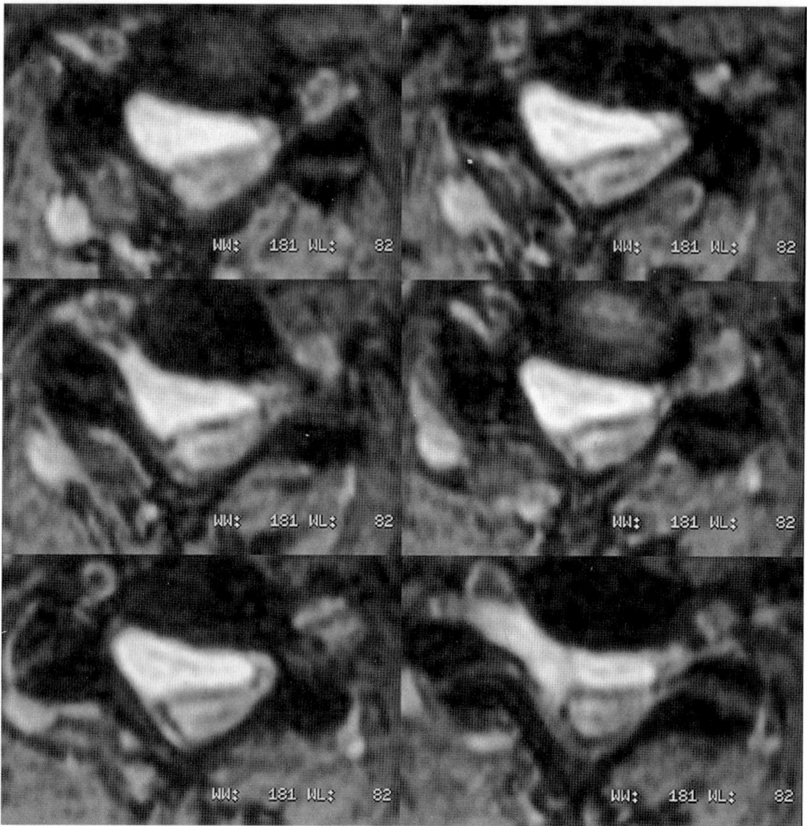

Fig. 3.66. Nerve root avulsion. Transverse T2-weighted images with fat saturation showing a dural leak in the right anterior aspect of the spinal canal. The spinal cord is displaced posteriorly to the left. Myelomalacia lesions in the spinal cord on the right. Avulsion of the right C5 to C8 nerve roots

4 Degenerative Disorders

4.1 Osteochondrosis

Anatomy

Spinal osteochondrosis is defined as degeneration of the anterior components of the spinal motion segments. The motion segments are functional articular units consisting of several anatomically distinct components. Except for the first two cervical motion segments (atlanto-occipital, C0-1; and atlantoaxial, C1-2), the spinal motion segments have a uniform structure comprising the following components:

- the intervertebral disc consisting of a pulpy center (nucleus pulposus) and a fibrous ring (annulus fibrosus) interposed between two adjacent vertebral bodies,
- the vertebral body enclosed above and below by cartilaginous endplates,
- the anterior and posterior longitudinal ligaments, and
- the posterior structures comprising
  - the ligamentum flavum,
  - the facet joints, and
  - the soft tissue structures (such as ligaments and muscles) between the spinous and transverse processes.

The intervertebral disc is an elastic plate that functions as a colloid osmotic system and serves to resist pressure. The circumferential ringlike portion (annulus fibrosus) provides tensile strength and is attached to the two adjacent vertebral bodies at the site of the fused epiphyseal ring by so-called Sharpey fibers. The annulus consists of concentric lamellae composed of fibers that run obliquely from one vertebra to another, the fibers of one lamella typically running at right angles to those of the adjacent ones. The inner connective tissue layers of the annulus gradually blend into a zone of fibrocartilage. This fibrocartilage is the limiting capsule of the pulpy center, the nucleus pulposus, which also contains some remnants of the embryonic notochord. The well-hydrated gelatinous core is under internal pressure and swells when the disc is cut.

The vertebral bodies are delimited from the intervertebral discs by cartilaginous plates covering the inferior and superior vertebral body surfaces central to the site of fusion of the former epiphyseal ring. In adults, the vertebral endplates consist of hyaline cartilage. The vertebral bodies grow from the cartilaginous plate, which is why they contain a typical proliferation and transitional zone in children and juveniles. At that age, the ridges likewise consist of cartilage and are part of the cartilaginous plate.

Until about four years of age, the annulus fibrosis is supplied by blood vessels from the adjacent vertebral bodies. Thereafter, the annulus, like the nucleus pulposus, is avascular and the medullary spaces of the vertebrae communicate with the intervertebral discs via the cartilaginous endplate through pores in the vertebral surface.

Anterior and posterior to the vertebral bodies, the intervertebral disc spaces are bridged by the longitudinal ligaments. The anterior longitudinal ligament is firmly attached to the ventral surfaces of the vertebral bodies and loosely to the intervertebral discs. It becomes wider from top to bottom.

The posterior longitudinal ligament becomes narrower as it courses downward. It fans out at the disc levels but without completely covering the posterior aspects of the discs. The posterior longitudinal ligament is firmly bound to the upper and lower edges of the vertebral bodies and to the intervertebral discs.

Radiographic Findings

The hallmark radiographic finding in intervertebral disc degeneration is narrowing of the disc space due to a loss of disc bulk (water). This process may be associated with the formation of gas-filled spaces or clefts within the disc (vacuum phenomenon). Narrowing of the disc space causes relative instability of the affected motion segment (relative loosening of the ligamentous apparatus) – which may become apparent as backward/forward slippage on flexion and extension views. The loss of function (load transmission, shock absorption) caused by degenerative changes of the disc leads to secondary sclerotic induration in adjacent vertebral segments (transition from intervertebral chondrosis to osteochondrosis) with subsequent erosion of the sclerotic bone.

Another secondary phenomenon commonly seen in intervertebral disc degeneration, but also in other conditions, is spondylosis or uncovertebral spondylosis of the cervical spine.

Besides a height reduction of the degenerated disc, radiographs typically show zones of densification in adjacent vertebral bodies. These are most prominent in load-bearing areas with osteophytic outgrowths at the margins. Vertebral osteophytes typically form around the unstable disc space from both sides in a mirror-image-like fashion. Finally, in acute/erosive osteochondrosis, radiographs may show destructive changes of the adjacent endplates, which are sometimes difficult to differentiate from the changes seen in vertebral destruction by an inflammatory or tumorous process.

Pathomechanism

The intervertebral discs are the largest avascular structures in the human body. The main mechanisms underlying general disc degeneration are premature aging of bradytrophic tissues and the high load to which the discs are exposed. Motion-related stress is greatest in the cervical region, while the pressure load predominates in the lumbar region.

The pressure to which the lowermost lumbar discs are exposed is about 150–250 N when lying and about 1500 N when standing and may increase to over 2500 N when lifting a heavy object.

MR Technique

The reactive bony changes associated with disc degeneration are best appreciated on sagittal and coronal T1- and T2-weighted images, supplemented by T2-weighted images with fat saturation (STIR technique) as required.

MR Findings

Besides signs of intervertebral disc degeneration, acute osteochondrosis is characterized by the depiction on T2-weighted images of band-like hyperintensities of the vertebral bodies near the endplates on either side of the degenerated disc. The signal alterations vary with the imaging parameters used and the amount of fatty marrow in the vertebrae. The signal increase is most conspicuous on STIR images.

The MRI changes of the vertebral bodies associated with degenerative disc disease are classified into three distinct types according to Modic.

Type 1 changes are characterized by a decreased signal intensity on T1-weighted images and are due to excessive fluid obscuring the normally bright fatty marrow. Following contrast administration, the signal intensity will approach that of the unchanged fatty marrow on T1.

In chronic disc degeneration the changes of the affected discs become more pronounced. There is narrowing of the disc and dehydration, seen as a change in signal intensity.

At this stage, the adjacent vertebrae show bands of increased signal intensity at the endplates on both T1- and T2-weighted images. On fat-saturated images, these areas are dark. This appearance is consistent with fatty degeneration. There is only minimal enhancement after contrast administration. These changes are classified as Modic type 2 and correspond to the densification zones on radiographs.

Type 3 osteochondrotic changes consist of decreased signal intensity on both T1- and T2-weighted images and correlate with bony sclerosis at the vertebral endplates bordering a degenerated disc.

The erosive stage shows all signs of acute osteochondrosis with additional destructions of the endplates. The erosive changes are indistinct from early vertebral body destruction in spondylodiscitis. Better differentiation is achieved in conjunction with the clinical findings or follow-up examination (Fig. 4.1).

Clinical Significance

In cases of disc space narrowing, MRI can differentiate between loss of disc mass (chondrosis) and herniation as the underlying cause but not between acute (activated) osteochondrosis and primary inflammatory disease of a spinal motion segment (e.g. bacterial spondylitis – spondylodiscitis, spondylodiscitis in chronic polyarthritis). Patients with inconclusive MR findings in whom the clinical symptoms do not require immediate diagnostic workup may undergo follow-up MRI (transition from Modic stage 1 to stage 2/3).

In patients with proven intervertebral chondrosis/osteochondrosis, only additional flexion and extension views (radiography or MRI) will identify associated instability.

The MRI diagnosis of intervertebral chondrosis/osteochondrosis leads to therapeutic consequences only in conjunction with the patient's clinical findings. No therapy is required in asymptomatic patients. The severity of the clinical symptoms determines whether conservative therapy or surgery is indicated.

4.2 Spondyloarthrosis

Pathoanatomy

Spondyloarthrosis is the progressive destruction of the facet joints by primary noninflammatory processes and is characterized by the loss of articular cartilage and formation of osteophytes. This reactive repair process of the bony structures may lead to hypertrophy of the entire facet joint and the formation of degenerative synovial cysts as the disease progresses. The underlying processes include reactive changes of the synovial membrane, hypertrophic proliferation with inclusion of small foci of chondroid metaplasia, and formation of foci of ossification. A large osteophyte may form a nearthrosis with an adjacent vertebral arch.

Advanced facet joint degeneration may cause narrowing of the neural foramina, especially in the cervical and lumbar regions. Spondyloarthrosis is also the main cause of secondary stenosis of the spinal canal or a lateral recess.

Pathogenesis

As with other forms of arthrosis, spondyloarthrosis is caused by a combination of exogenous and endogenous mechanical and biological processes that contribute to the dysregulation of cartilage metabolism of the cartilaginous matrix.

The most important exogenous factor contributing to facet joint degeneration is malalignment and asymmetry of the joints secondary to disc degeneration with narrowing of the interspace. This is why the more severe forms of spondyloarthrosis are rarely seen when the corresponding disc is intact and of normal height.

MR Technique

Axial images, usually acquired with T1- and T2-weighting, are most suitable for evaluating degenerative changes of the facet joints. Sagittal and coronal images may provide additional information in some cases.

MR Findings

Degeneration of the facet joints is characterized by narrowing of the joint space. More advanced disease is characterized by bony hypertrophy with enlargement of the vertebral arch and focal osteophyte formation extending anteromedially and posterolaterally. This can cause secondary narrowing of the spinal canal at the level of the degenerated facet joints and is seen as T-shaped deformity of the spinal cord on axial images in severe cases.

Bony outgrowths are visualized on T1-weighted images as low-signal-intensity expansions of the normal bone structures. Depending on disease activity, T2-weighted sequences depict edema as slight increases in signal intensity directly adjacent to the joint space. In most cases, fluid collections are present in the joint space and are visible as bright bands on T2-weighted images. The ligamenta flava may be displaced by osteophytes and show reactive thickening, indicated by a rather low signal intensity on T1 and T2. There may be clinically significant secondary spinal canal stenosis, especially when facet joint degeneration occurs in conjunction with intervertebral disc degeneration (Figs. 4.2–4.5).

MR Pitfalls

When there is severe hypertrophy of the facet joints, the MR appearance may be similar to the changes seen in spondylolysis, especially on axial images.

Clinical Significance

While facet joint degeneration itself can also be diagnosed and evaluated by conventional radiography and

CT, MRI also identifies signs of secondary inflammation (activated arthrosis) and is thus suited to correlate the imaging findings with the patient's clinical symptoms (so-called facet syndrome). The most important contribution of MRI, however, lies in the direct visualization of secondary stenoses of the spinal canal, lateral recesses, and neural foramina with irritation or compression of neural structures.

4.3 Synovial Cysts

Pathoanatomy

Synovial cysts are ganglion-like outpouchings of a synovial membrane. Spinal synovial cysts are found in the area of a facet joint and grow inside or outside the spinal canal. In spondylolisthesis synovial cysts may also arise from a neosynovial membrane of a pseudarthrosis.

Pathomechanism

Hyperplastic proliferation of a synovial membrane through chronic irritation, e.g. in the area of a pseudarthrosis of the pars interarticularis (spondylolysis), or, more commonly, in association with spondyloarthrosis.

MR Technique

Axial T1- and T2-weighted images are most suitable for evaluating the mass effect of a synovial cyst. Additional coronal and sagittal images are helpful in selected cases.

MR Findings

MRI shows a tumor that is contiguous to the joint space of a facet joint, from where the cyst usually extends anteromedially. Increased signal intensity in the adjacent joint indicates joint effusion. On contrast-enhanced images, cysts have an unchanged, homogeneous appearance with only the wall showing slight enhancement. Large synovial cysts may cause spinal canal stenosis. Occasionally, bilateral synovial cysts are seen (Figs. 4.6–4.13).

MR Pitfalls

Synovial cysts must be differentiated from other cyst-like lesions. A synovial cyst is characterized by its proximity to a facet joint. Cystically degenerated disc herniations typically have thicker walls than synovial cysts and are rarely found near a facet joint.

Clinical Significance

Synovial cysts occurring secondary to other conditions become clinically relevant only when they develop close to neural structures or in the spinal canal, a lateral recess, or a neural foramen.

4.4 Spinal Stenosis

Anatomy and Pathoanatomy

Narrowing of the spinal canal is defined as a discrepancy between the width of the canal and that of its contents (Epstein 1987). There have been numerous attempts to establish precise numerical thresholds (for diameters, cross-sectional areas, or volumes), but none of them is satisfactory due to interindividual normal variation.

The most widely used measure is the sagittal diameter with a threshold of about 13 mm for the cervical canal below C4 and about 12 mm for the lumbar canal. The threshold for stenosis of a lateral recess in the lumbar region is 3 mm.

The term spinal canal stenosis encompasses all forms of narrowing of the spinal canal that are not caused by inflammation (spondylitis), tumors, or disc herniation. Etiologically, stenosis can be divided into two major categories: developmental or congenital spinal stenosis and acquired stenosis. The specific pathoanatomic changes vary with the underlying condition causing the stenosis. Another distinction is made between static and dynamic stenosis. Hyperlordosis reduces the width of the spinal canal in several segments. Moreover, any segmental or multisegmental instability can cause a circumscribed subcritical spinal stenosis during inclination or reclination. With few exceptions (e.g. posttraumatic stenosis), spinal stenoses occur in the cervical and lumbar regions but not in the thoracic spine. The cervical canal decreases in size from C1 to C3 and has a fairly uniform dimension from C4 through C7. The lumbar canal shows some physiologic narrowing at the L3 and L4 levels.

Degenerative disease is by far the most common cause of spinal canal stenosis and may be superimposed on developmental narrowing. Both abnormal bone and soft tissue structures may encroach on the spinal canal, in particular osteophytes from the facet joints, herniated intervertebral discs, posterior spondylophytes, hypertrophic proliferations of the synovial membrane, and a markedly thickened ligamentum flavum.

Pathomechanism

Narrowing of the spinal canal may be due to congenital or acquired conditions. Great care is required in patients with mild forms of segmental instability (e.g. instability due to disc degeneration, inflammatory instability in the upper cervical region in rheumatoid arthritis) because a dynamic spinal canal stenosis may not be apparent clinically or on imaging unless flexion and extension views are obtained.

MR Technique

Spinal canal stenosis is best seen on axial images. A T2-weighted 3D myelography sequence is a useful adjunct in individual cases. Additional sequences in coronal and sagittal planes may be helpful depending on the underlying cause of the stenosis.

MR Findings

Abnormal narrowing of the spinal canal primarily affects the subarachnoid space. Depending on the individual width of the spinal canal, spinal stenosis is assumed when the anteroposterior diameter is less than 13 mm in the cervical region and less than 12 mm in the lumbar region. The structures encroaching on the canal displace CSF and often obscure the epidural fatty tissue. Long-standing chronic compression of the spinal cord causes myelomalacia, which is identified on MRI by intraspinal signal changes. Myelomalacia of the cauda equina, which cannot be detected by MRI, is less relevant because the cauda is much more pliable and will adjust to a narrowed spinal canal (Figs. 4.14–4.27).

Clinical Significance

Absolute spinal stenosis causing clinical symptoms or neurophysiologic changes requires prompt surgical management tailored to the individual patient's pathomorphologic findings. Adequate surgical treatment is important precisely because the neurologic deficits typically progress only slowly, which is why the changes are not perceived as abnormal by the mostly elderly patients. Surgical decompression will lead to a 50-60% reduction of neurologic deficits. There is a highly negative correlation between the success of surgical measures and the duration of symptoms.

MRI (including flexion and extension views) is currently the most suitable imaging modality for a comprehensive evaluation of the pathomorphologic changes underlying a patient's clinical and neurologic symptoms and thus for identifying those patients who will benefit from surgical treatment. MR imaging provides detailed information on the underlying pathomorphologic changes, the exact width of the residual spinal canal, and the level of the pathology (affected segment) as well as prognostic information (spinal cord abnormalities). In the cervical (and thoracic) region, MRI is helpful in establishing the indication for surgery (timing of the intervention) by showing whether or not an uninterrupted CSF column is present in patients who have not yet developed neurologic/neurophysiologic deficits (imminent cervical myelopathy).

4.5 Foraminal Stenosis

MR Technique

Sagittal and axial images are best suited to evaluate the neural foramina for stenosis. Additional coronal T2-weighted images may be helpful.

T1-weighted images before and after contrast administration are acquired in patients with foraminal stenosis to exclude/detect contrast-enhancing lesions such as neurofibroma, neurinoma, metastasis, or bone tumors.

MR Findings

The structure narrowing the neural foramen may be depicted with a high or low signal intensity. Characteristically, the mass displaces the fatty tissue that normally surrounds the low-signal-intensity nerve root in the foramen. Compression or irritation of the root is indicated by a signal increase on T2-weighted images and a decrease on T1-weighted images.

Parenchymal tumors are characterized by contrast enhancement, which distinguishes them from cystic or cortical lesions. On contrast-enhanced images, disc fragments exhibit virtually no enhancement, whereas postoperative scars can be identified for many years by mild signal enhancement. Tumors typically show pronounced enhancement, while cyst enhancement is confined to the wall with otherwise low signal intensity on T1-weighted images (Figs. 4.28–4.32).

4.6 Atlantoaxial Arthrosis

Pathoanatomy

Articular degeneration predominantly affects the atlantodental joint, less commonly the lateral atlantoaxial joints.

Pathomechanism

Degenerative damage of the joint. There may be an association with prearthrotic deformity or a congenital or developmental variant in individual cases.

MR Technique

Sagittal and axial T1- and T2-weighted images should be obtained. Contrast-enhanced images are useful to exclude/identify inflammatory changes (pannus). Acute irritation is visualized on T2-weighted images with fat saturation (STIR sequence) as high-signal-intensity zones in the bone marrow.

MR Findings

Narrowing of the joint space and hypertrophy of bony structures are best appreciated on sagittal and axial images. Reactive edema is identified by an intramedullary increase in signal intensity and is most conspicuous on STIR images.

In patients with atlantoaxial joint degeneration, it is important to evaluate the width of the spinal canal, which is best accomplished on axial images. T2-weighted axial images are most suitable for identifying compression of the medulla oblongata and proximal spinal cord. Concomitant myelomalacia is identified by its high signal intensity on T2-weighted images (Figs. 4.33 and 4.34).

Clinical Significance

Advanced atlantoaxial joint degeneration, which is rare and associated with pronounced functional losses, in particular reduced rotational mobility, may cause severe posture- and movement-related headache. Moreover, it has been postulated that degeneration of this area may cause cervical vertigo because the upper cervical spine and the afferent fibers from its joints are connected to the vestibular and oculomotor nuclei.

4.7 Disc Herniation

Anatomy and Pathoanatomy

The intervertebral discs are fibrocartilaginous plates that establish mobile connections between the bodies of adjacent vertebrae. With the two uppermost motion segments (C0-1 and C1-C2) having no intervertebral discs, the normal spine comprises 23 discs. Clinically, the intervertebral discs at the junctions are assigned to the region above, resulting in six cervical discs, twelve thoracic discs, and five lumbar discs.

The intervertebral disc height increases from the cervical to the lumbar region. Altogether, the discs account for about 20–30% of the overall length of the vertebral column. The discs are oval with a greater transverse diameter in the cervical region, circular in the thoracic region, and nearly kidney-shaped in the lumbar spine.

In the sagittal plane, the thoracic discs are rectangular while the cervical and lumbar discs are wedge-shaped and higher anteriorly. The disc shape produces the normal curvature (lordosis) of the cervical and lumbar spine while the thoracic kyphosis is caused by the shape of the vertebral bodies.

An intervertebral disc consists of the nucleus pulposus at its center and the ringlike annulus fibrosus. It is functionally closely related to the cartilaginous endplates of the adjacent vertebral bodies.

The endplates are bound firmly to the annulus fibrosus but only loosely to the vertebral body. In adults, the cartilaginous endplates are delimited by the rounded epiphyseal ring.

The nucleus pulposus consists of a cellular, gelatinous ground substance and makes up about 30% to 50% of the cross-sectional area of the disc. It is located more posteriorly than centrally.

The annulus fibrosus is arranged in concentric layers of parallel collagen fibers that crisscross those of the next layer. Because the nucleus pulposus is more posteriorly placed, the annulus is thinner posteriorly. Anteriorly, the annulus blends imperceptibly with the nucleus. Superiorly and inferiorly, it is firmly anchored to the vertebral bodies.

Disc herniation is the most widely used term to refer to different degrees of disc material displaced beyond the intervertebral disc space. The simplest form of unphysiologic displacement of disc material is known as intradiscal displacement of the nucleus pulposus, which occurs with a fully intact fiber ring and without any visible change in the configuration of the disc. Disc protrusion describes a circumscribed herniation with partial rupture of the annulus fibrosus while disc extrusion is defined as complete rupture of the annulus.

Herniated discs may extend beyond the normal boundaries of the interspace in all directions: anteriorly, laterally, posterolaterally toward a lateral recess or neural foramen, and posteriorly toward the spinal canal (central type).

The anterior and posterior surfaces of the intervertebral discs are covered by the longitudinal ligaments which are loosely attached to the annulus anteriorly and firmly posteriorly. Clinically, an inner and outer annulus are distinguished.

Two grades of intervertebral disc protrusion are distinguished according to Kraemer. Grade 1 refers to unphysiologic intradiscal mass displacement with protrusion of the intact annulus while the inner ring is torn in grade 2 protrusion.

When there is complete rupture of the annulus fibrosus (disc extrusion), the herniated tissue may become separated from the parent disc (free fragment or sequester). An extruded disc or sequester may be contained by the posterior longitudinal ligament or anterior epidural membrane (subligamentous/submembraneous herniations) or rupture through these structures. A free disc fragment can migrate into the anterior epidural space or, less frequently, into the posterior epidural space. Even true intradural disc herniations with extension of free disc fragments into the thecal sac have been reported in the literature.

In severe disc herniation, it is not only nucleus material that is displaced toward the spinal canal but also portions of annulus and of the adjacent cartilaginous endplate.

A special type of disc herniation is intraforaminal herniation.

Furthermore, from both a pathogenetic and clinical perspective, true disc herniation (focal) must be differentiated from circumferential disc bulging, which is characterized by diffuse extension of the disc beyond the adjacent vertebral margins in all directions and is due to disc space narrowing secondary to progressive degeneration.

Specific features of the discs in the three spinal regions and how they affect patterns of disc herniation are described below.

Cervical Disc Herniation

The cervical discs are wedge-shaped and higher anteriorly. They do not extend as far laterally as in other spinal regions because they are confined by the uncinate processes projecting from the lateral margins of the vertebral bodies. Also the cervical discs develop horizontal clefts at the level of the uncinate processes, which already occur in childhood and are considered normal because they are not associated with disc degeneration. Rather, they function as additional joints, commonly referred to as the uncovertebral joints of Luschka.

Disc degeneration can cause widening of the joint-like clefts, predisposing the disc to interdiscal mass displacement, bulging, and herniation. Being additional functional joints, they can also contribute to progressive degeneration of the motion segment. Extension of the clefts toward the center can lead to complete splitting of the disc with corresponding instability.

The unique bony confinement of the cervical discs explains why true herniation of a cervical disc (soft herniation) is rare despite the increased movement necessary in the cervical region and the high pressure per unit area. On the other hand, so-called hard disc herniation due to degeneration of the uncinate processes (uncovertebral arthrosis) is rather common and may further compromise an already narrow intervertebral foramen in the cervical region.

Thoracic Disc Herniation

The thoracic spinal canal is narrow and has only a small epidural space with the narrowest portion extending from T4 through T9. The thoracic intervertebral discs are thinner relative to the height of the vertebral bodies compared with the cervical and lumbar spine. Due to the normal kyphotic curvature of the thoracic spine, the axial load is exclusively transmitted by the vertebral bodies and intervertebral discs (and not by the facet joints). These unique characteristics predispose the thoracic spine to early and severe regressive changes, predominantly involving the anterior elements (spondylosis, osteochondrosis).

The intervertebral foramina in the thoracic region are relatively large and differ from the cervical and lumbar foramina in that they do not lie at the level of the intervertebral discs but somewhat higher behind the vertebral bodies. This is why a laterally herniated thoracic disc rarely impinges on a nerve root.

Lumbar Disc Herniation

The lumbar discs decrease in height from top to bottom. They are biconvex in shape with a thicker anterior portion. The lumbosacral disc is about 30% narrower than the adjacent discs. The lumbar neural foramina come to lie progressively lower toward the inferior end of the spinal column and are at the levels of the disc spaces in the lower lumbar region. This is why laterally herniated lumbar discs are more likely to impinge on the nerve roots. Also, the foraminal opening is rather small at the lumbosacral junction due to the narrow interspace and the orientation of the articular facets.

Pathomechanism

Disc herniation occurs when there is a mismatch between intradiscal pressure and the tensile strength of the annulus fibrosus. As both the mechanical strength of the annulus and the ability of the nucleus pulposus to rebound after compression decrease with age, the incidence of intervertebral disc herniation does not increase steadily but peaks between 30 and 50 years of age.

Disc Protrusion

MR Technique

Sagittal and axial T1- and T2-weighted sequences are most suitable for evaluating the intervertebral disc space and identifying protruded discs. Images in coronal orientation are useful when looking for foraminal narrowing. Contrast-enhanced imaging is usually necessary only in patients with prior back surgery.

MR Findings

Disc protrusion is typically seen as a generalized extension of the disc margin beyond the boundaries of the adjacent vertebral bodies. There is no rupture of the annulus fibrosus with extrusion of nuclear material. Typically, the herniated disc material is confined by osteophytes from adjacent vertebral bodies. Disc degeneration is common and is best seen as decreased signal intensity on T2-weighted images (Fig. 4.35).

MR Pitfalls

Postoperative scars may mimic a protruded disc on unenhanced images.

Disc Extrusion

MR Technique

Again, T1- and T2-weighted axial and sagittal sequences are most widely used, while coronal images may be helpful to better evaluate narrowing of the neural foramina. Moreover, coronal T2-weighted images may improve the identification of free disc fragments.

MR myelography may be indicated in cases where the degree of spinal narrowing needs to be determined.

MR Findings

Degenerated discs with low signal intensity on T2-weighted images often contain a hyperintensity representing a tear of the annulus fibrosus. Disc extrusion is usually seen as focal extension of disc material. Depending on the site of extrusion, the disc material may narrow the spinal canal and/or a neural foramen. Contrast-enhanced imaging is required to exclude a scar in patients with a history of back surgery.

As avascular structures, the intervertebral discs will not enhance after contrast administration. T2-weighted images often enable better evaluation of encroachment on the dural sac than T1-weighted images because they depict CSF with high signal intensity. Extruded disc material remains contiguous with the interspace of origin. The herniated disc may extend above or below the disc level. This is most conspicuous in subligamentous disc herniation, where the disc tissue typically extends upward and looks like a hockey stick on sagittal images, while a herniated disc extruding both cranially and caudally looks like a mushroom.

An extruded disc has low signal intensity on T1- and T2-weighted images and may indent the dural sac or displace intraforaminal fatty tissue (Figs. 4.36–4.56).

MR Pitfalls

Postoperative scars may mimic an extruded disc on unenhanced images. Inconclusive cases can be resolved by contrast-enhanced imaging because scars differ from disc tissue in that they show fairly clear enhancement. The mass effect of a scar is usually much smaller than that of disc extrusion.

Free Disc Fragments

MR Technique

The standard sequences are T1 and T2 in axial and sagittal planes, supplemented by a coronal T2-weighted sequence to evaluate foraminal narrowing and to better appreciate the size of a sequester and its relationship to the parent disc. Contrast administration is not needed because the free fragment is avascular but may be helpful to exclude a scar or tumor.

MR Findings

A sequester is a free disc fragment that is separated from its parent disc and is typically found near the interspace of origin but may also migrate after detachment. A free disc fragment is depicted epidurally as a mass of low signal intensity on T1- and T2-weighted images and will not show enhancement after contrast administration. The signal intensity of a disc fragment is typically similar to that of the parent disc, but a longstanding sequester that has undergone further degeneration or calcification may show marked signal alterations (cervical disc sequestration: Figs. 4.57–4.59; lumbar sequestration: Figs. 4.60–4.78).

MR Pitfalls

Free disc fragments must be differentiated from tumors or scar tissue in postoperative patients. Contrast-enhanced MRI is required in patients with inconclusive findings. Occasionally, it is difficult to differentiate a sequester located near a nerve root from conjoined roots. In such cases, the examiner must carefully search the disc levels below and above the sequester for "missing roots" in order not to overlook conjoined roots.

Clinical Significance

The ability of MRI to directly visualize or exclude intervertebral disc herniation and associated changes offers the unique opportunity to directly correlate a patient's clinical symptoms with the underlying anatomic pathology, which is not possible with other diagnostic modalities such as myelography.

Whether and how to treat a patient with proven disc herniation depends on a variety of factors. These include the clinical symptoms such as severity and duration of pain and type and severity of motor deficits. Anterior and anterolateral disc herniations have no clinical relevance. When a disc herniation extends toward the spinal canal, a lateral recess or a neural foramen, however, the distinction between disc protrusion and expulsion is practically relevant with regard to the indication for invasive (surgical) treatment. Another clinically relevant parameter is the reserve space around the spinal cord (congenitally narrow spinal canal, narrow lateral recess, extension of herniated disc into neural foramen). Finally, the need for therapy depends on the topographic relationship of the disc herniation to other spinal structures: patients with imminent spinal cord compression (posterior protrusion) require a more aggressive therapeutic approach than patients with contact or imminent contact of the herniated disc to a nerve root.

4.8 Muscular Dystrophy

Pathoanatomy

Atrophy of muscle with a compensatory increase in fatty and connective tissue.

Pathomechanism

Myopathies of unclear pathogenesis with a genetic predisposition.

MR Technique

Muscular dystrophy is a rare indication for requesting an MRI examination. The condition is typically detected as an incidental finding. The extent of spinal muscle atrophy varies with the type of muscular dystrophy. The basic protocol comprises axial T1- and T2-weighted images. Coronal and sagittal images may provide useful additional information on specific muscles.

MR Findings

Muscular dystrophy is characterized by a loss of striated muscle and fatty involution. In patients with muscular dystrophy, the mass of striated muscle is markedly decreased and the muscle shows marked fatty involution. This is seen on T1- and T2-weighted images as hyperintense areas replacing the low-signal-intensity striated muscle.

Muscular dystrophy is differentiated from muscular atrophy in bedridden patients or patients after stroke on the basis of the history (Figs. 4.79 and 4.80).

Clinical Significance

The MRI findings may point to the correct diagnosis in some forms of muscular dystrophy with a favorable prognosis.

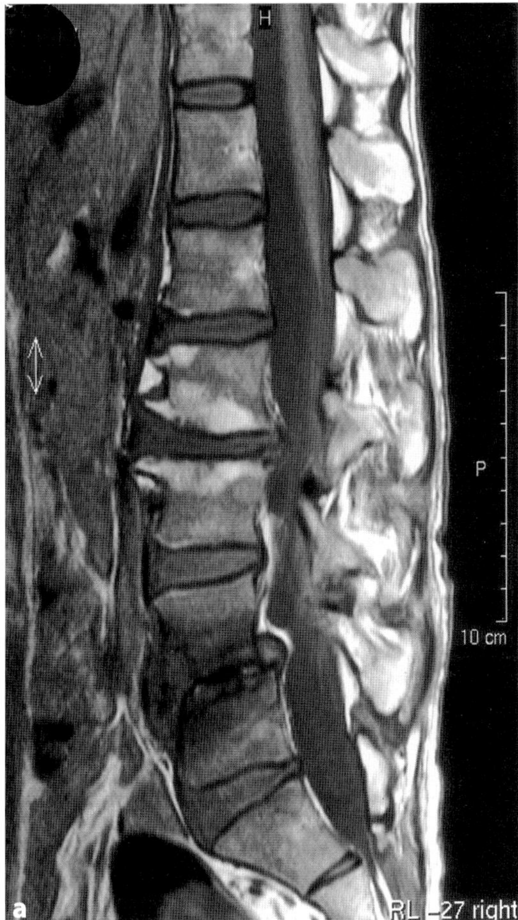

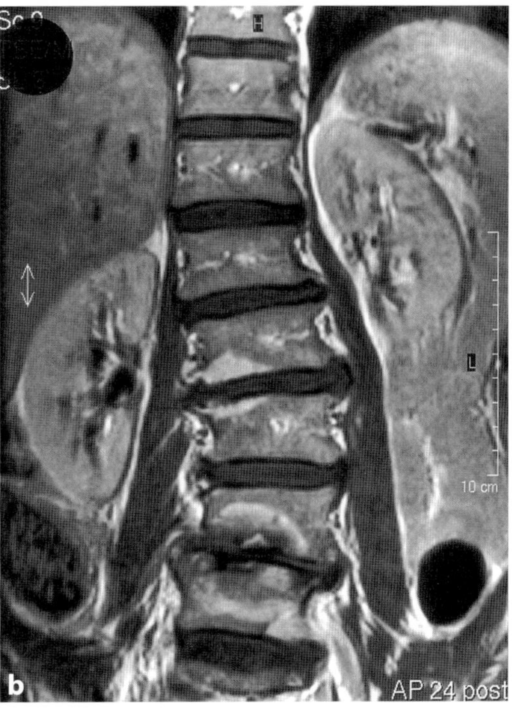

Fig. 4.1a, b. Chronic and acute osteochondrosis. Chronic osteochondrotic changes in the L2-3 segment are indicated by increased signal intensities in the anterior vertebral portions on T1-weighted image (**a**) and T2-weighted image (**b**). In contrast, acute osteochondrosis, seen here at the L4-5 level, is characterized by a decrease in signal intensity on T1 and an increase on T2

Fig. 4.2. Axial T2-weighted image through the level of L3-4 showing degenerative hypertrophy of the facet joints. The changes are more pronounced on the right, where the signal intensity also suggests increased fluid. In addition, there is minimal indentation of the dural sac on the right. The appearance is consistent with severe spondyloarthrosis. No signs of irritation of surrounding soft tissue structures

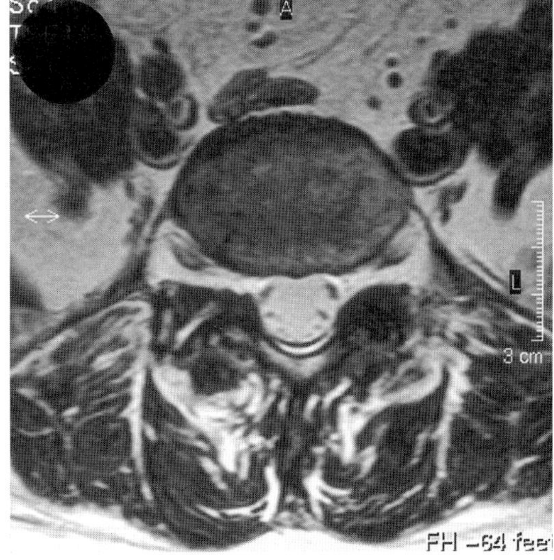

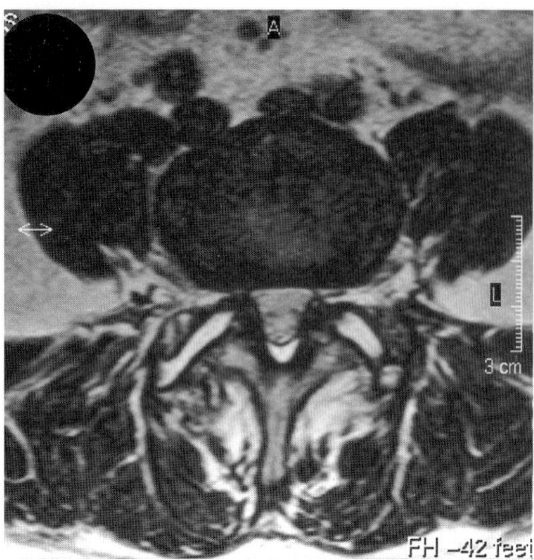

Fig. 4.3. Axial T2-weighted image through the L4-5 level showing high-signal-intensity fluid collections distending the facet joints. In addition, there is moderate hypertrophy of the bony structures on both sides. The diagnosis is bilateral spondyloarthrosis

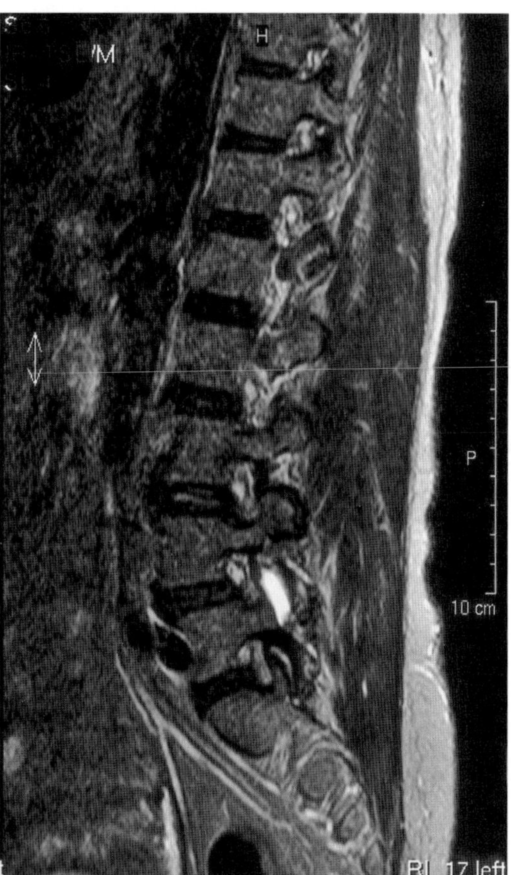

Fig. 4.4. Sagittal T2-weighted image with fat saturation showing the fluid collection in the left facet joint at L4-5

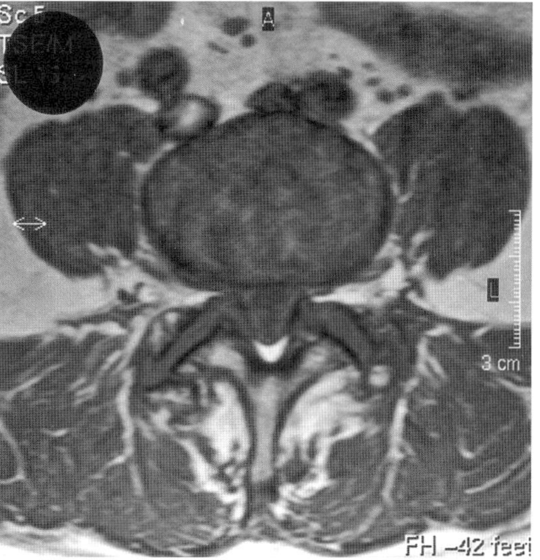

Fig. 4.5. Same patient as Figs. 4.3 and 4.4 (spondyloarthrosis). Axial T1-weighted image showing cystic widening of the L4-5 facet joint as a low-signal-intensity lesion with well-defined margins. Bilateral joint effusion

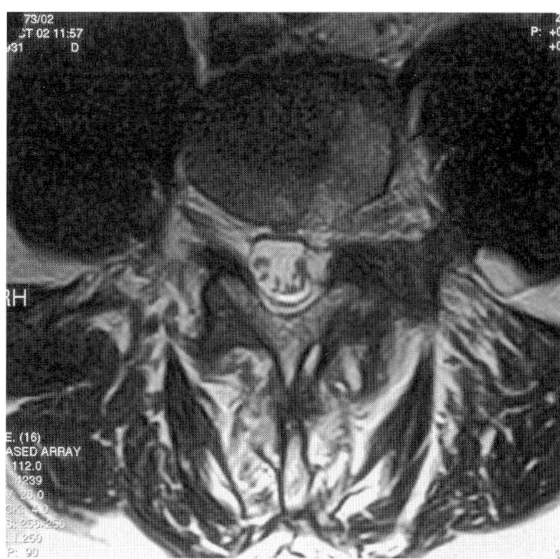

Fig. 4.6. Axial T2-weighted image through the L4-5 level in this patient showing a cystic lesion with smooth margins in the immediate vicinity of the left facet joint and slightly indenting the dural sac

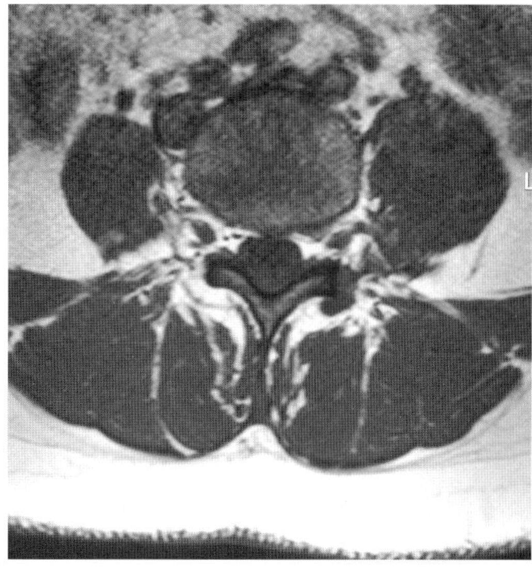

Fig. 4.7. Axial T1-weighted image through the L3-4 level showing a well-defined, low-signal-intensity mass extending posteriorly from the left facet joint. The appearance is consistent with a synovial cyst

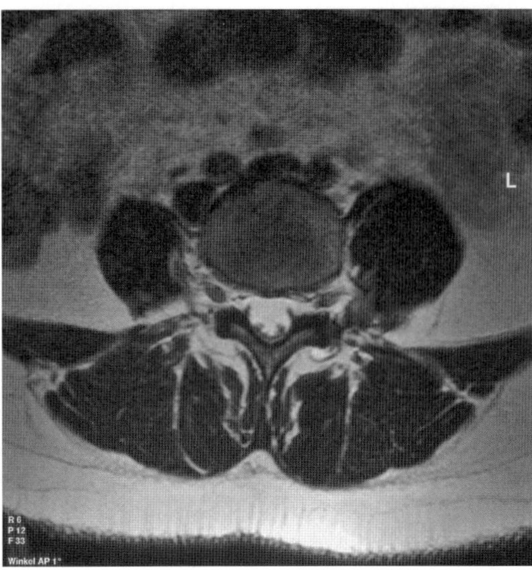

Fig. 4.8. Same patient. Axial T2-weighted image through the L3-4 level showing the synovial cyst posterior to the left L3-4 facet joint

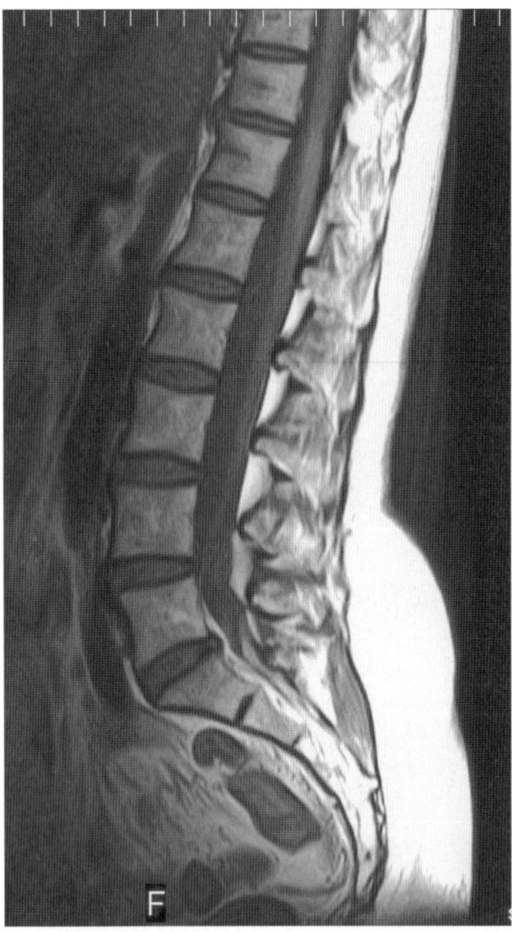

Fig. 4.9. 59-year-old patient with unspecific back pain. Sagittal T1-weighted image of the lumbar region and thoracolumbar junction without any significant degenerative changes or a mass lesion

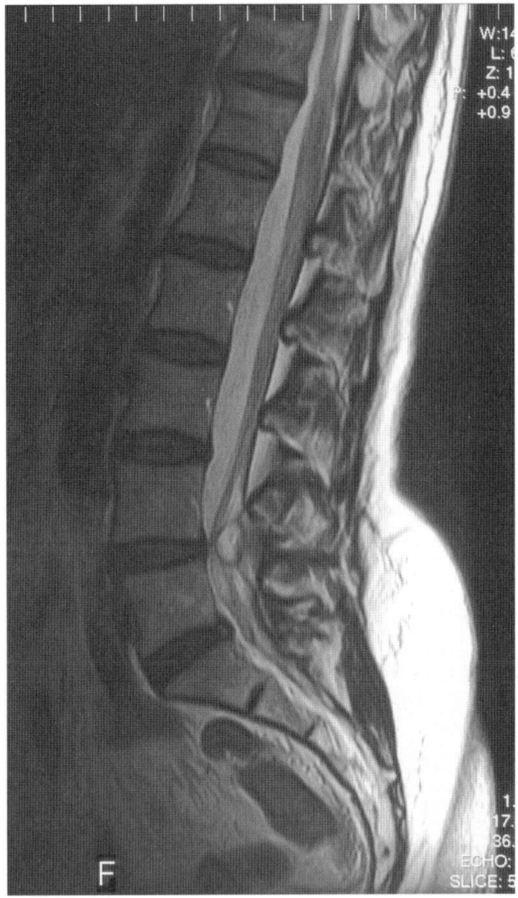

Fig. 4.10. Same patient. Sagittal T2-weighted image showing a cystic lesion at the L4-5 level on the right. The lesion is sharply demarcated with a central signal intensity isointense to CSF

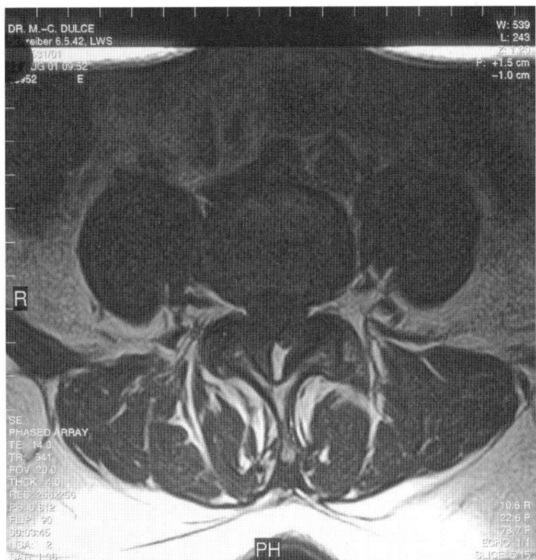

Fig. 4.11. Axial T1-weighted image showing widening of the right facet joint and slight deformity of the dural sac. There is no clear sign of a mass effect

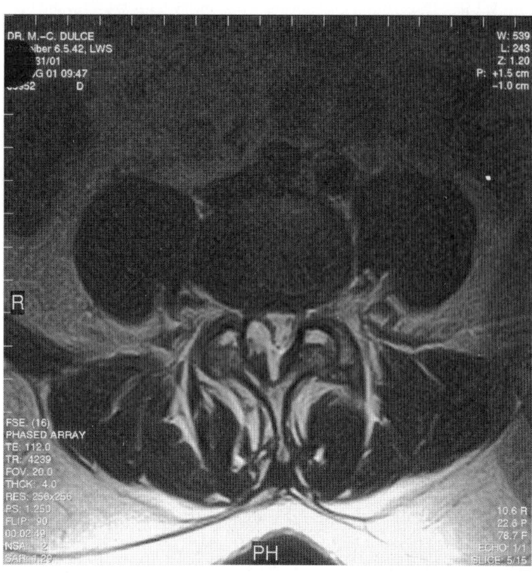

Fig. 4.12. Same patient. Axial T2-weighted image through the L4-5 level. Cystic lesion contiguous with the right facet joint, consistent with a synovial cyst. Indentation of the dural sac

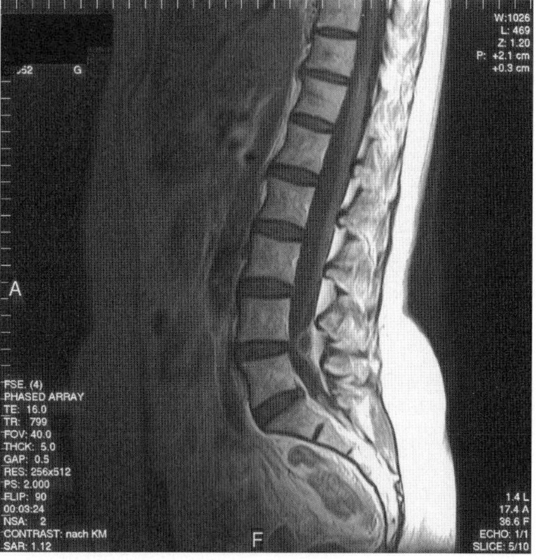

Fig. 4.13. Sagittal T1-weighted image after contrast administration showing wall enhancement of the synovial cyst at the L4-5 level on the right

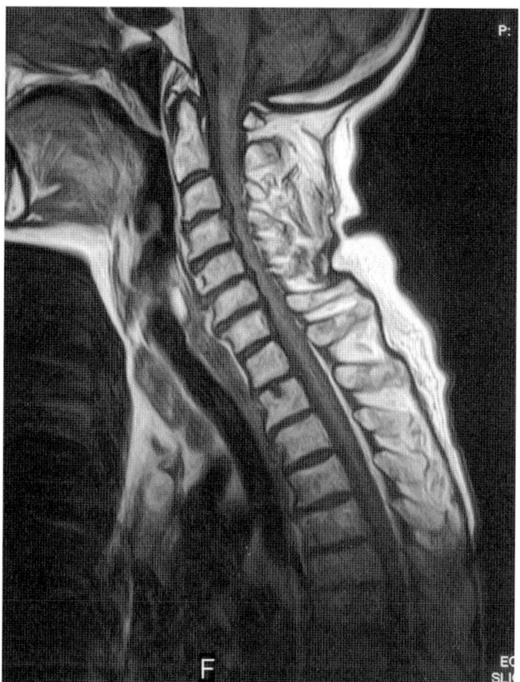

Fig. 4.14. 83-year-old patient presenting with paresthesia of both arms. Sagittal T1-weighted image showing severe degenerative changes of the cervical spine from C3-4 through C6-7 with posterior disc herniations at these levels. Congenitally narrow spinal canal with a width well below the anteroposterior diameters of the vertebral bodies

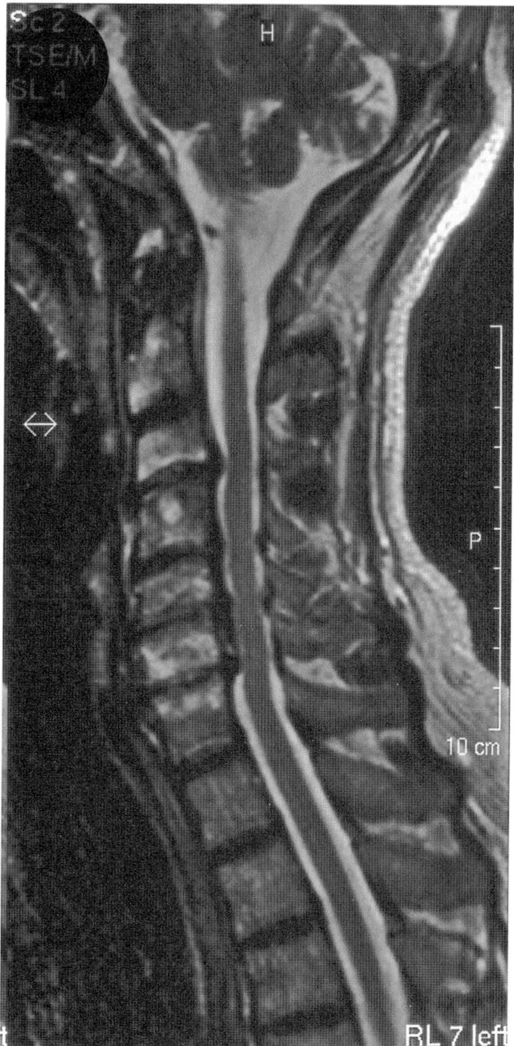

Fig. 4.15. Sagittal T2-weighted image showing high-grade narrowing of the anterior subarachnoid space from C3 through C6-7 with prominent spinal cord indentation at C3-4 and C5-6. Normal cord signal. The anteroposterior diameter of the spinal canal is markedly smaller than that of the corresponding vertebral bodies, suggesting spinal canal stenosis

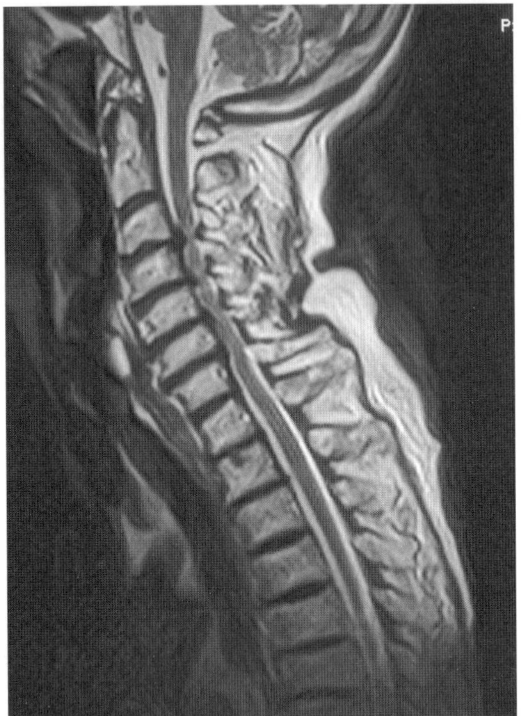

Fig. 4.16. Same patient as Fig. 4.14. Sagittal T2-weighted image of the high-grade spinal stenosis showing the large intervertebral disc protrusions and the decreased anteroposterior diameter of the spinal canal

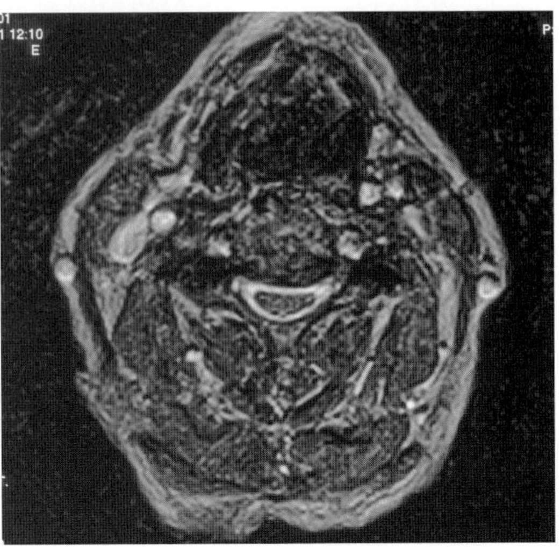

Fig. 4.17. Axial T2-weighted image at the C3-4 level confirming high-grade narrowing of the spinal canal with deformity of the spinal cord. The diagnosis is cervical spinal stenosis

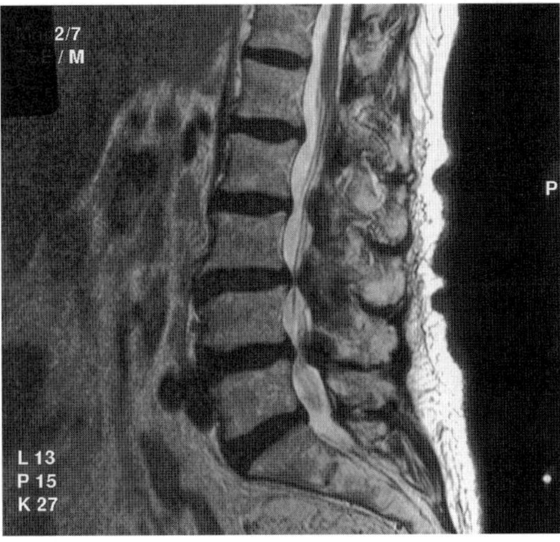

Fig. 4.18. Sagittal T2-weighted image showing high-grade narrowing of the spinal canal at L3-4 and L4-5 due to marked hypertrophy of the facet joints and moderate disc herniation in a patient with a congenitally narrow spinal canal

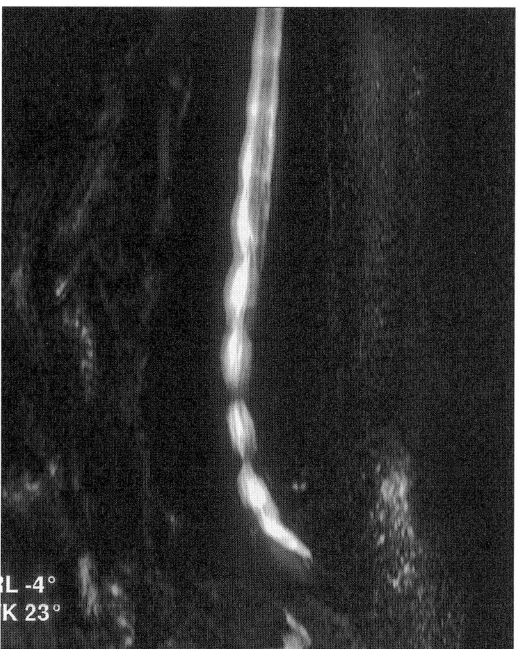

Fig. 4.19. Same patient as Fig. 4.18. Heavily T2-weighted 3D slab MR myelography shows almost complete absence of CSF signal at the levels of the L3-4 and L4-5 disc herniations, confirming marked narrowing of the spinal canal at these levels

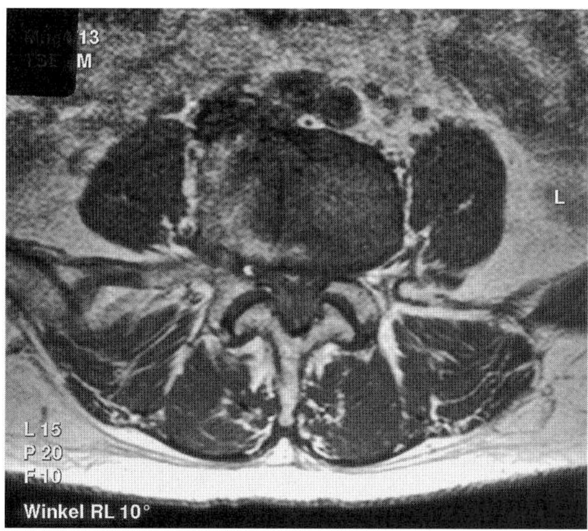

Fig. 4.20. Axial T2-weighted image through the L3-4 level showing nearly complete loss of fluid signal at this level, consistent with severe spinal stenosis

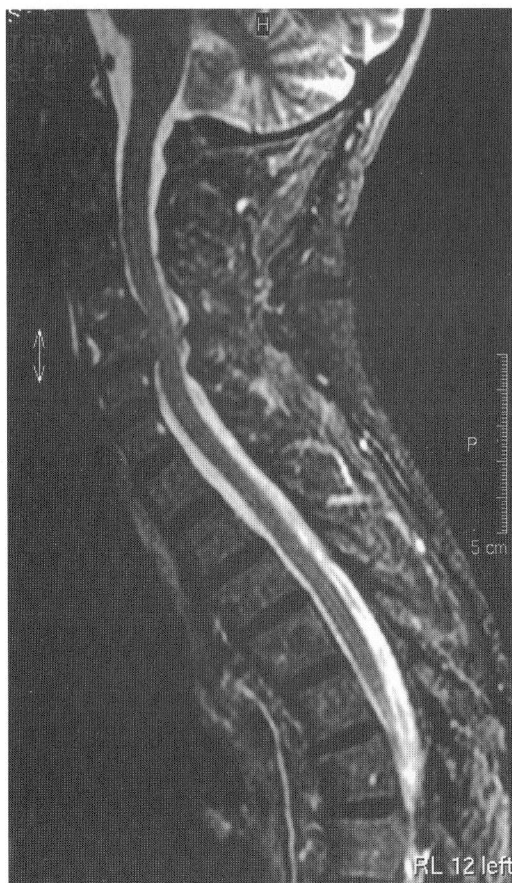

Fig. 4.21. Sagittal T2-weighted image with fat saturation of the cervical region and cervicothoracic junction showing spinal stenosis at C5-6. Kyphosis with the apex at this level and slight posterior displacement of the C5 vertebra. The body of the C5 vertebra is slightly reduced in height. The bone marrow signal is homogeneous and there are no signs of a fresh lesion

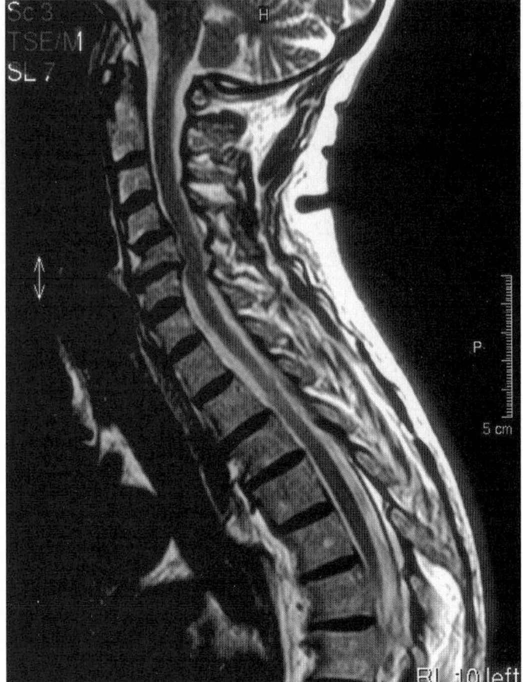

Fig. 4.22. Sagittal T2-weighted image without fat saturation of the patient with C5-6 spinal stenosis, postural kyphosis, and degenerative changes. An older compression fracture of the anterior portion of C5 is suggested. Slight posterior displacement of C5 relative to C4 and C6. No evidence of myelomalacia

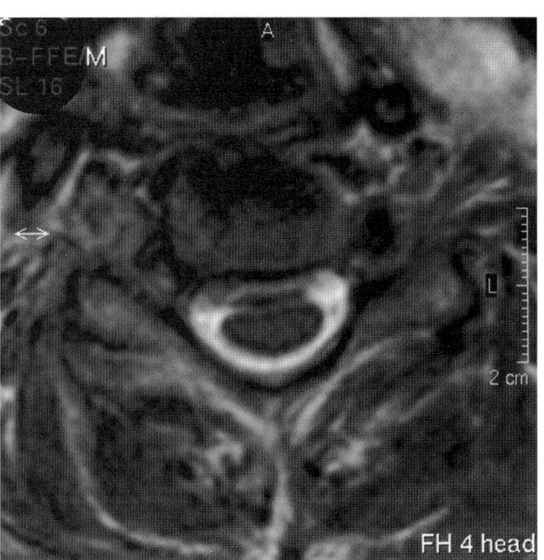

Fig. 4.23. Same patient. Axial T2-weighted image through the C5-6 level showing narrowing of the anterior subarachnoid space by kyphotic curvature. The spinal cord is displaced posteriorly but again shows no signs of myelomalacia

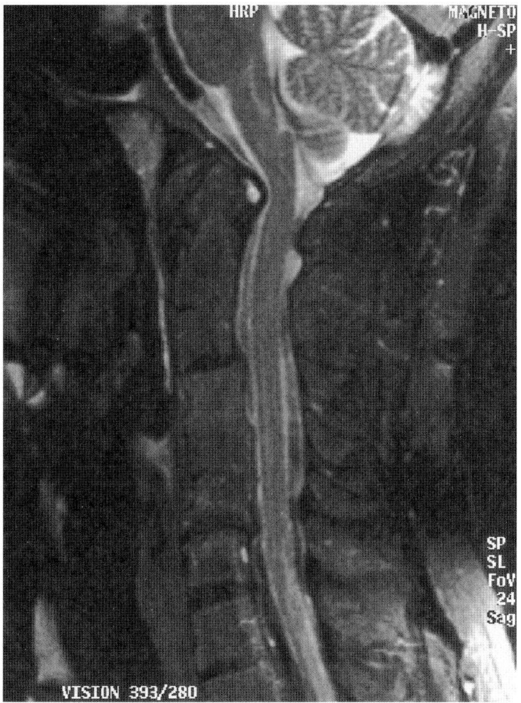

Fig. 4.24. Sagittal T2-weighted image of the cervical region and craniocervical junction in a 76-year-old patient with chronic polyarthritis. The image shows synostoses between C2 and C3 and from C4 to C6. There is marked hypertrophy of the atlantoaxial joint causing spinal stenosis at the C1 level as well as slight indentation and marked posterior displacement of the spinal cord

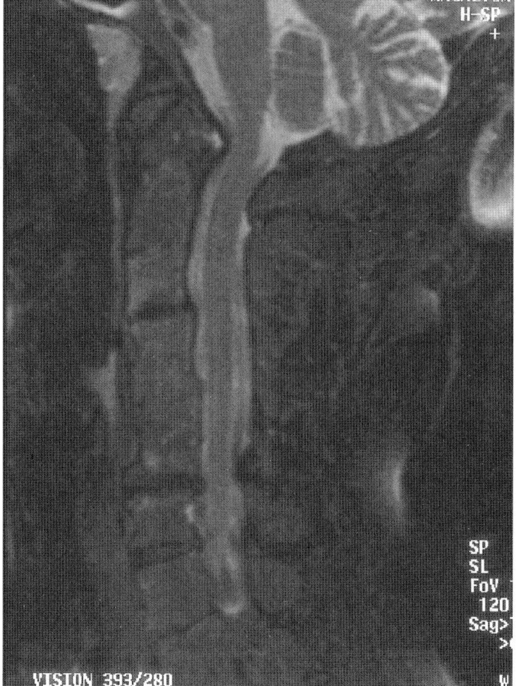

Fig. 4.25. Sagittal T2-weighted image showing the C1 spinal stenosis during maximum reclination. There is no significant increase in the stenosis grade in this position

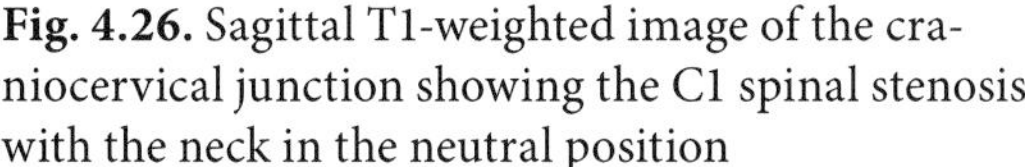

Fig. 4.26. Sagittal T1-weighted image of the craniocervical junction showing the C1 spinal stenosis with the neck in the neutral position

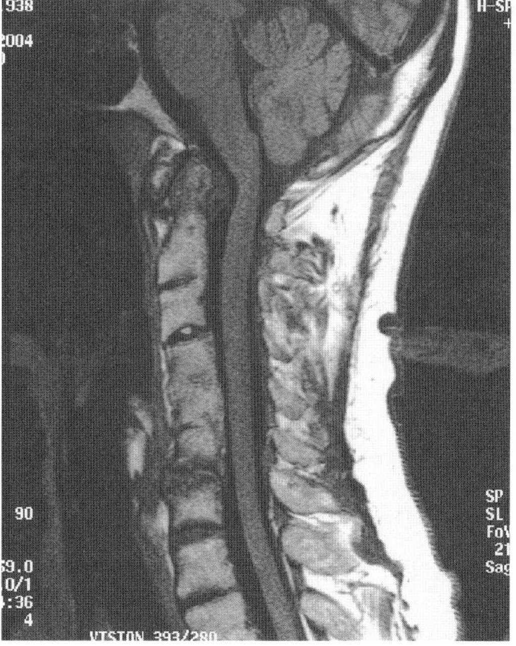

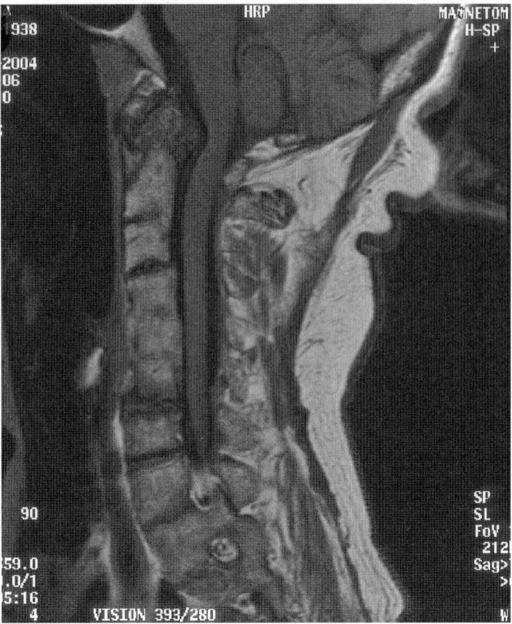

Fig. 4.27. Same patient. Sagittal T1-weighted image of the craniocervical junction, again showing the almost unchanged stenosis during maximum reclination

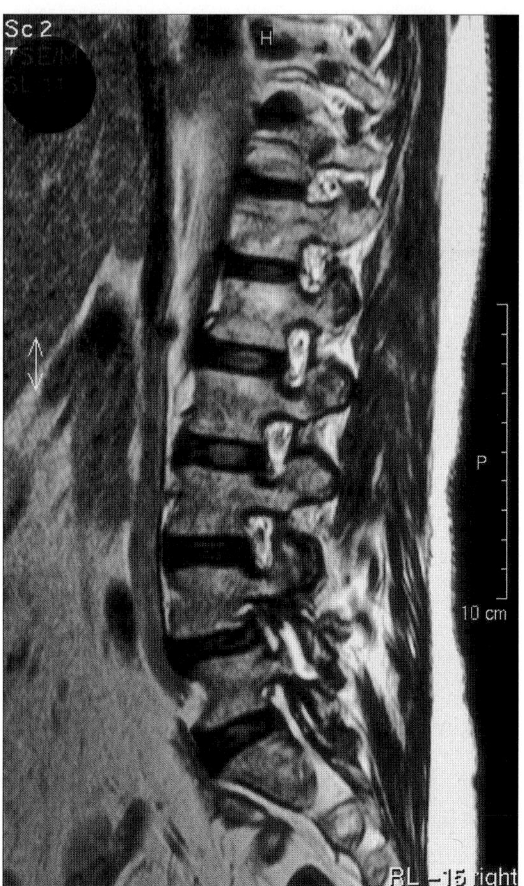

Fig. 4.28. Sagittal T2-weighted image of the lumbar region. High-grade narrowing of the L4 neural foramen in a patient with spondyloarthrosis and mild disc herniation. Normal appearance of the L1 to L3 foramina

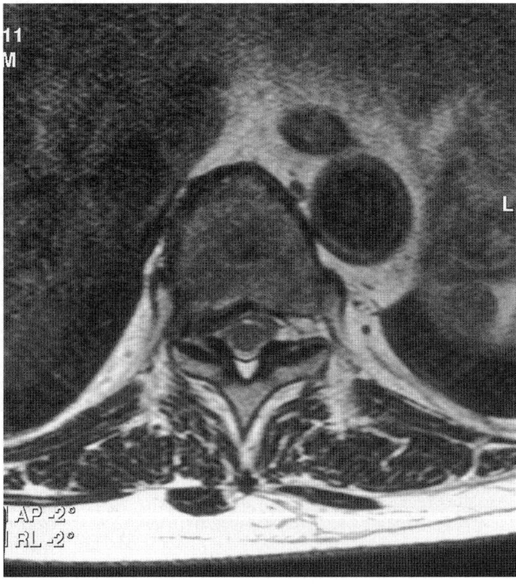

Fig. 4.29. Axial T2-weighted image of the lower thoracic spine showing narrowing of the right T9 foramen. Broad-based posterolateral disc herniation and hypertrophy of the facet joints

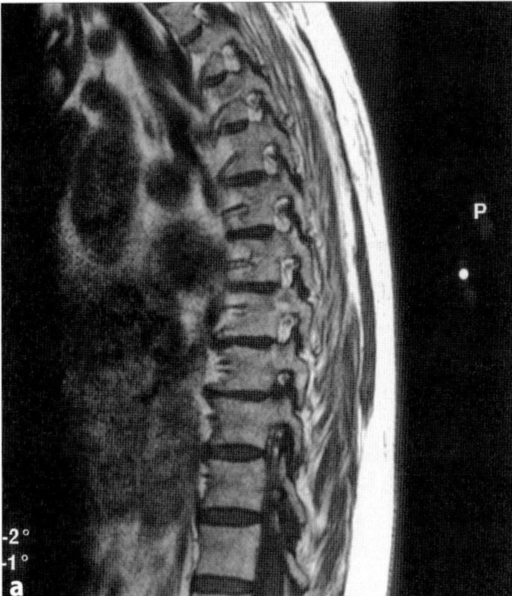

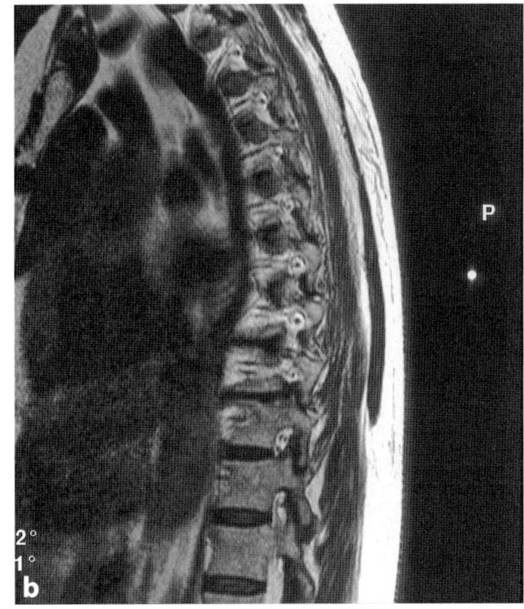

Fig. 4.30a, b. Sagittal images of the same patient showing narrowing of the lower third of the right T9 foramen by herniated disc material

Fig. 4.31. Sagittal T2-weighted image of the lumbar region. High-grade narrowing of the right L4 foramen due to severe disc herniation and slight hypertrophy of the facet joints

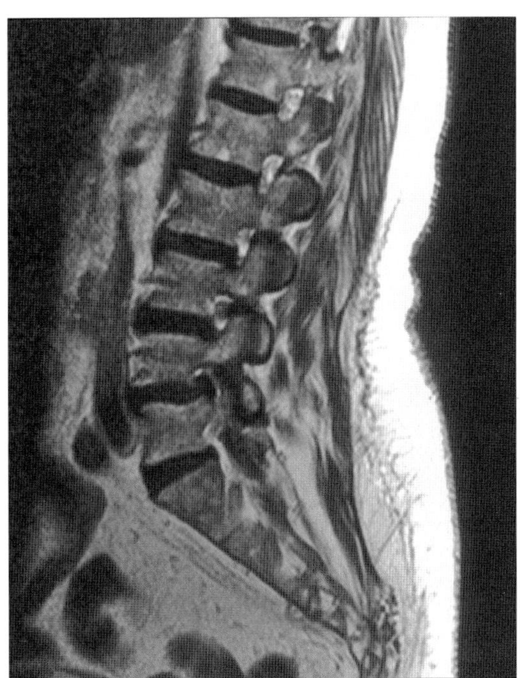

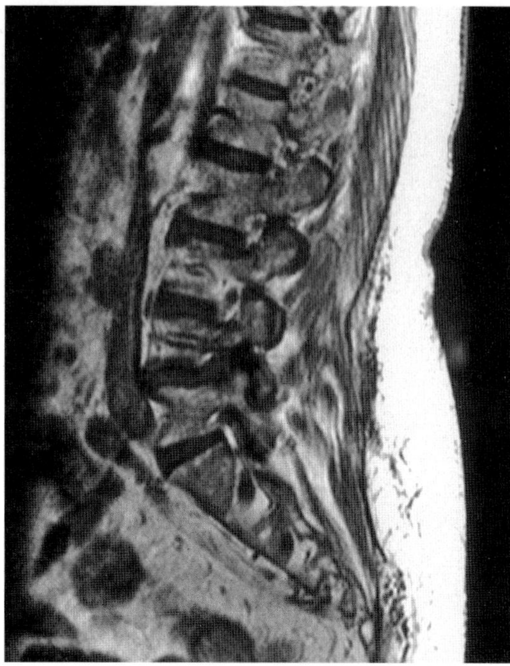

Fig. 4.32. Same patient. Corresponding sagittal T1-weighted image confirming presence of low-signal-intensity disc tissue in the right L4 foramen

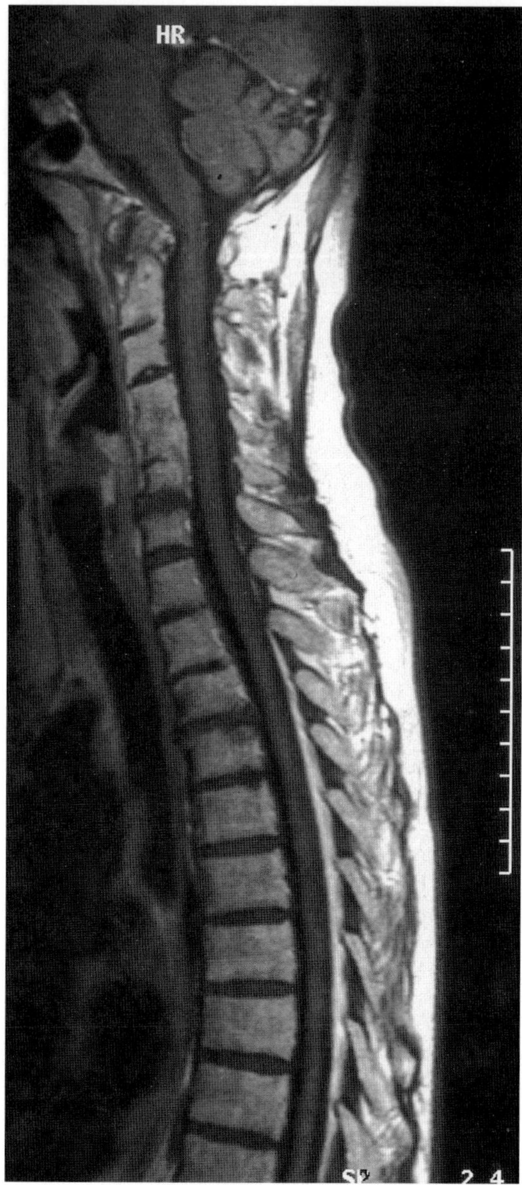

Fig. 4.33. Sagittal T1-weighted image of the cervical and thoracic regions showing synostoses between C2 and C3 and from C4 to C6 in severe atlantoaxial arthrosis. Osteophytic outgrowths from the atlas ring and arthrotic deformity of the dens axis with narrowing of the joint cleft. Spinal stenosis at the C1-2 level with posterior displacement of the spinal cord due to hypertrophy of the C1-2 joint

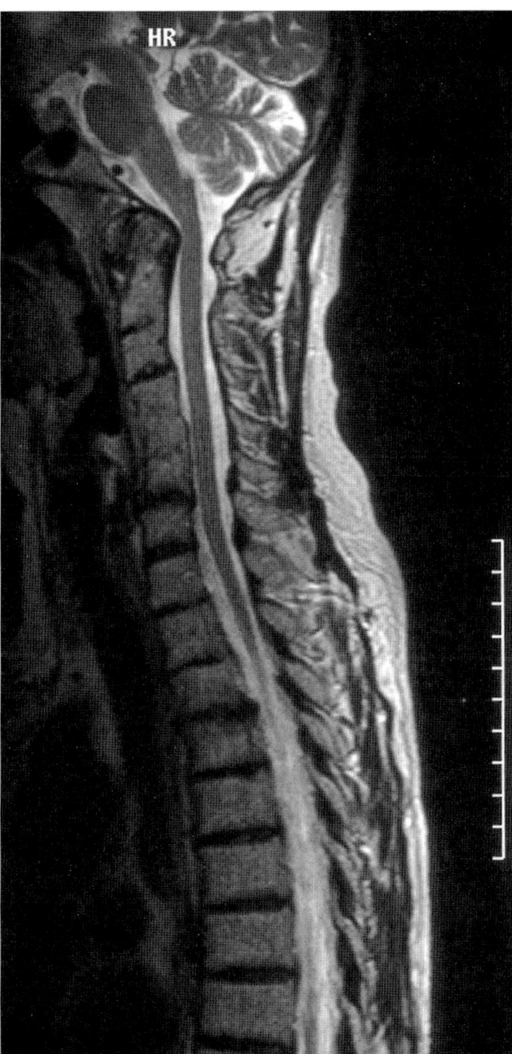

Fig. 4.34. Same patient. Sagittal T2-weighted image of the cervical and thoracic spine. The fluid signal posterior to the dens axis indicates joint effusion due to severe arthrosis of the C1-2 joint. The fluid displaces and compresses the upper cervical cord

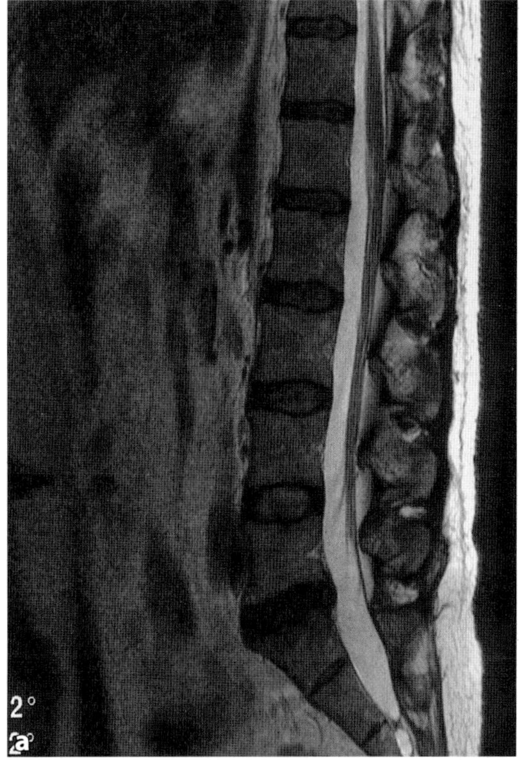

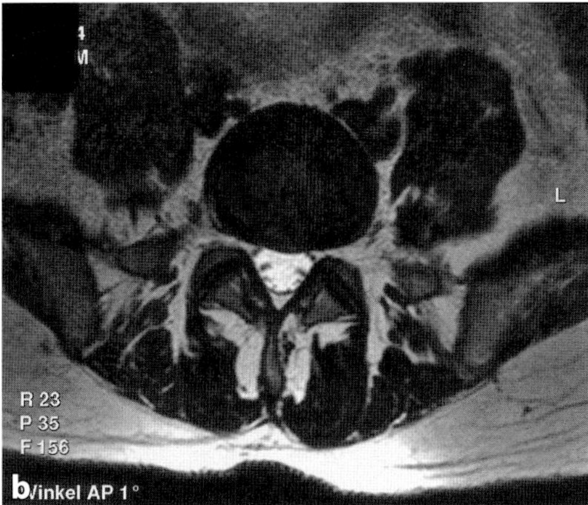

Fig. 4.35a,b. Disc herniation. Sagittal and axial T2-weighted images of the lumbar region. Changed signal intensity of the L5-S1 disc with posterior protrusion. The axial image shows broad-based herniation with slight indentation of the dural sac

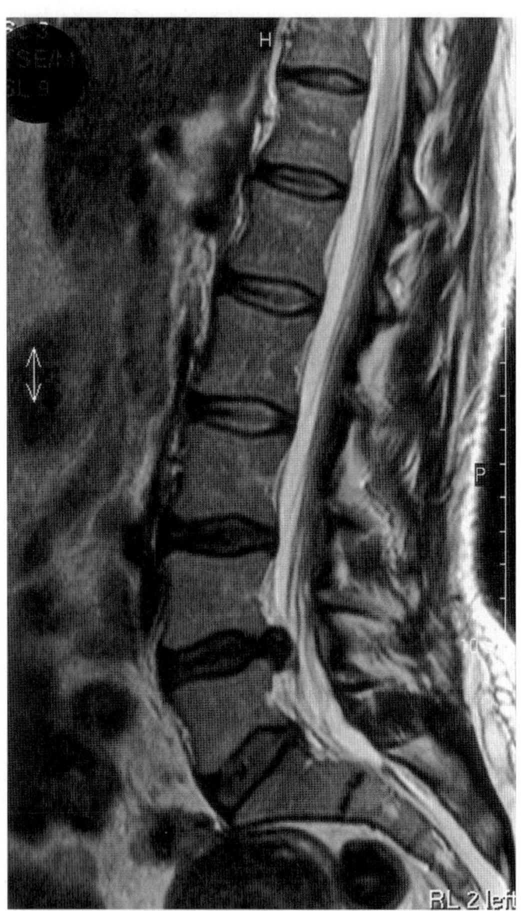

Fig. 4.36. Sagittal T2-weighted image showing low-signal-intensity disc herniation posterior to the L4-5 vertebrae with dural sac indentation

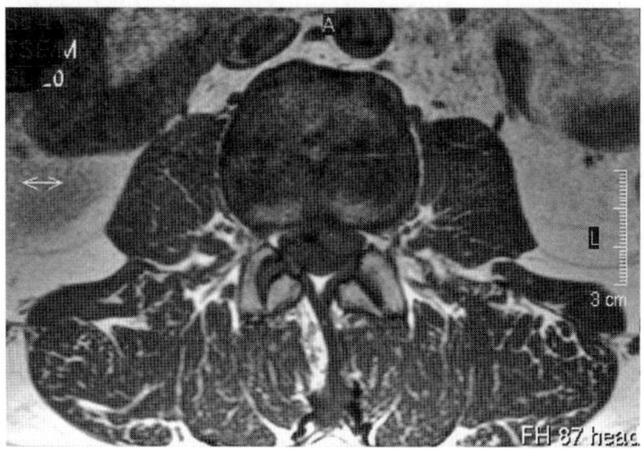

Fig. 4.37. Axial T1-weighted image through the L4-5 level depicting the left mediolateral disc herniation with indentation of the dural sac, which is of a slightly lower signal intensity

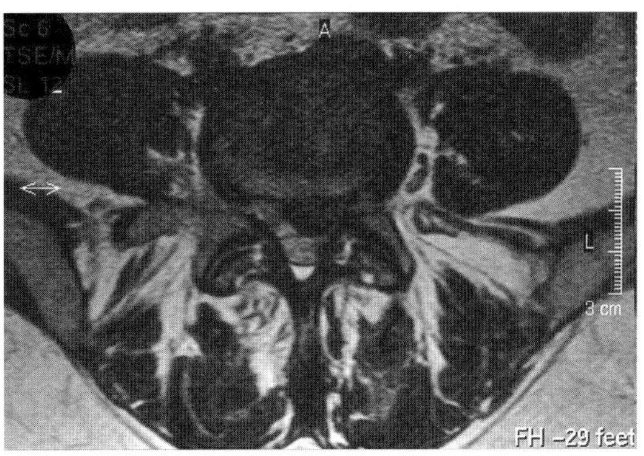

Fig. 4.38. Axial T2-weighted image through the L4-5 level depicting the low-signal-intensity disc herniation extending posteriorly to the left. In addition, there is degenerative hypertrophy of the facet joints. These two factors together cause slight narrowing of the spinal canal

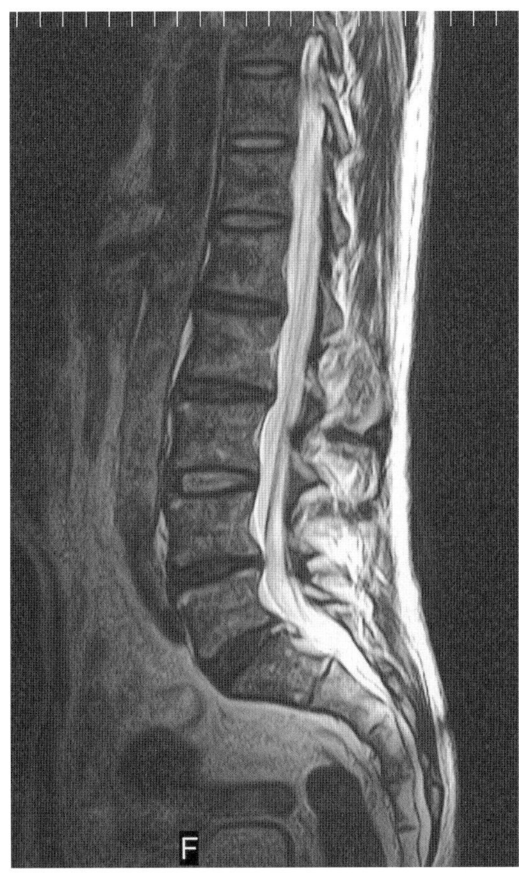

Fig. 4.39. Sagittal T2-weighted image of the lumbar region. Cyst-like lesion extending posteriorly and inferiorly from the L5-S1 disc with a slight mass effect. This appearance suggests an old disc herniation with cystic degeneration of the herniated disc material. Focal signal changes of the L4-5 and L5-S1 discs

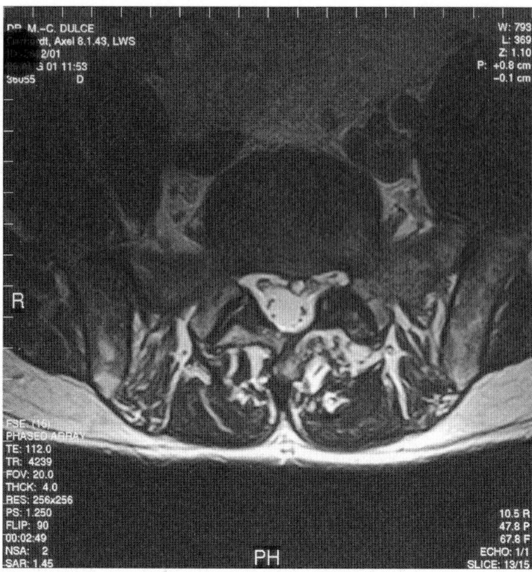

Fig. 4.40. Same patient. Axial T2-weighted image showing the cystic lesion posteromedially, consistent with cystic degeneration of an old disc herniation with slight indentation of the dural sac

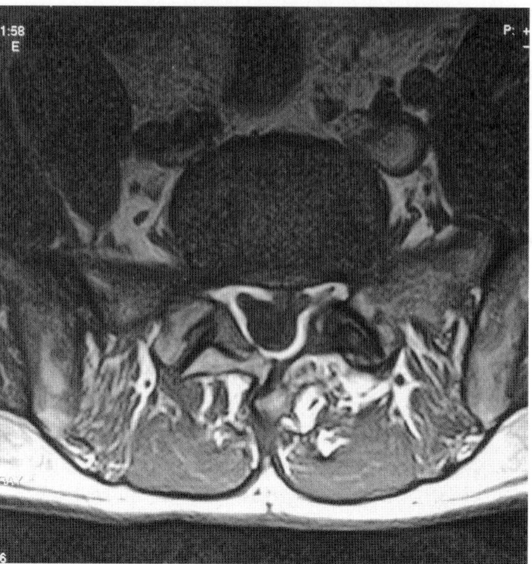

Fig. 4.41. Axial T1-weighted image depicting the old disc herniation with the same signal intensity as the disc. There is slight displacement of the left S1 root and dural sac indentation

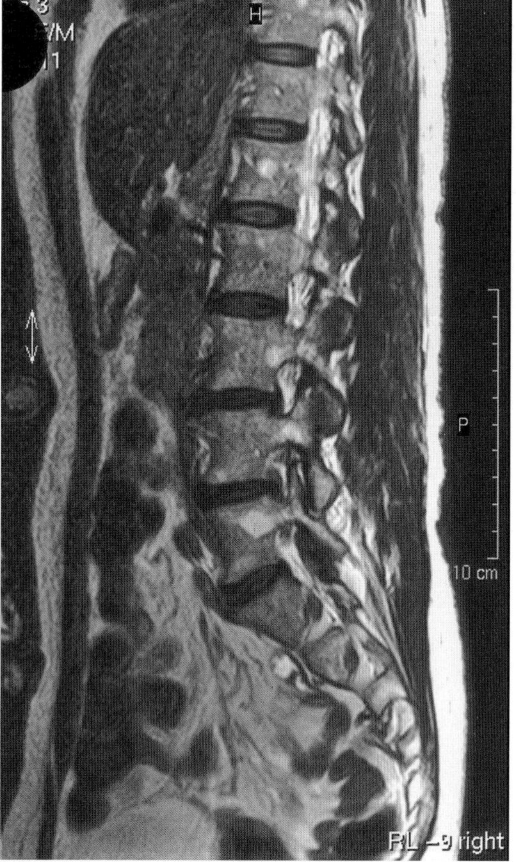

Fig. 4.42. Right paramedian T2-weighted image at the level of the neural foramina showing a focal mass in the L4 foramen with cranial displacement of the nerve root and replacement of the perineural fat in the lower part of the L4 foramen

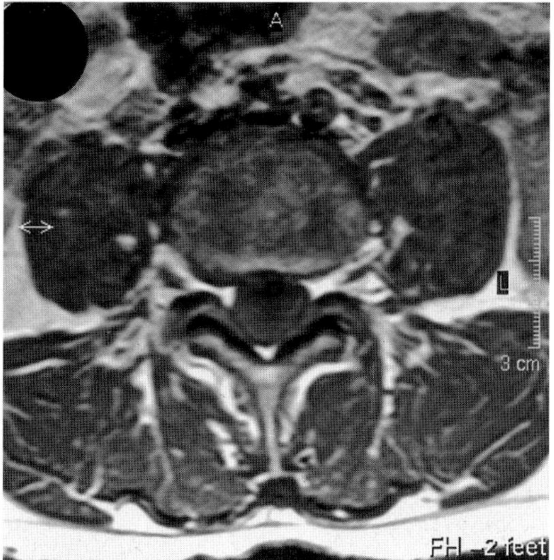

Fig. 4.43. Axial T1-weighted image of a patient with right-sided symptoms. Image through the L4-5 level showing a focal mass in the right foramen, consistent with small intraforaminal disc herniation

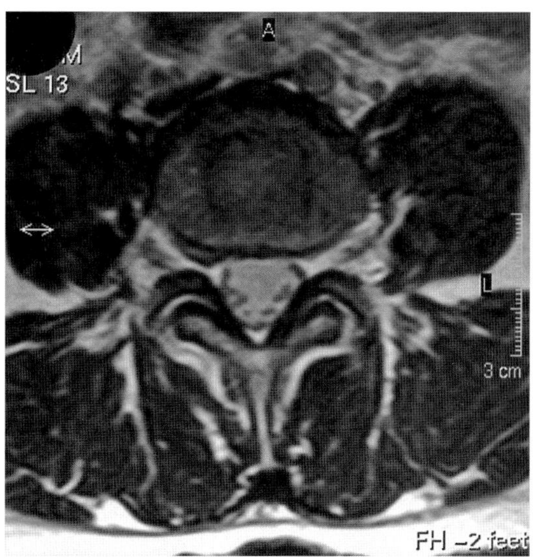

Fig. 4.44. Axial T2-weighted image of the same patient showing the herniated disc material in the right neural foramen without deformity of the dural sac

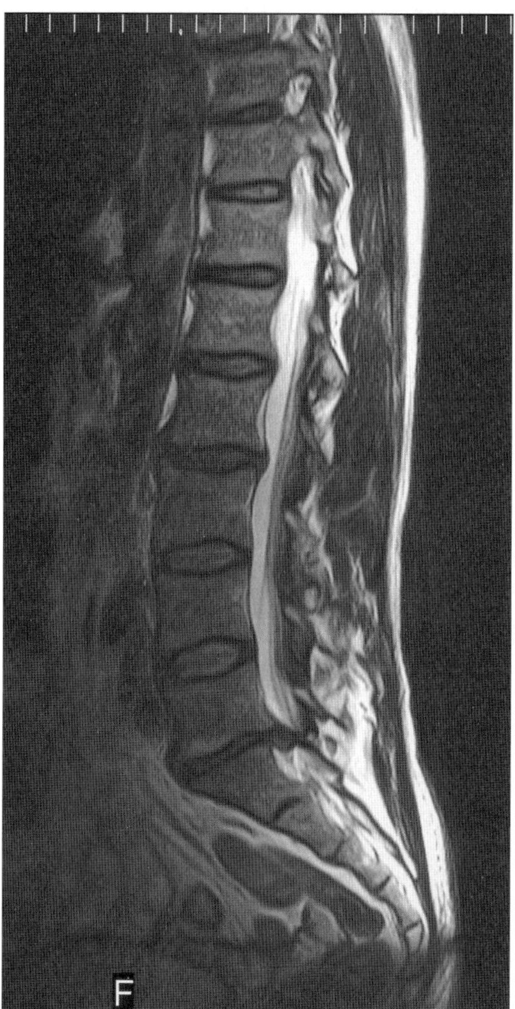

Fig. 4.45. Sagittal T2-weighted image of the lumbar spine and thoracolumbar junction showing narrowing of the L5-S1 disc space and a posterior mass of the same signal intensity as the disc causing marked dural sac deformity

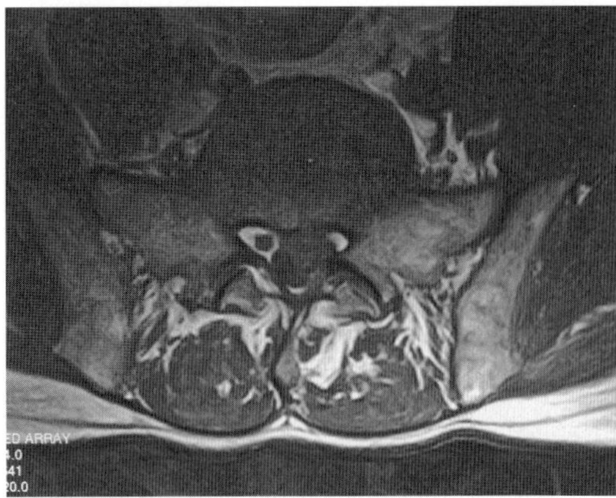

Fig. 4.46. Same patient. Axial T1-weighted image of the L5-S1 level showing the large extruded mass posteriorly and to the left of the disc space. The proximal S1 root seems to be markedly displaced and is not clearly demarcated from the large disc herniation. In addition, there is moderate hypertrophy of the facet joints

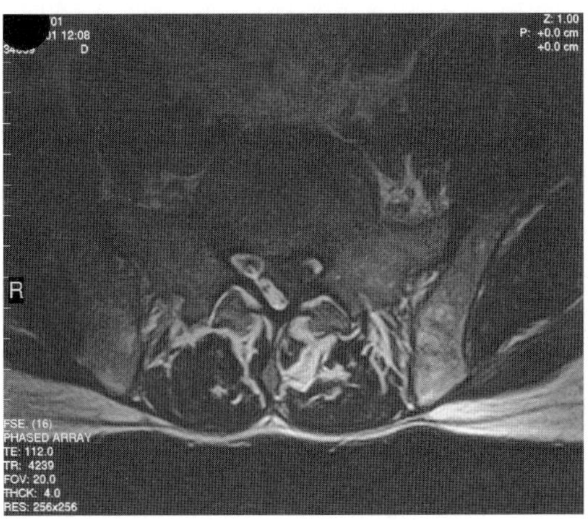

Fig. 4.47. Axial T2-weighted image through the L5-S1 level depicting the low-signal-intensity disc extrusion posteriorly and in the left lateral recess. The S1 root is displaced and somewhat more conspicuous than on the T1-weighted image. Pronounced compression of the dural sac by the herniated disc

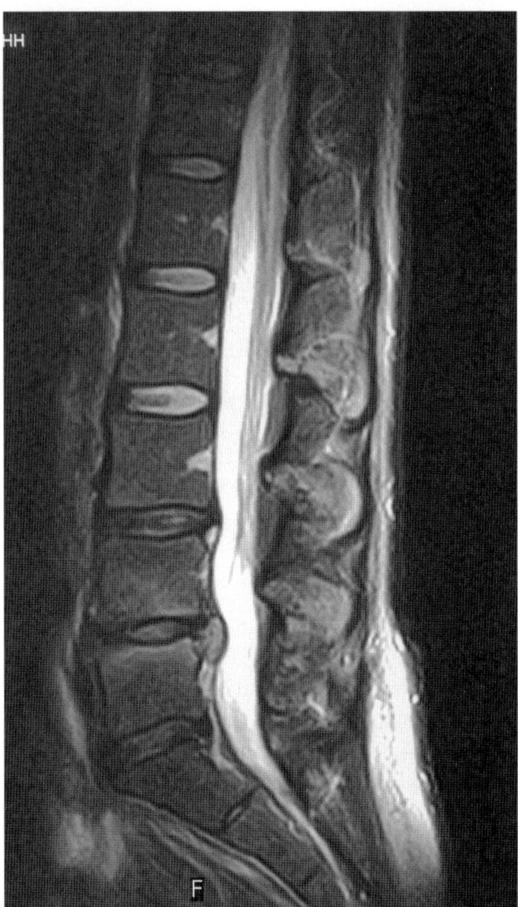

Fig. 4.48. Sagittal T2-weighted image of the lumbar region showing an epidural mass at the level of L4-5 and a less obvious mass at L3-4. Signal alterations of the L3-4, L4-5, and L5-S1 interspaces consistent with disc dehydration and degeneration

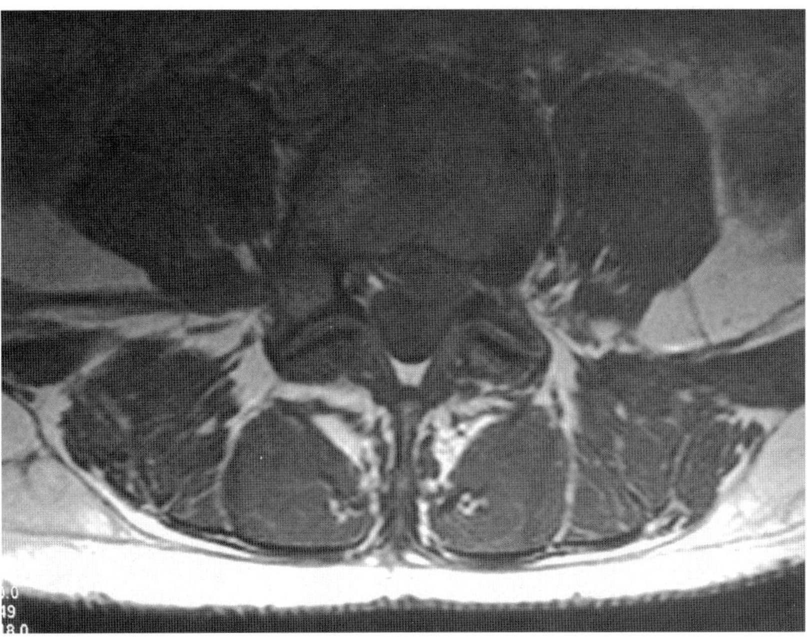

Fig. 4.49. Same patient. Axial T1-weighted image through the L4-5 level with conspicuous dural sac indentation and epidural tissue of disc signal intensity posteromedially and on the left

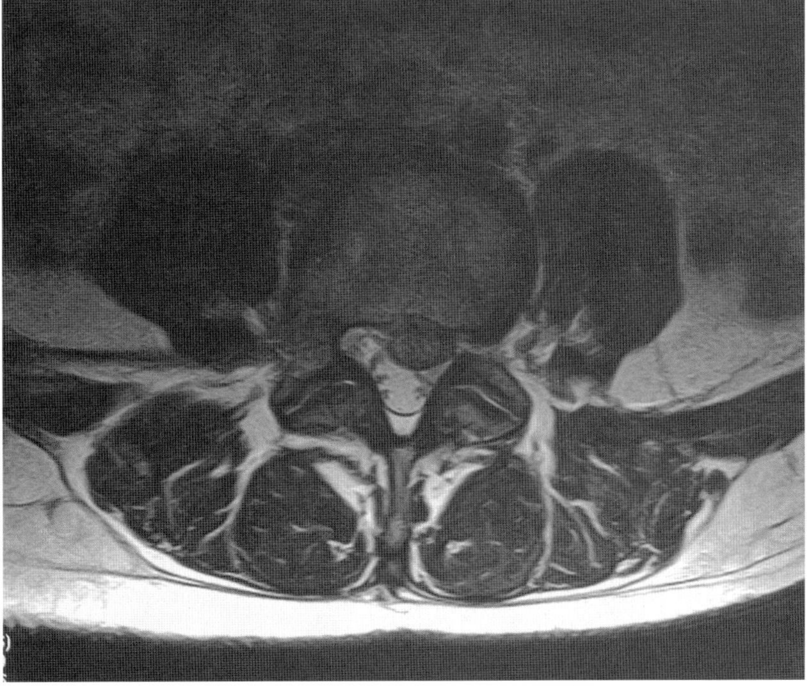

Fig. 4.50. Axial T2-weighted image through the L4-5 level with good delineation of the herniated disc posteriorly and in the left lateral recess. The image confirms marked dural sac indentation

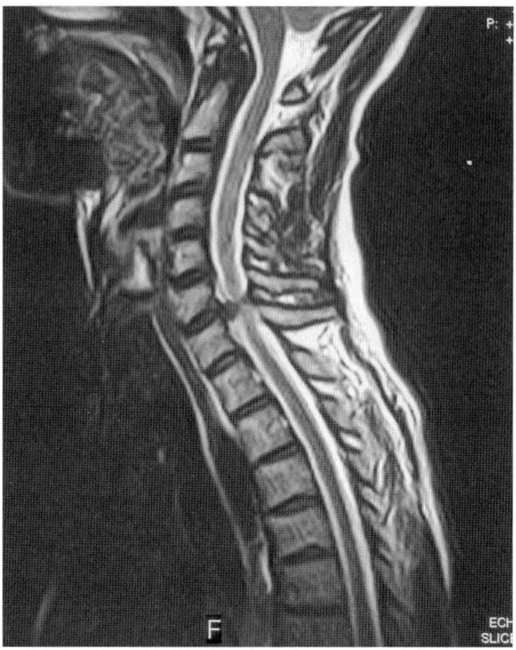

Fig. 4.51. Sagittal T2-weighted image of the cervical region and cervicothoracic junction showing tissue isointense with the disc posterior to the C6-7 interspace. There is pronounced indentation of the dural sac and posterior displacement of the spinal cord

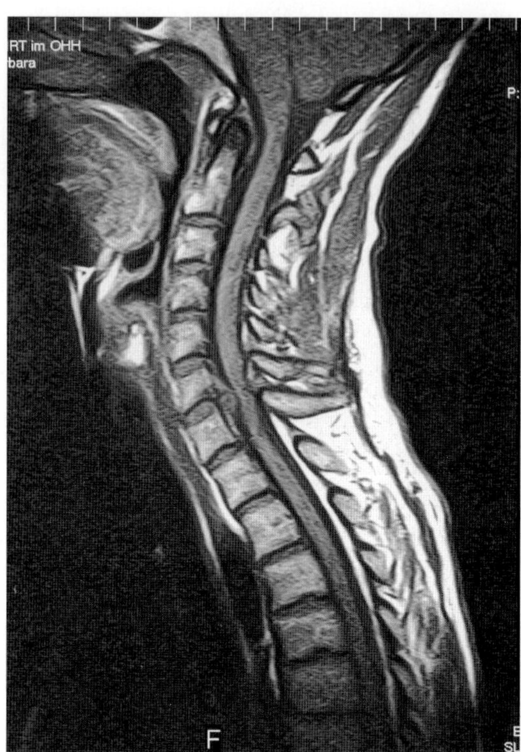

Fig. 4.52. Sagittal T1-weighted image showing the large herniation posterior to the C6-7 interspace with displacement of the spinal cord

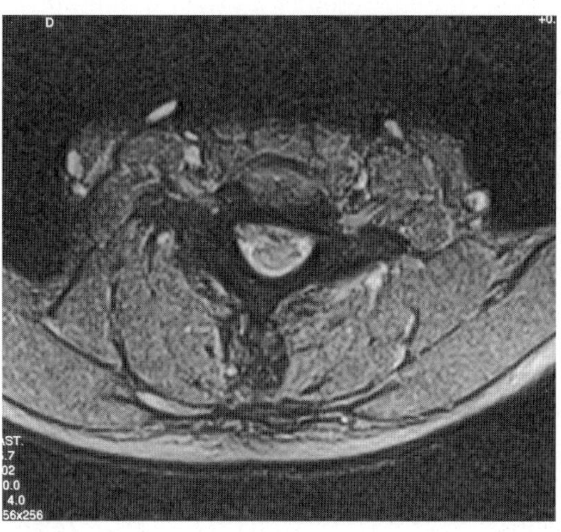

Fig. 4.53. Axial T2-weighted image through the C6-7 level showing the disc herniation posteriorly and posterolaterally on the right. There is obstruction and displacement of the dural sac and CSF as well as slight posterior displacement and deformity of the cervical cord without signs of myelomalacia

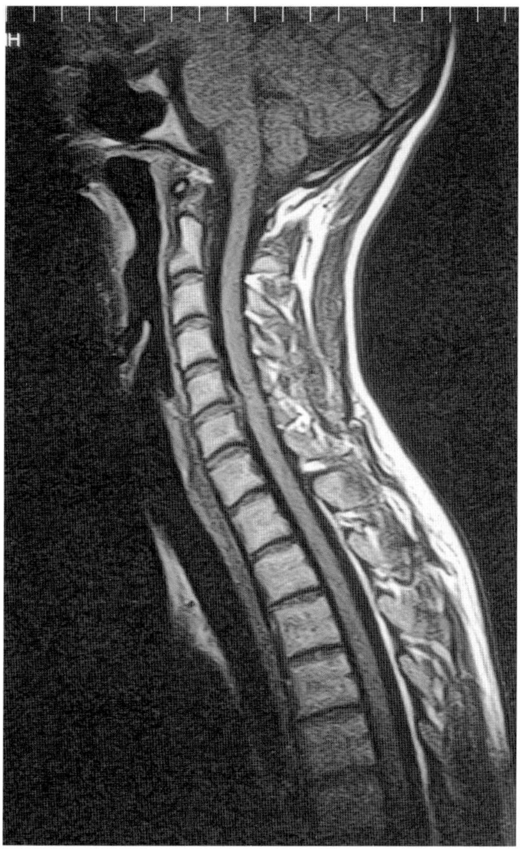

Fig. 4.54. Sagittal T1-weighted image showing herniation of disc signal intensity posterior to the C5-6 interspace. The subarachnoid space is obstructed while there is only minimal spinal cord displacement

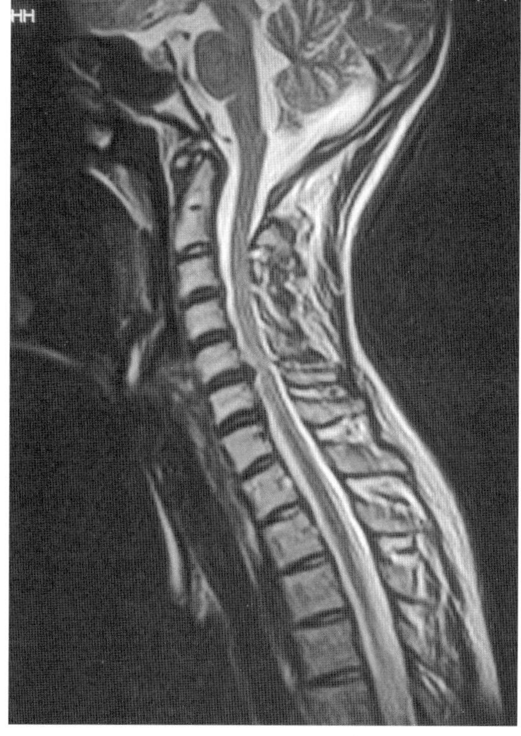

Fig. 4.55. Sagittal T2-weighted image showing the disc herniation at C5-6 with narrowing of the anterior subarachnoid space and mild spinal cord deformity. The cord appears unremarkable while the discs from C3-4 through C6-7 show marked degeneration

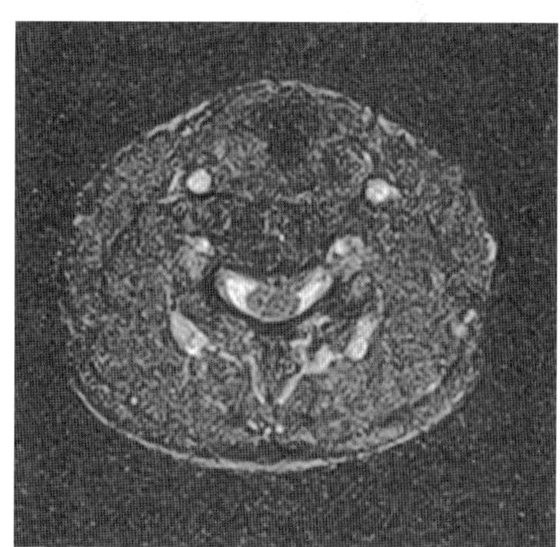

Fig. 4.56. Axial T2-weighted image with fat saturation through the C5-6 level showing the herniated disc posteromedially and slightly paramedially on the left. Subarachnoid space obstruction and slight cervical cord deformity

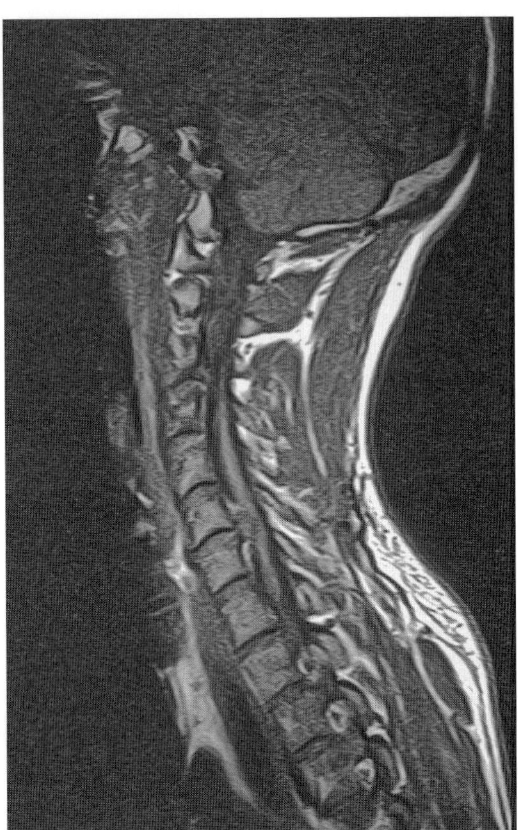

Fig. 4.57. 36-year-old patient with cervical spine complaints. Sagittal T1-weighted image of the cervical region and cervicothoracic junction close to midline. Depiction of a mass with soft-tissue-intensity posterior to the C7-T1 disc. There is tenting of the posterior longitudinal ligament, and slightly hyperintense structures are depicted anterior to the anterior longitudinal ligament above and below the C7-T1 interspace. Posterior displacement of the cervical spinal cord

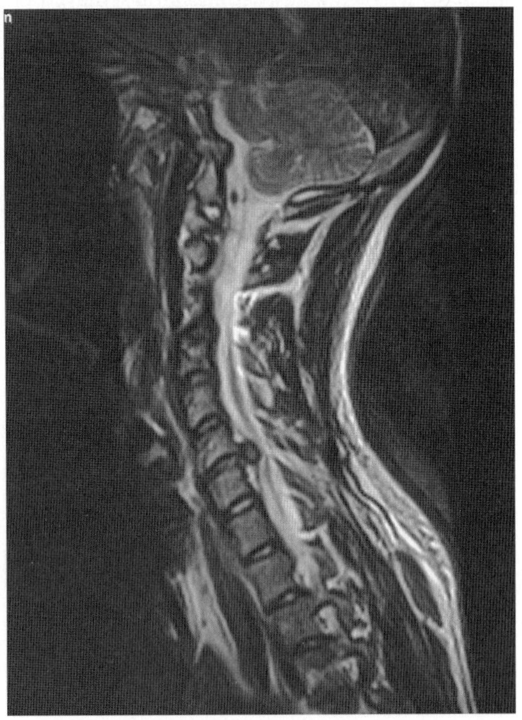

Fig. 4.58. Sagittal T2-weighted image demonstrating a disc fragment slightly above the C7-T1 disc level. The signal intensity of the disc is nearly the same as that of the other discs. The tented posterior longitudinal ligament is clearly visualized as a band-like structure. Marked posterior displacement of the cervical spinal cord

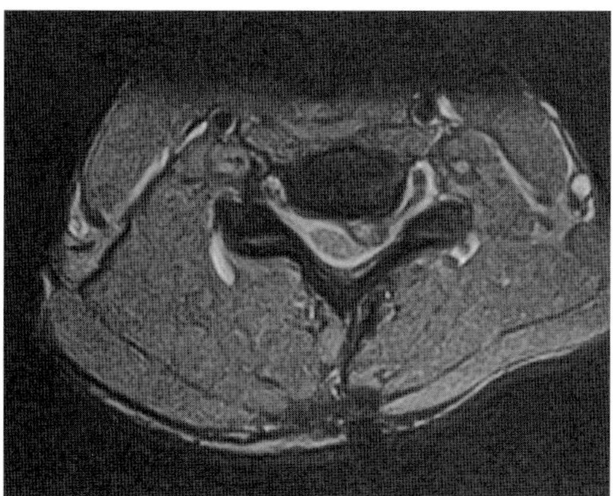

Fig. 4.59. Same patient. Axial T2-weighted image through the C7-T1 level showing the disc fragment posteriorly on the left side. There is clear indentation of the dural sac with right posterior displacement of the cervical cord. No focal signal alterations of the cord

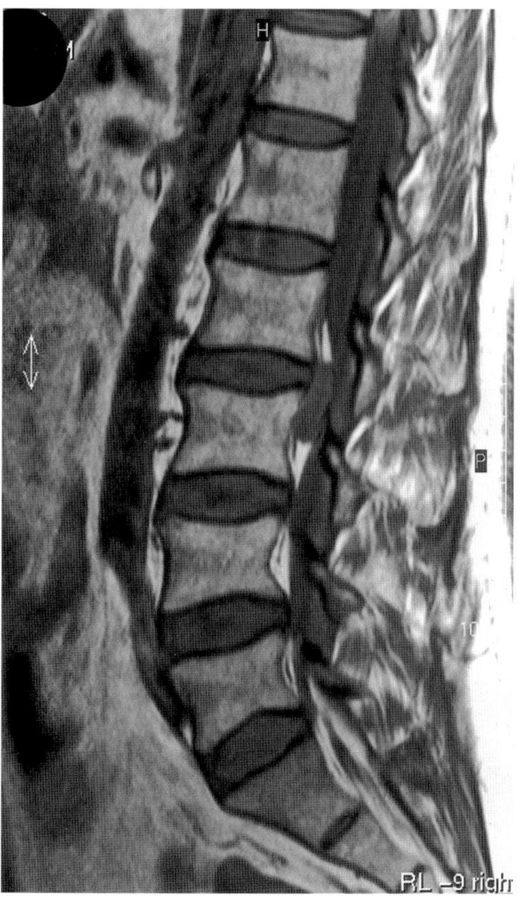

Fig. 4.60. Left paramedian T1-weighted image of the lumbar spine. Focal mass of the same signal intensity as the disc posterior to the L2-3 interspace and the upper aspect of the L3 vertebral body. The posterior longitudinal ligament is tented and there is deformity of the dural sac. Unremarkable appearance of the vertebrae

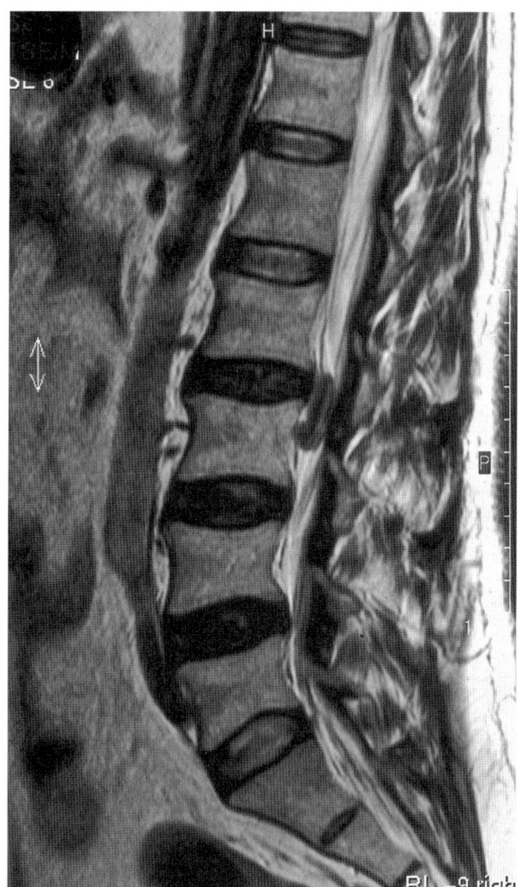

Fig. 4.61. Disc fragment posterior to the L2-3 interspace. The fragment is of nearly the same signal intensity as the L2-3 disc and causes marked indentation of the dural sac

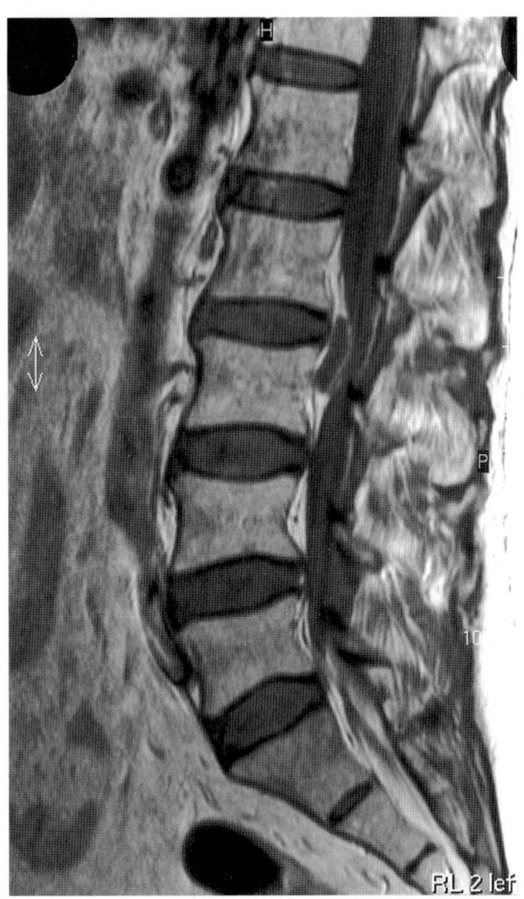

Fig. 4.62. Same patient. Sagittal T1-weighted image after contrast administration showing a ring of enhancement around the epidural disc fragment at the L2-3 level

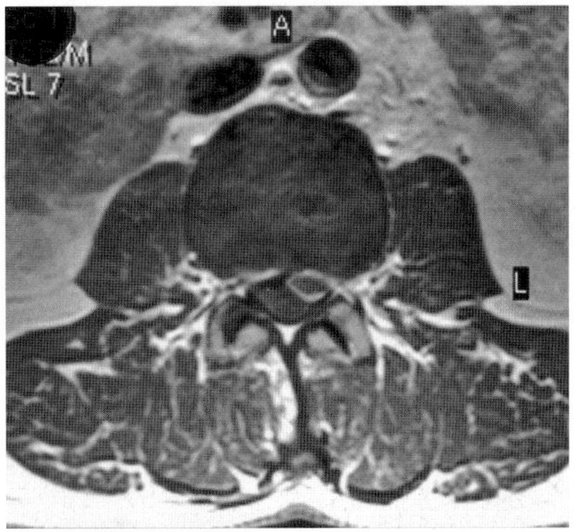

Fig. 4.63. Axial T1-weighted image through the L2-3 level after contrast administration showing circular enhancement of the disc fragment, consistent with peripheral perfusion and absence of central perfusion

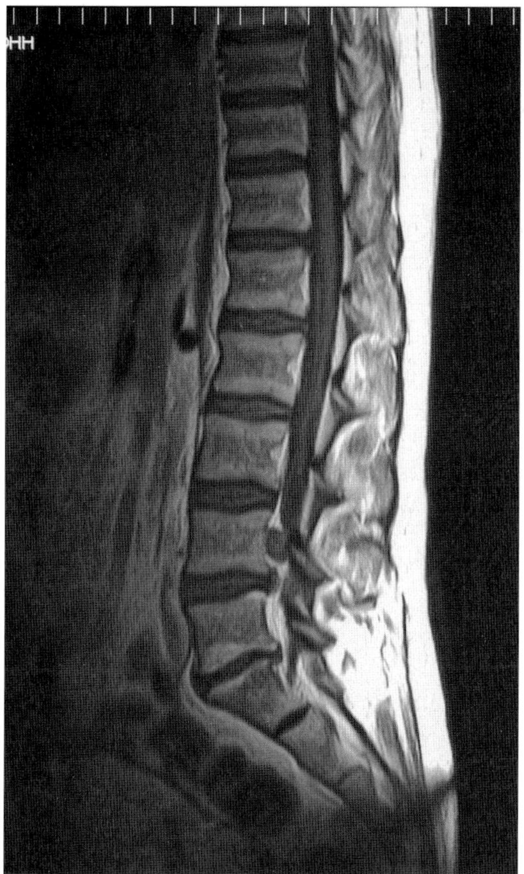

Fig. 4.64. Slightly parasagittal T1-weighted image showing a round mass with disc signal intensity posterior to the L4 vertebra. There is marked degeneration of the two lowest discs, L4-5 and L5-S1, with narrowing of the L5-S1 interspace. Chronic osteochondrosis (Modic type 2)

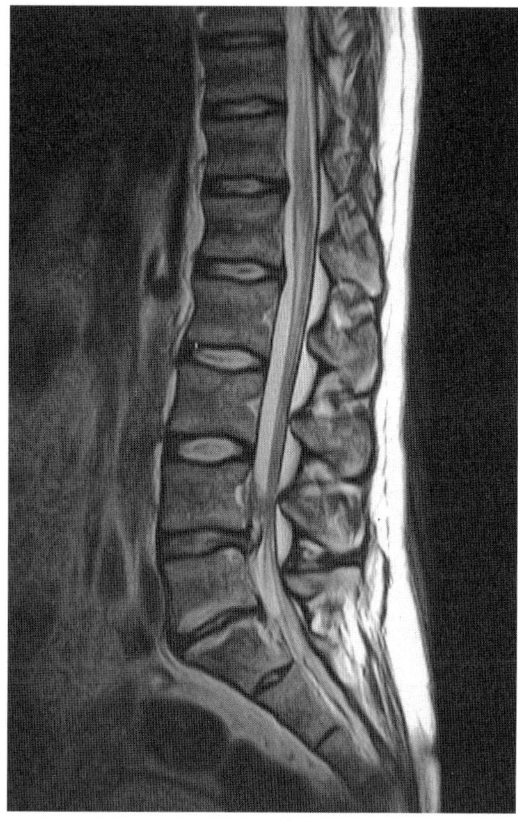

Fig. 4.65. Sagittal T2-weighted image showing a tongue-shaped mass extending superiorly from the L4-5 level. Signal alteration of the L4-5 and L5-S1 interspaces consistent with dehydration. Narrowing of L5-S1

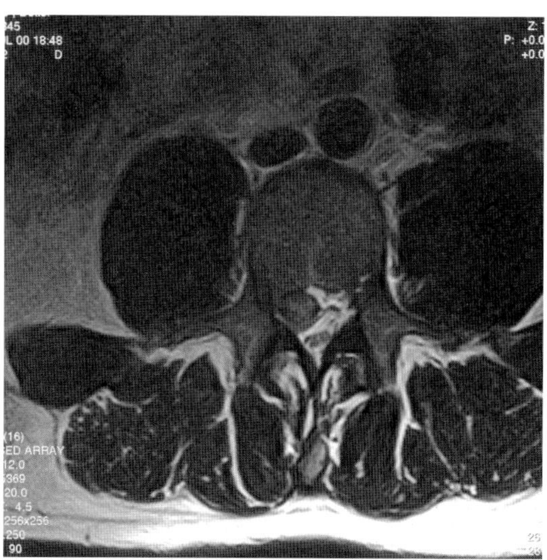

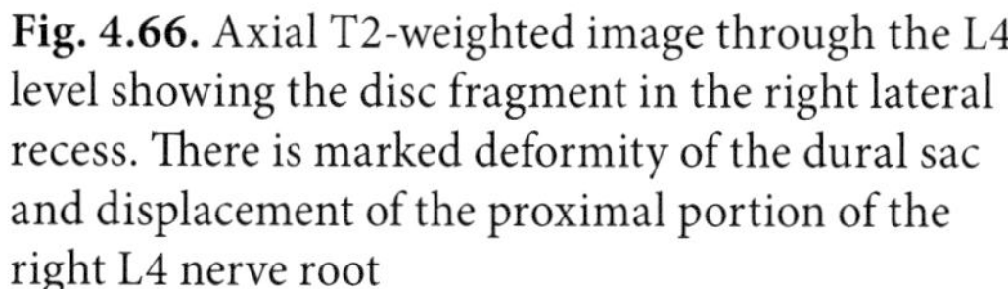

Fig. 4.66. Axial T2-weighted image through the L4 level showing the disc fragment in the right lateral recess. There is marked deformity of the dural sac and displacement of the proximal portion of the right L4 nerve root

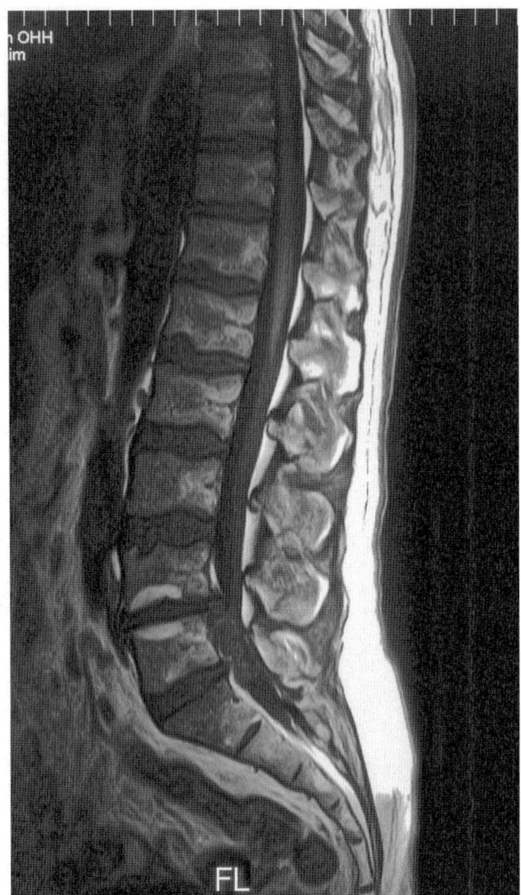

Fig. 4.67. 48-year-old patient with low back problems. Left paramedian T1-weighted image of the lumbar region and thoracolumbar junction. Note irregularities of the endplates of all vertebral bodies shown. This appearance is consistent with status post Scheuermann's disease. The signal alterations at the L4 inferior endplate and L5 superior endplate indicate Modic type 2 osteochondrosis. Focal mass posterior to the L4-5 interspace and possibly also posterior to L5, suggesting disc herniation

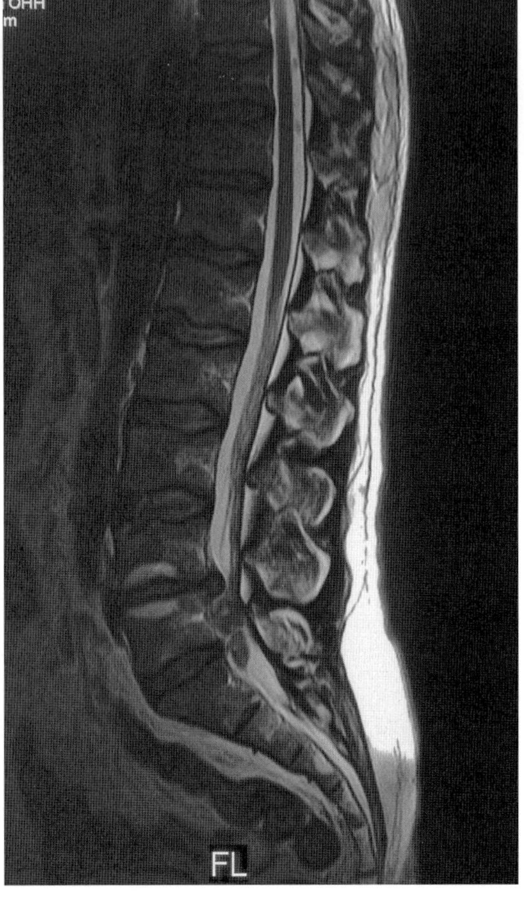

Fig. 4.68. Left paramedian T2-weighted image of the lumbar region showing disc herniation posterior to the L4-5 disc space with a slightly hyperintense structure relative to the disc located posterior to the L5 vertebral body, from where it extends down to the L5-S1 level. The appearance suggests a sequestered disc

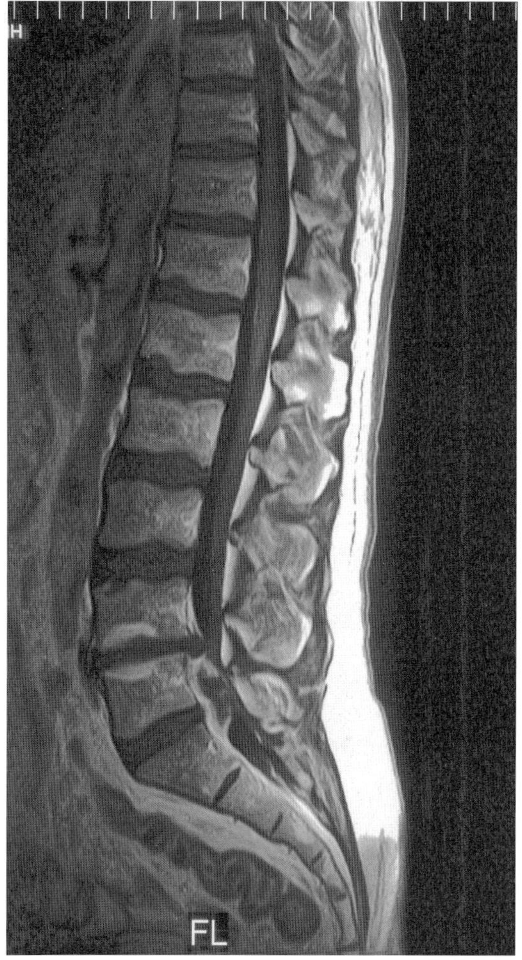

Fig. 4.69. Same patient. Sagittal T1-weighted image after contrast administration depicting the disc sequester posterior to the L5 vertebra and L5-S1 interspace. In addition, there is residual postero-medial herniation of the parent disc. A ring of enhancement is seen around the disc fragment while there is no enhancement of the fragment itself

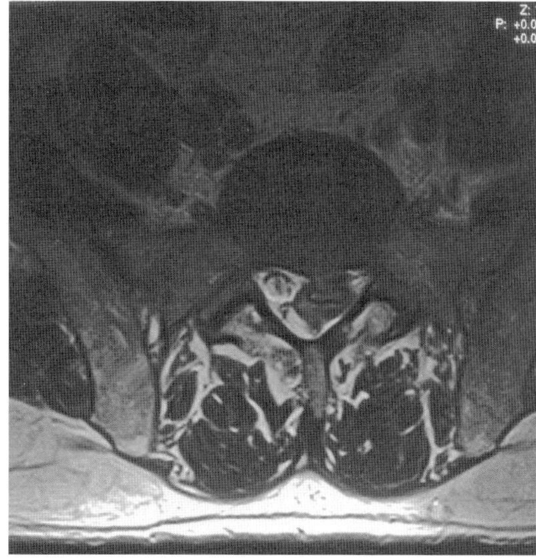

Fig. 4.70. Axial T2-weighted image through the L5-S1 level showing the disc fragment in the left lateral recess with marked deformity of the dural sac. Conjoined nerve roots on the right. The exit of the left root is difficult to identify and displaced by the disc fragment

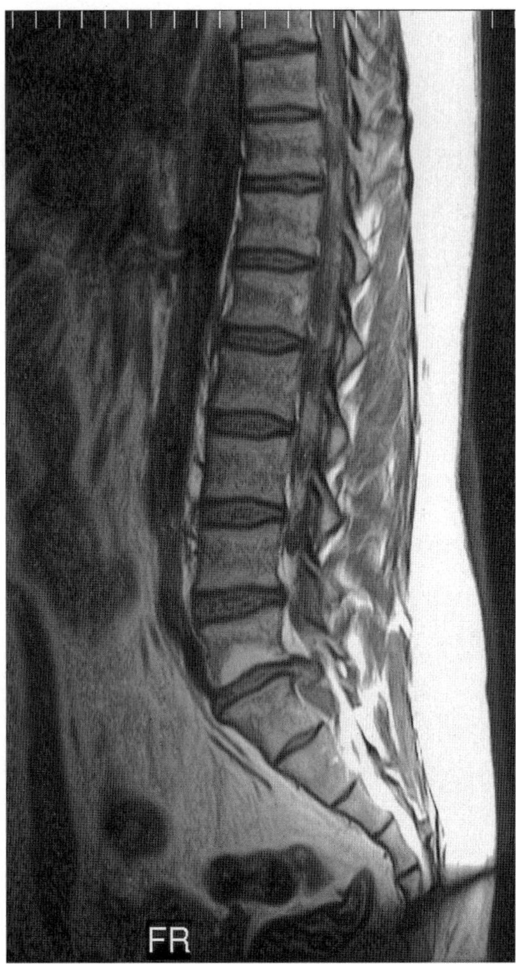

Fig. 4.71. 33-year-old patient with low back problems. Left paramedian T1-weighted image of the lumbar region. Tongue-shaped disc herniation at L5-S1 with a mass of soft-tissue-signal-intensity located epidurally below the herniation

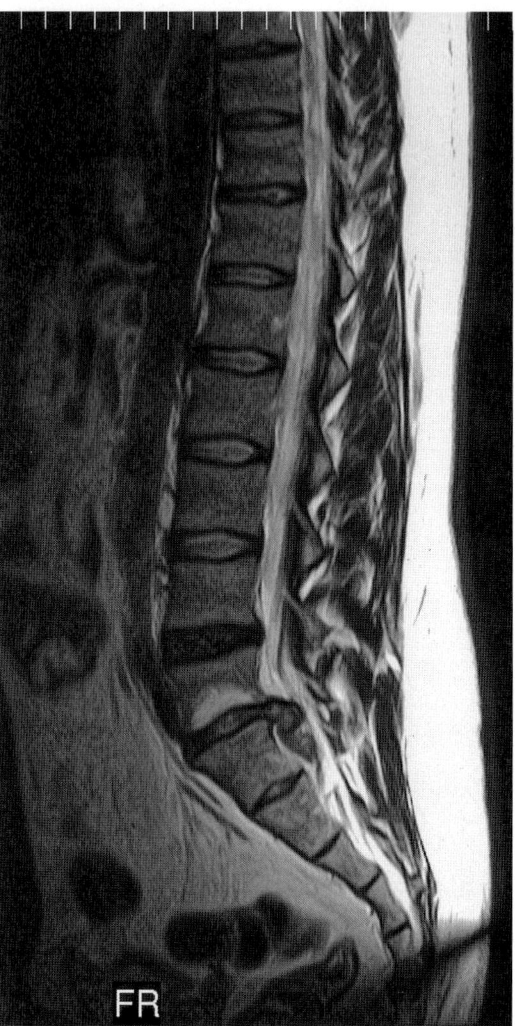

Fig. 4.72. Sagittal T2-weighted image of the lumbar region showing the large herniation and a sequester posterior to S1. Increased signal intensity of L5 at the inferior endplate, consistent with chronic osteochondrosis

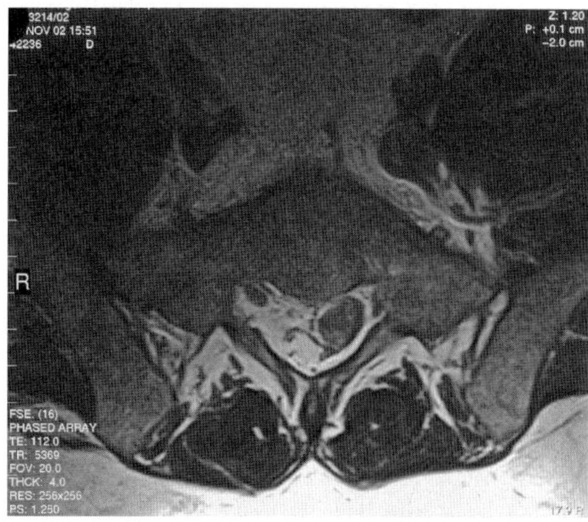

Fig. 4.73. Same patient. Axial T2-weighted image through the L5-S1 level showing the disc sequester in the left lateral recess with deformity of the dural sac. The two proximal S1 nerve roots are not contiguous with the herniated disc

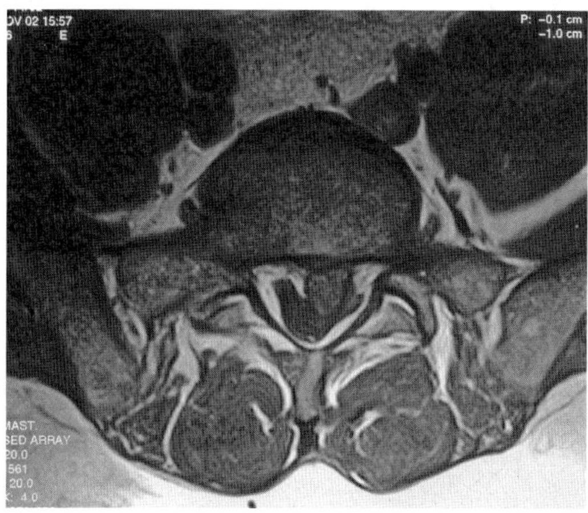

Fig. 4.74. Axial T1-weighted image after contrast administration showing only slight enhancement around the sequester in the left lateral recess without signs of perfusion of the herniation/fragment. Deformity of the dural sac

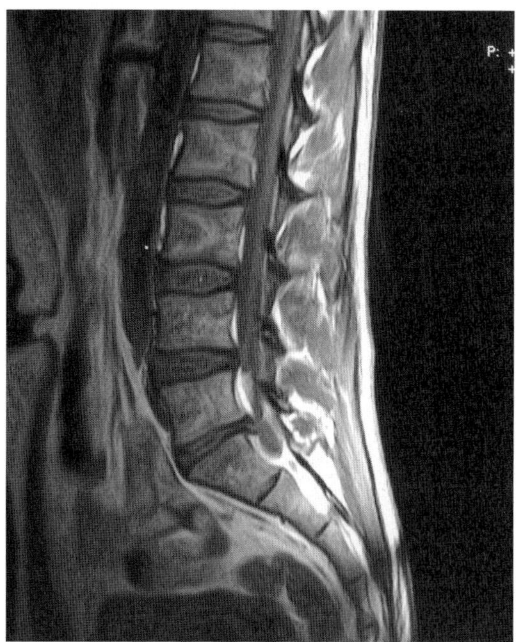

Fig. 4.75. 33-year-old patient with low back problems. Left paramedian T1-weighted image of the lumbar region showing a mass nearly isointense with muscle below the herniated L5-S1 disc

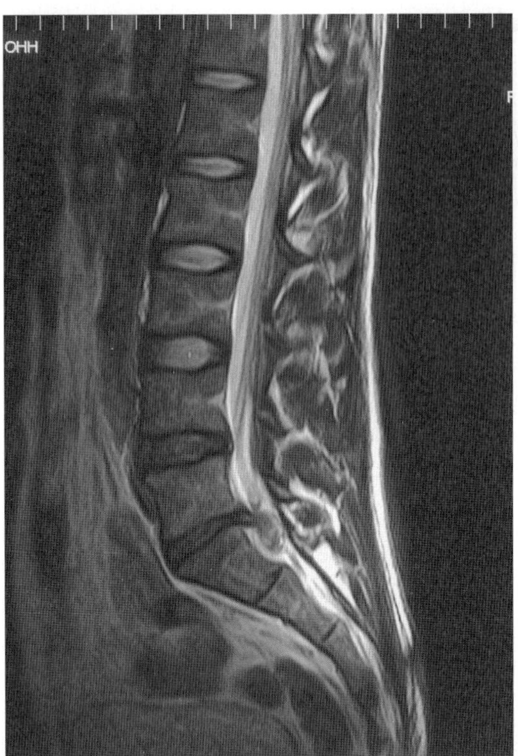

Fig. 4.76. Same patient. Sagittal T2-weighted image of the lumbar region showing marked signal changes of the L4-5 and L5-S1 discs consistent with dehydration. In addition, there is moderate narrowing of the L5-S1 disc space. A mass separated from the L5-S1 disc and nearly isointense with the disc is seen posterior to S1. The punctate hyperintensity in the L4-5 disc suggests a small tear of the annulus fibrosus

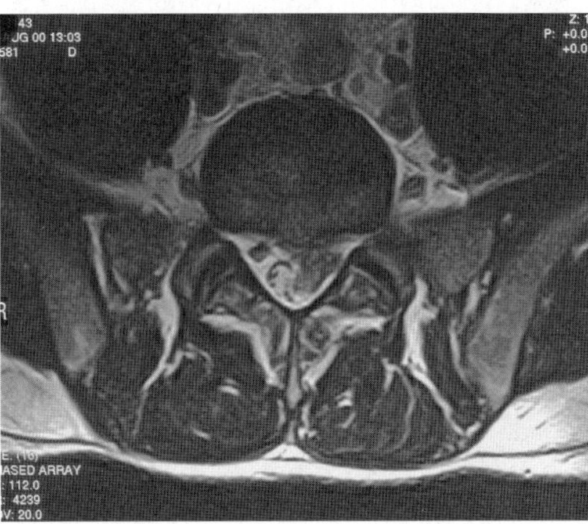

Fig. 4.77. Same patient. Axial T2-weighted image through the L5-S1 disc level depicting the disc fragment posteriorly on the left with deformity of the dural sac. The proximal portion of the left S1 nerve root is obscured by the disc fragment

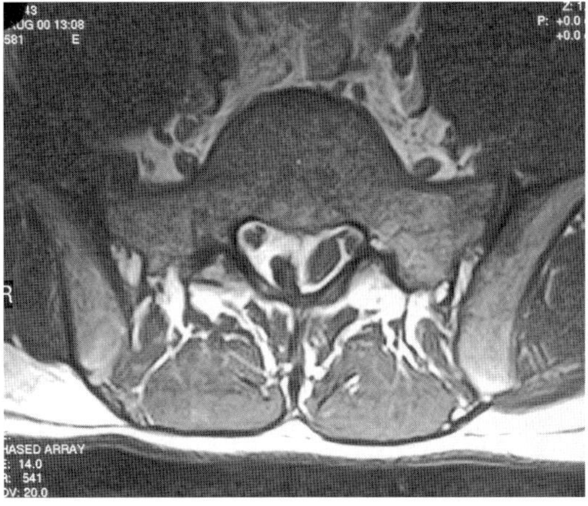

Fig. 4.78. Same patient. Axial T1-weighted image just below the L5-S1 level showing the disc fragment posterolaterally on the left between the proximal S2 root and the dural sac, which is slightly displaced posteriorly

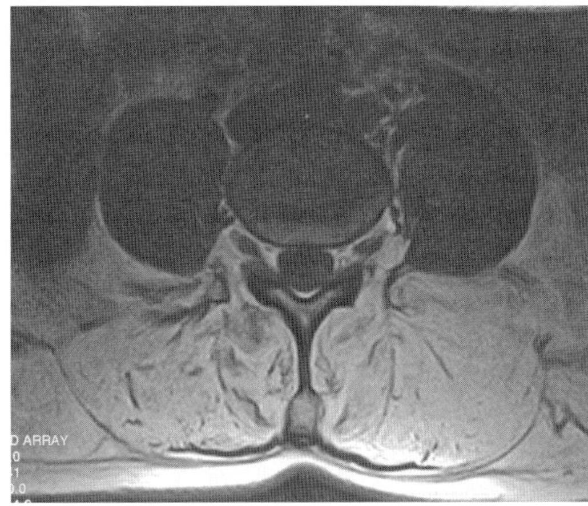

Fig. 4.79. 60-year-old patient with known muscular dystrophy. Axial T1-weighted image of the mid-lumbar spine through the L3 level. Note the conspicuous signal alteration of the extensor muscles suggesting complete fatty degeneration of the muscle. Normal signal of the paravertebral psoas muscles and unremarkable appearance of the vertebrae and spinal canal

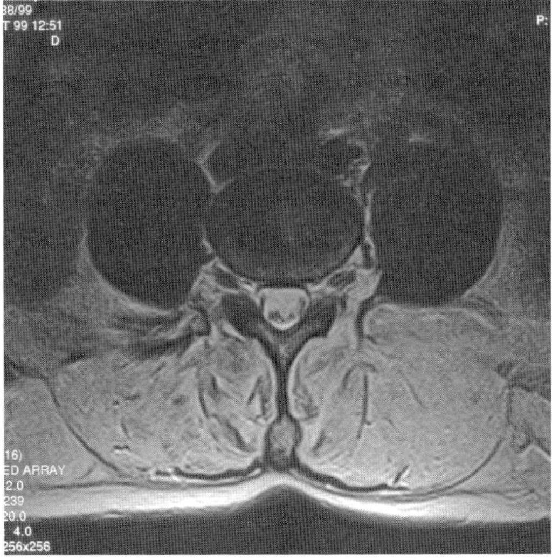

Fig. 4.80. Axial T2-weighted image through the L3 level. Fatty degeneration of the extensor muscles with unremarkable appearance and signal intensity of the paravertebral psoas muscles on both sides

5 Inflammatory Conditions

5.1 Spondylitis/Spondylodiscitis

Pathoanatomy

Spondylitis is used loosely to encompass all forms of inflammatory conditions affecting a spinal motion segment. Because of their rarity, all circumscribed inflammatory processes involving the vertebral processes (posterior spondylitis, almost exclusively in tuberculous spondylitis where its incidence is approximately 2‰) or the facet joints (nearly always iatrogenic or in conjunction with inflammatory systemic disorders such as chronic polyarthritis or ankylosing spondylitis) are also grouped together. Typical spondylitis/spondylodiscitis is an inflammatory condition of a spinal motion segment characterized by the destruction of two adjacent vertebral bodies and the interposed disc. Early subchondral defects are seen at the two adjacent endplates of the involved vertebral bodies. Prolonged inflammation is associated with irregular zones of bone densification at the margins of the inflammatory lesions.

Anterior spondylitis is considered a special subtype that predominantly occurs in the thoracic spine. It is characterized by anterior subligamentous spread of the inflammatory process and causes concave deformities of the anterior surfaces of one or more vertebral bodies.

Spondylitis is virtually always associated with concomitant inflammation of surrounding soft tissue structures, predominantly at the level of the affected disc space. Severity ranges from a diffuse inflammatory reaction to extensive abscess formation. The inflammation can spread in all directions: posteriorly (subligamentous/epidural), anteriorly (retropharyngeal abscess in the cervical region, anterior spondylitis in the thoracic region), and laterally or into adjacent structures (e.g. psoas abscess).

Pathogenesis

Most spinal infections are caused by bacteria while localized inflammation of nonbacterial origin is rare and is typically associated with inflammatory systemic diseases such as chronic polyarthritis or ankylosing spondylitis. A distinction is made between hematogenous spread and exogenous infection (e.g. after surgery). The most common pathogen causing spondylitis worldwide is M. tuberculosis, while nontuberculous types of spondylitis are more common in Europe with S. aureus accounting for most cases (about 50-70%). The ratio of nontuberculous to tuberculous spondylitis is about 20:1 in Europe. Fungi (e.g. Candida spondylitis) or parasites are occasionally found.

In the most common type, primary hematogenous bacterial spondylitis, the inflammatory process starts at the endplates, where the vascular network is densest. Primary spread to an intervertebral disc does not seem to be possible in adults (primary discitis) because the discs are not vascularized. Nevertheless, there is early involvement of the adjacent disc in the destructive inflammatory process of the endplate. Endplate defects allow disc material to enter the vertebral body and the resulting narrowing of the disc space is seen as an early (unspecific) radiologic sign of spondylitis, while vertebral defects become apparent on radiographs only with progressive bone destruction.

MR Technique

Evaluating patients with suspected spondylitis requires T1-weighted imaging in all three planes (sagittal, axial, and coronal) with and without fat saturation before and after contrast administration. Additional T2-weighted images should ideally be obtained with fat saturation.

Fat saturation and contrast administration improve the delineation of inflammatory lesions.

Intraspinal lesions displacing the CSF are often more conspicuous on T2-weighted images, which in most cases also allow better evaluation of the degree of liquefaction of focal inflammatory lesions.

MR Findings

Inflammatory tissue has relatively high signal intensity on T2-weighted images, although there is some variation depending on the amount of fluid present. T1-weighted images allow better evaluation because they depict an abscess/focal inflammatory lesion as a low-signal-intensity structure displacing and infiltrating surrounding fatty tissue structures. Most inflammatory lesions show contrast enhancement, which is typically more pronounced in the periphery. It is important to depict the entire inflammatory process including its borders to accurately evaluate its extent. The examiner should also consider a gravitation abscess which may extend down to the pelvic level or even into the legs.

In most cases, longitudinal images (coronal and sagittal, both T1 and T2) are somewhat more suitable for evaluating damage to the bony structures and intervertebral disc. Typical vertebral changes are destruction of the normal cortical bone and edematous signal alterations of the adjacent bone marrow space.

In evaluating an inflammatory process and/or abscess formation, it is important to carefully determine the extent of the changes in relation to adjacent organs and the great vessels. Detailed information on the topographic relationships is important when surgery or drainage is planned. Finally, the radiologist should also report vascular pathology (e.g. aneurysm) (Figs. 5.1–5.49).

MR Pitfalls

Old hematomas or seromas after surgery or trauma may resemble cystic lesions. An abscess will show more pronounced peripheral enhancement than these entities after contrast administration. Moreover, the examiner must take into account the patient's laboratory results.

The differential diagnosis of an inflammatory condition includes bone marrow edema (traumatic) and isolated tumor manifestations. Involvement of the disc space suggests an inflammatory process.

Clinical Significance

A microbiologic diagnosis should be obtained in all patients with isolated spondylodiscites without systemic inflammatory disease. All patients with spondylodiscitis require tailored therapy. The therapeutic approach in uncomplicated bacterial spondylitis combines operative and conservative measures including local excision of the inflammatory tissue and suitable antimicrobial chemotherapy. Additional operative measures vary with the severity and extent of local destruction (defect filling, correction of deformity, stabilization in patients with manifest or impending instability).

Inflammatory invasion of the spinal canal (subligamentous abscess, epidural abscess) is an indication for emergency surgery. Concomitant abscess – which may predominate both the clinical manifestation and the MR appearance – must be taken into account in planning the surgical procedure because its localization may be crucial for selecting the operative access (e.g. right versus left access in patients with paravertebral spinal abscess or psoas abscess).

5.2 Chronic Polyarthritis

Pathoanatomy and Pathomechanism

Destruction of the atlantoaxial, atlanto-occipital, and/or atlantodental joints usually occurs in patients with chronic polyarthritis and less commonly in individuals with a subtype of juvenile ankylosing spondylitis (so-called bipolar manifestation).

Destruction of the atlanto-occipital joint, and less commonly destruction of the atlantoaxial joint, will cause both horizontal and vertical instability, resulting in a high dens and progressive translocation into the foramen magnum, where it may encroach on the medulla oblongata.

Other vertebral structures may be involved as well (in particular the facet joints and rarely the intervertebral disc space) but this has no clinical implications in most cases.

MR Technique

T1- and T2-weighted images in all three planes with and without contrast administration; occasionally unenhanced and enhanced T1-weighted images with fat saturation may be helpful.

MR Findings

Chronic polyarthritis/rheumatoid arthritis is a systemic connective tissue disease characterized histologically by an excessive growth of synovial cells and degradation of cartilage, predominantly in the vicinity of the inflammatory synovial membrane or pannus. Correspondingly, the only MR change seen in early disease is mild contrast enhancement of the synovial membrane. The presence of pannus is depicted as thickening of the synovial structures, which will also show marked contrast enhancement.

Rheumatoid arthritis of the spine most commonly affects the cervical region and the craniocervical junction while thoracic and lumbar manifestations are fairly uncommon. Inflammatory processes involving the craniocervical junction typically cause erosion of the dens axis, which is seen on coronal and sagittal images as irregularities and signal alterations of the cortical layer. Synovial proliferation is often present in the direct vicinity of these changes, which can be best appreciated on T1-weighted images before and after contrast administration.

Destruction of the transverse ligament by inflammation can be identified on axial images. There may be malalignment with narrowing of the intervertebral disc spaces in the middle and lower cervical region. If no osteophytes are present, subchondral irregularities as well as sclerosis and erosion will be seen.

Spinal narrowing resulting from instabilities or mass effects of inflammatory lesions can be demonstrated by MRI on sagittal and axial images. Compression of the spinal cord with reactive changes (myelomalacia) is best appreciated on T2-weighted images (Figs. 5.50–5.78).

MR Pitfalls

Chronic polyarthritis must be differentiated from unspecific inflammatory conditions (inflammatory solid pannus without abscess formation, spondyloarthropathy).

Clinical Significance

In patients with inflammatory rheumatoid disease involving the upper cervical spine, MR imaging can provide important supplementary information, while dislocation or instability can also be demonstrated with other imaging modalities including flexion-extension radiographs. Based on current standards, surgery is indicated when the anterior atlantodental distance is 6 mm or more. MRI is the only diagnostic modality that enables direct evaluation of the reserve space between the upper cervical cord and adjacent bony structures (posterior surface of dens, posterior arch of atlas, and posterior bony margin of foramen magnum) or between the cord and abnormal soft tissue such as retrodental pannus. MR findings are not only crucial for establishing the indication for surgery but also for planning details of the surgical procedure, e.g. posterior stabilization alone or with posterior decompression, resection of the posterior arch of atlas, widening of the foramen magnum, and additional anterior (transoral) decompression with resection of the dens.

5.3 Ankylosing Spondylitis (Bechterew's Disease)

Anatomy and Pathoanatomy

Ankylosing spondylitis causes progressive stiffening of the axial skeleton and patients are likely to develop kyphosis of all spinal segments. Bridging syndesmophytes across all disc spaces connect the cortical bone of adjacent vertebrae, resulting in the classic bamboo spine. Syndesmophytes predominantly arise from the margins of the endplates and less commonly from the prediscal loose connective tissue, thus differing from spondylophytes, which are ossifications of the anterior longitudinal ligament. Except for regressive changes, the discs remain largely intact but ossifications in the area of the annulus fibrosus may occasionally be seen in patients with end-stage disease. The facet joints are generally involved and may eventually become ankylosed.

The discovertebral junction sometimes exhibits destructive foci that resemble the inflammatory lesions in abacterial spondylodiscitis (so-called Andersson 1 lesions).

Vertebral fractures in ankylosing spondylitis have characteristic pathomorphologic and clinical features. Fractures are most commonly caused by hyperextension and run through the ankylosed disc space. They typically occur in the cervical region but can also involve the thoracolumbar spine.

Pathogenesis

Based on current knowledge, ankylosing spondylitis is an inflammatory enthesopathy with a genetic predisposition. There is a strong 95% association with HLA-B27. The initial inflammatory reaction induces chondroid metaplasia of connective tissue cells, which will eventually lead to endochondral ossification. Andersson 1 lesions (destructive foci of the discovertebral junction) are considered by some to represent discospondylitis caused by the spread of the primary inflammatory process to the disc spaces and vertebral endplates. Others attribute the lesions to pseudarthrosis secondary to a transdiscal fatigue fracture, resulting in a mobile segment that is exposed to mechanical overload due to the rigidity of the adjacent segments.

MR Technique

The standard MR protocol in patients with ankylosing spondylitis comprises sagittal and axial T1- and T2-weighted sequences, which may be supplemented by images in coronal orientation or a fat-saturated sequence (STIR technique).

MR Findings

Spinal fractures complicating ankylosing spondylitis are typically identified by a horizontal line of altered signal running through the disc space. In addition, MRI will show the characteristic changes of adjacent spinal motion segments associated with the underlying disease. Spinal fractures in an ankylosed spine tend to heal poorly due to excessive motion of the fractured segment in an otherwise rigid spine. Other changes such as edema at the endplates of adjacent vertebral bodies, irritation of surrounding soft tissue structures, and hemorrhage are the same as in traumatic spinal fractures and vary with the time since fracture. (Figs. 5.79–5.88).

Clinical Significance

Early disease in the majority of patients with ankylosing spondylitis (early adulthood) is associated with sciatic/pseudosciatic symptoms that are usually worse in the morning. The complaints are not disc-related but may be mistaken for disc herniation. These patients then fail to respond to initial therapy and may be submitted to unnecessary surgery.

Andersson 1 lesions in early ankylosing spondylitis may escape detection on conventional radiography while they will show the characteristic signs of spondylodiscitis on MR images. The lesions typically cause severe local pain, do not tend to heal spontaneously, and usually fail to respond to conservative measures.

As with Andersson 2 lesions, early surgical management is desirable. In most cases, internal fixation by posterior osteosynthesis is sufficient and induces rapid bony union.

The rate of spinal fractures that are initially overlooked in patients with ankylosing spondylitis is high for several reasons: minor trauma may be sufficient to cause fracture due to unfavorable biomechanical properties of the ankylosed spine and osteopenia; radiologic fracture signs are inconspicuous when the fracture line runs through the disc space and there is no dislocation; in addition, spinal fractures in the lower cervical region are difficult to evaluate radiographically due to immobility of the shoulder girdle and preexisting flexion deformity. The fact that fractures in a rigid spine may run through all stabilizing structures (including the ossified ligaments) makes them highly unstable, especially in the cervical region but also in the thoracolumbar spine. Spontaneous healing tends to be poor in patients treated conservatively.

In conclusion, patients developing spinal symptoms after minor trauma or casual injuries should undergo MRI if conventional radiologic methods fail to demonstrate a spinal fracture. When there is involvement of the cervical region, even emergency MRI is indicated and should be repeated within 24 to 48 hours if necessary.

5.4 Myelitis

Pathoanatomy and Pathophysiology

Transverse myelitis is an acute inflammatory demyelinating disorder of the spinal cord that is histomorphologically distinct from multiple sclerosis.

The etiology of myelitis is highly variable and comprises bacterial and viral infections, AIDS, paraneoplastic syndromes, vaccination, tuberculosis, toxoplasmosis, and systemic diseases such as lupus erythematosus (where there may be an association with the antiphospholipid antibody syndrome). Myelitis typically affects the thoracocervical region. In many cases, the underlying cause cannot be elucidated.

When there is involvement of the optic nerve, the condition is referred to as neuromyelitis optica or Devic's syndrome. This subtype mainly occurs in patients with multiple sclerosis but may also be observed in association with other systemic viral diseases.

MR Technique

T2-weighted imaging in sagittal and transverse planes and sagittal T1-weighted images, which may be supplemented by T1-weighted images in sagittal (and transverse) orientation after contrast administration.

MR Findings

Patchy appearance of the spinal cord with decreased signal intensity on T1-weighted images and increased intensity on T2. The diameter of the spinal cord is normal or slightly increased. Signs of diffuse edema may be seen and there is variable uptake of gadolinium-DTPA (Figs. 5.89–5.91).

MR Pitfalls

Myelitis may be difficult to differentiate from ischemic lesions, infarction, and venous congestion secondary to arteriovenous fistula.

Clinical Significance

The diagnosis can only be established in conjunction with the patient's clinical symptoms and the results of complementary diagnostic tests.

Spinal MRI reliably demonstrates extramedullary compression of the spinal cord, which may present with similar symptoms as myelitis.

5.5 Multiple Sclerosis

Pathoanatomy and Pathophysiology

Multiple sclerosis is an inflammatory condition characterized by multifocal destruction of myelin in the brain and spinal cord. The destroyed myelin sheaths are replaced with scar tissue consisting of astrocytes. Progression of the disease will eventually lead to partial destruction of the demyelinated axons. While genetic factors play an important role in the pathogenesis of multiple sclerosis, it is assumed that the individual autoimmune response is modulated by environmental factors. The inflammatory reaction in active foci of demyelination involves complex cytotoxic processes.

Because of the heterogeneity of immunopathogenetic factors involved, various subtypes of multiple sclerosis have been distinguished on the basis of clinical, neuroimmunologic, genetic, pathologic, and neuroradiologic features.

MR Technique

The conventional MR imaging techniques (T1 before and after contrast administration, fast STIR, T2, proton density imaging) are increasingly being supplemented by specialized techniques such as MR spectroscopy, magnetization transfer imaging, and diffusion-weighted imaging for more detailed analysis of MS lesions.

MR Findings

According to the Barkhof criteria, the MRI diagnosis of multiple sclerosis requires proof of dissemination in space (DIS) and dissemination in time (DIT).

Active MS lesions will show enhancement after contrast administration (Figs. 5.92–5.100).

MR Pitfalls

MS plaques must be differentiated from other myelitic lesions and also from tumors. Disseminated encephalomyelitis is suggested by multisegmental manifestation and eccentric localization of the lesions. Moreover, inflammatory swelling of the spinal cord is often absent in encephalomyelitis.

Clinical Significance

Spinal MRI should be performed routinely in all patients with suspected multiple sclerosis. Spinal MRI will help corroborate the diagnosis in cases where the cerebral MR findings are inconclusive or difficult to interpret. Spinal MS lesions have been reported to be present in 87% of patients with multiple sclerosis.

A series of criteria have been established for diagnosing multiple sclerosis by MRI.

The spatial distribution of MS lesions demonstrated by MRI does not correlate with the clinical symptoms.

Fig. 5.1. Sagittal T2-weighted image of the cervical region. Partial destruction and blurred appearance of the dens axis. High-signal-intensity mass predominantly located anterior to the spine where it extends from the clivus down to the C4-5 level. Slightly increased amount of soft tissue posterior to the dens with mass effect causing mild narrowing of the subarachnoid space anterior to the medulla oblongata. No signal changes of neural structures

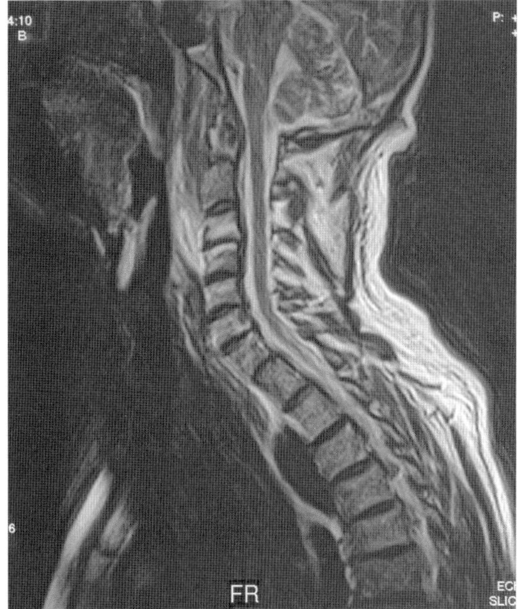

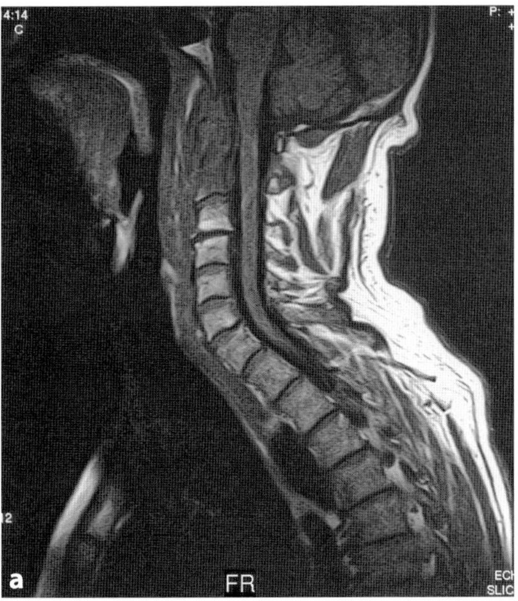

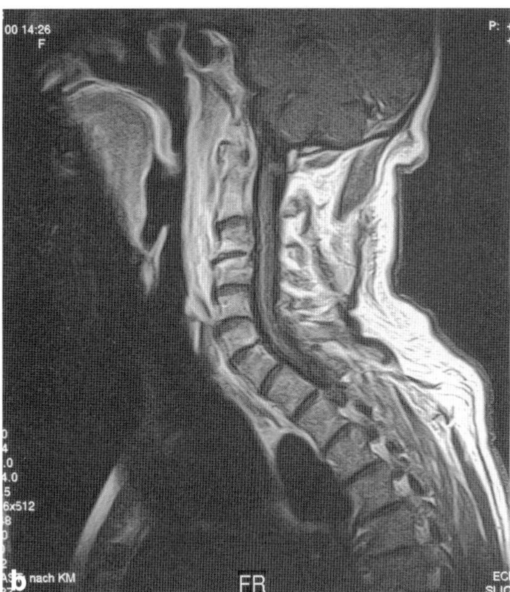

Fig. 5.2a, b. Sagittal T1-weighted images before and after contrast administration. The prespinal mass is nearly isointense to muscle, suggesting a high fluid content. Erosion of the dens is seen as blurring and cortical disruption anteriorly and at the tip. Following contrast administration, there is clear enhancement of the prespinal area from C5 to the clivus and less conspicuous enhancement posterior to the dens axis. The appearance is consistent with an extensive inflammatory process at the C1-2 level with paravertebral abscess formation predominantly anterior to the spine. Slight narrowing of the anterior subarachnoid space

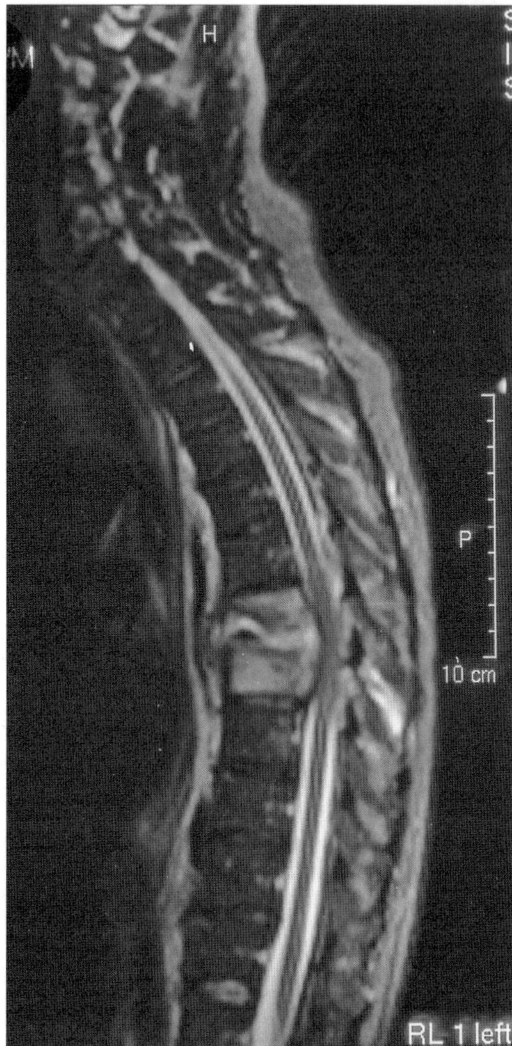

Fig. 5.3. Spondylodiscitis at T6-7. Sagittal T2-weighted image showing increased signal intensity of the T6-7 vertebral bodies and highly inhomogeneous appearance of the T6-7 interspace with higher signal intensity of its posterior portion. Posterior displacement and deformity of the spinal canal with obstruction of the anterior subarachnoid space. Prespinal area of increased signal intensity extending from T3 through T9. Slightly tilted appearance of the T6 vertebral body due to loss of height with partial destruction of inferior and anterior edges

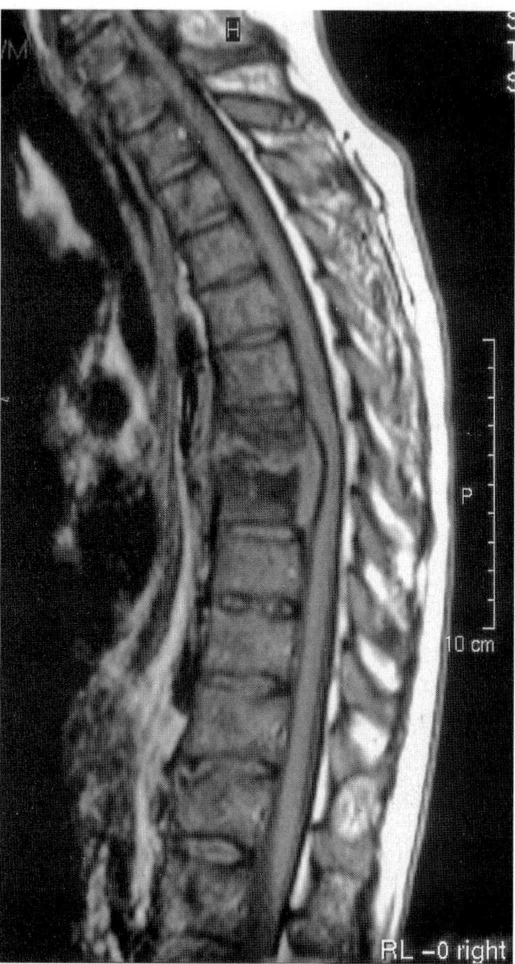

Fig. 5.4. Sagittal T1-weighted image showing reduced signal intensity of the T6-7 vertebral bodies and posterior epidural mass, consistent with spondylodiscitis at T6-7

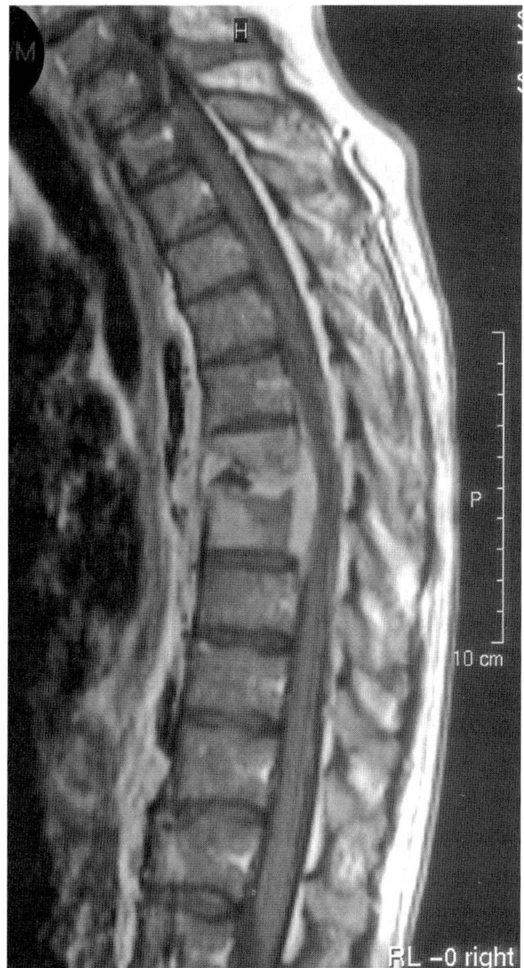

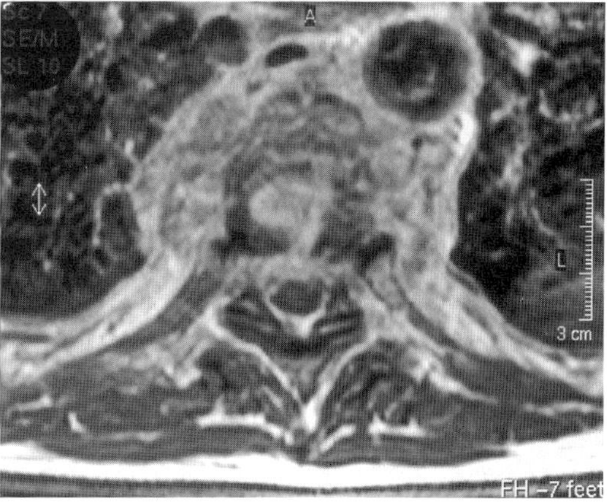

Fig. 5.6. Contrast-enhanced axial T1-weighted image through the T6-7 level showing destruction of the inferior T6 endplate and a nearly circular abscess with anterolateral extension to the aorta on the left and intraspinal extension with dural sac displacement. Marked narrowing of both T6 neural foramina

Fig. 5.5. Same patient as in Figs. 5.3 and 5.4. Sagittal T1-weighted image after contrast administration showing clear enhancement of the epidural abscess at the T6-7 level with additional enhancement anterior to the T3 through T9 vertebrae. Narrowing of the spinal canal without increased signal intensity of the spinal cord

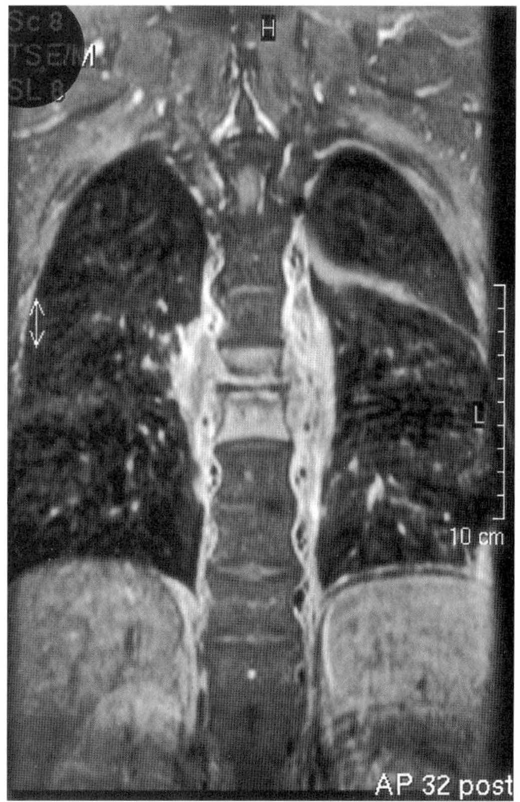

Fig. 5.7. Coronal T1-weighted fat-saturated image after contrast administration showing the large paravertebral abscess formations in T6-7 spondylodiscitis as masses with slightly inhomogeneous contrast enhancement. Larger abscess on the left than on the right

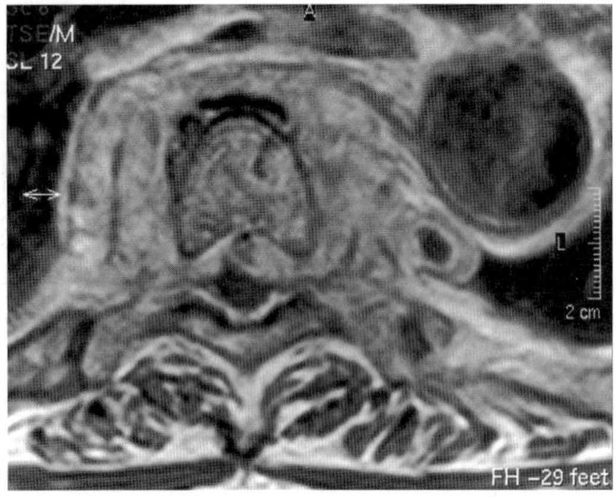

Fig. 5.8. Same patient as in preceding figures. Axial T1-weighted image through the T5-6 level with large paravertebral abscess and depiction of areas of liquefaction posteriorly and to the right of the aorta. There is invasion of the abscess into the spinal canal with narrowing, which is more pronounced on the left than on the right

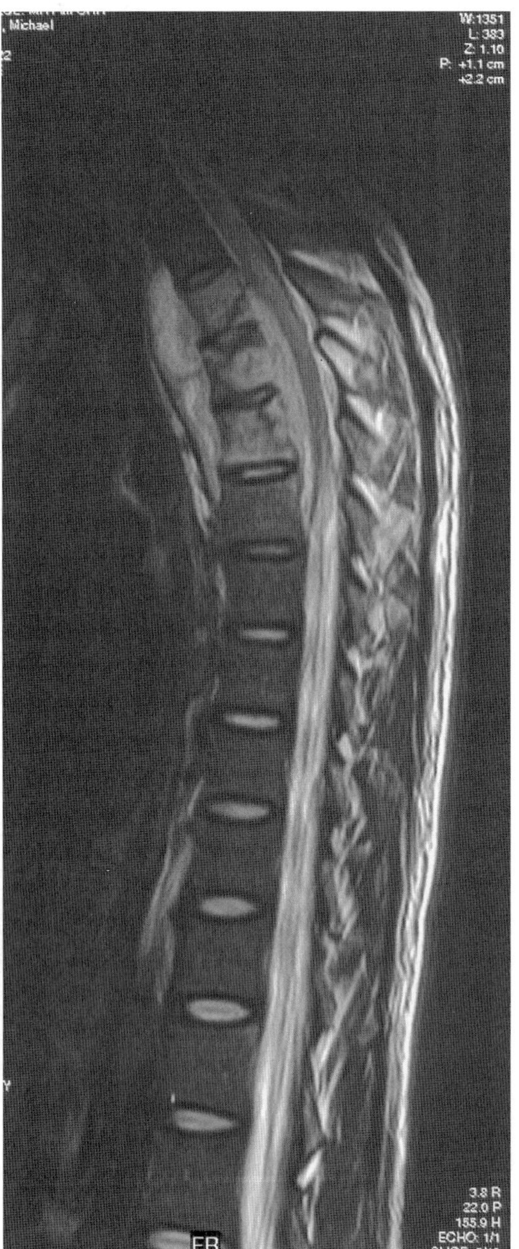

Fig. 5.9. Sagittal T2-weighted image of the thoracic region showing increased signal intensity of the T3 to T5 vertebral bodies and high-signal-intensity masses anteriorly and posteriorly. No definitive evidence of bony destructive changes in the vertebrae. Narrowing of the spinal canal

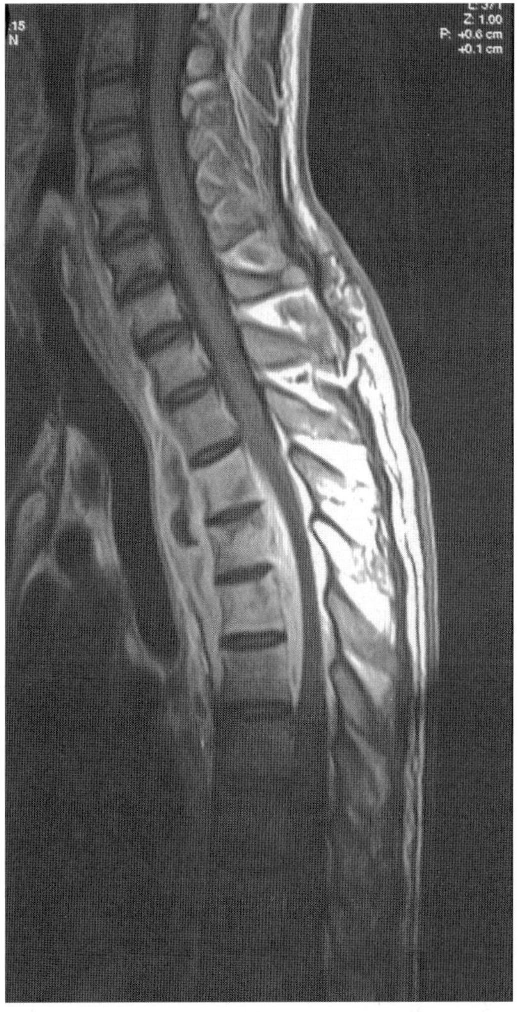

Fig. 5.10. Same patient as Fig. 5.9. Contrast-enhanced sagittal T1-weighted image of the cervical and upper thoracic spine showing the abscess extending from T2 through T5 anteriorly and from T3 through T5 posteriorly. A small area of liquefaction is depicted anterior to T3. Narrowing of the spinal canal

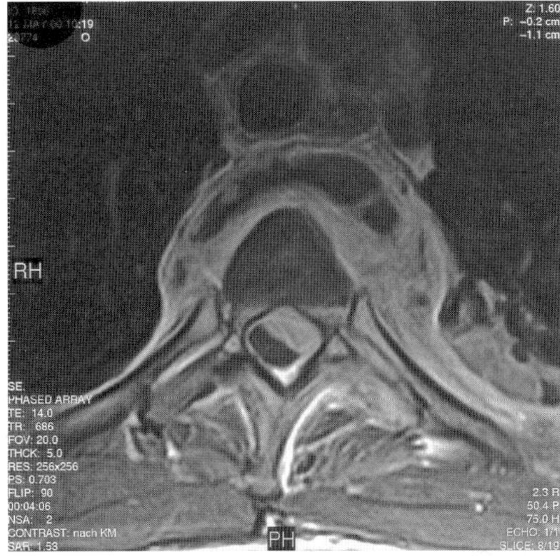

Fig. 5.11. Axial T1-weighted image after contrast administration showing the large prevertebral abscess extending to the aorta and inflammation in the left anterior aspect of the spinal canal. The spinal cord is markedly displaced but has normal signal intensity. Focal areas of liquefaction within the prevertebral abscess. The appearance is consistent with tuberculous spondylitis

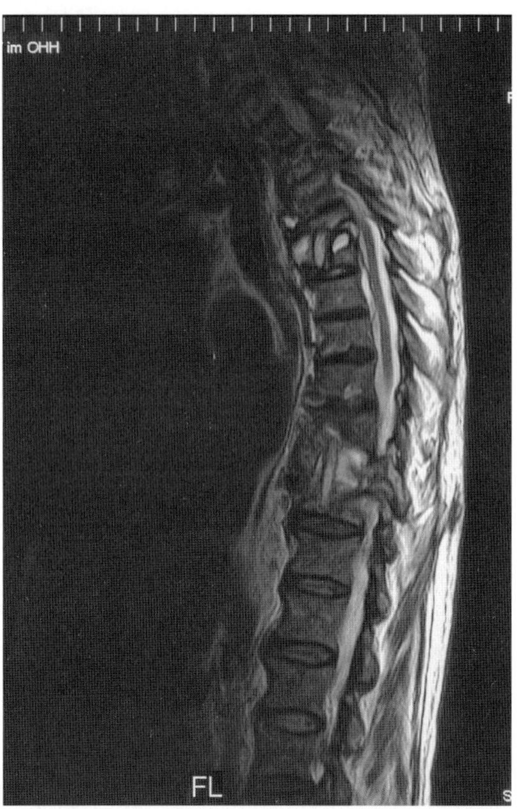

Fig. 5.12. 80-year-old patient after spondylodesis from T9 through T11 and at T5. Sagittal T2-weighted image of the thoracic region and thoracolumbar junction depicting the interposed bone chip extending from T9 to T11 with signal enhancement in the area of the former T10 vertebral body. The vertebral body itself is no longer discernible. Destruction of the inferior endplate of T9 and superior endplate of T11. High-signal-intensity epidural mass at the T6 level, consistent with hemorrhage

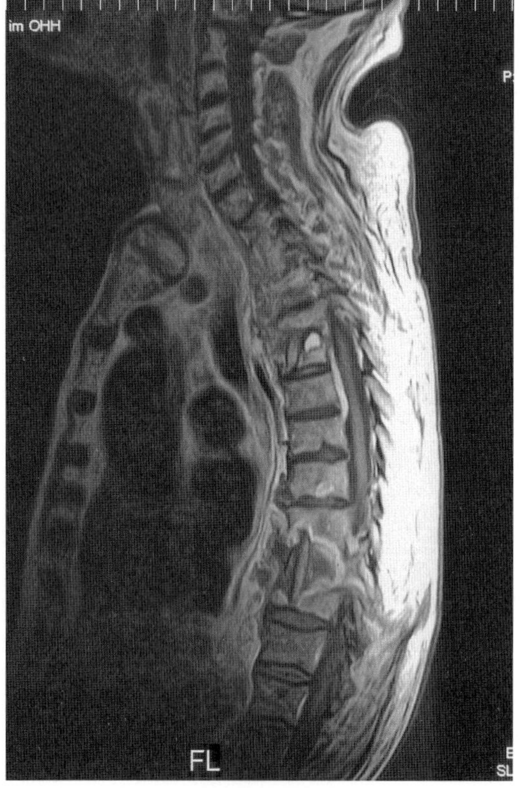

Fig. 5.13. Sagittal T1-weighted image after contrast administration showing peripheral enhancement in the area of the former T9 vertebra, at the tip of the interposed bone, and less conspicuous enhancement anterior to the former T10 vertebra. The appearance suggests large abscess formation with destruction of the T10 vertebral body, T9 inferior endplate, and T11 superior endplate

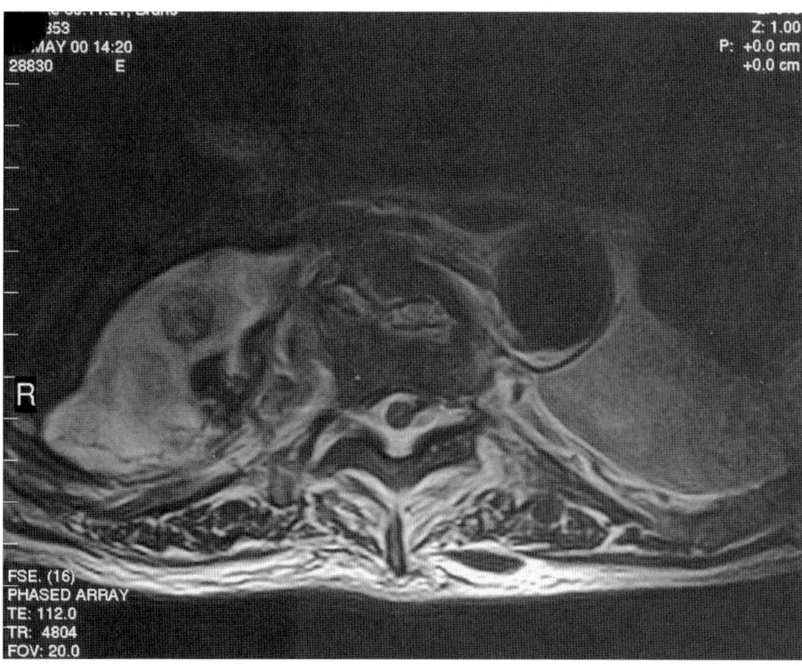

Fig. 5.14. Same patient. Axial T2-weighted image through the T9-10 level. Large inhomogeneous mass, mostly of high signal intensity, to the left and right of the vertebral body and surrounding the thoracic aorta, consistent with a large abscess with intraspinal extension. There is only partial vertebral destruction at this level. The dense oval structure seen within the vertebral body is the bone chip

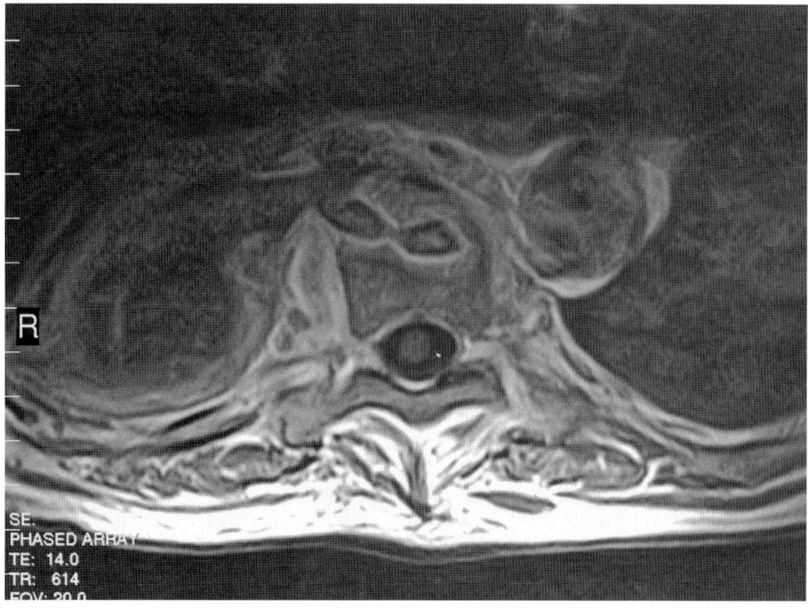

Fig. 5.15. Axial T1-weighted image through the T9-10 level after contrast administration with depiction of the bone chip. Extensive abnormal contrast enhancement in the immediate vicinity of the vertebra and peripheral enhancement of the large paravertebral abscess. The bulk of the paravertebral abscess is located on the right and extends epidurally

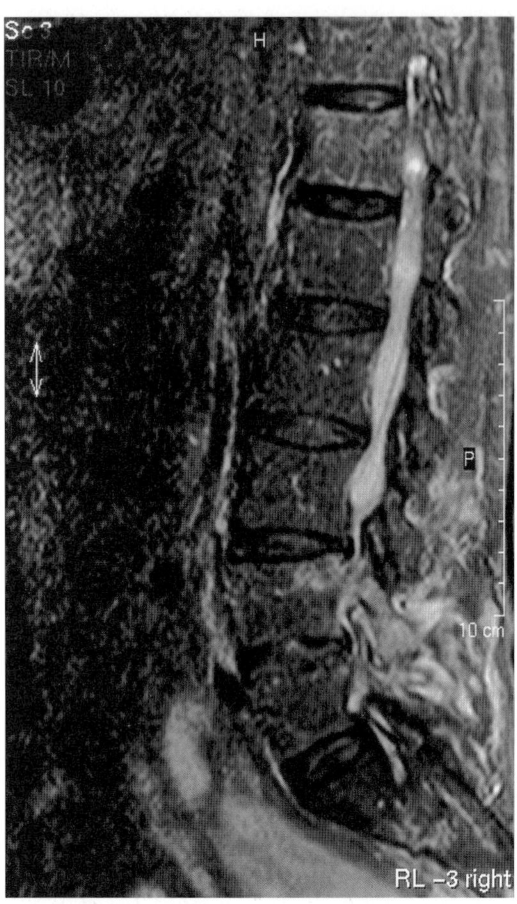

Fig. 5.16. Sagittal T2-weighted image with fat saturation of the lower lumbar region in a patient with spondylitis of L4-5 on the right. High-signal-intensity of the soft tissue structures posterior and to the right of L4-5 including the area of the transverse and spinous processes as well as posterior portions of L4 and L5

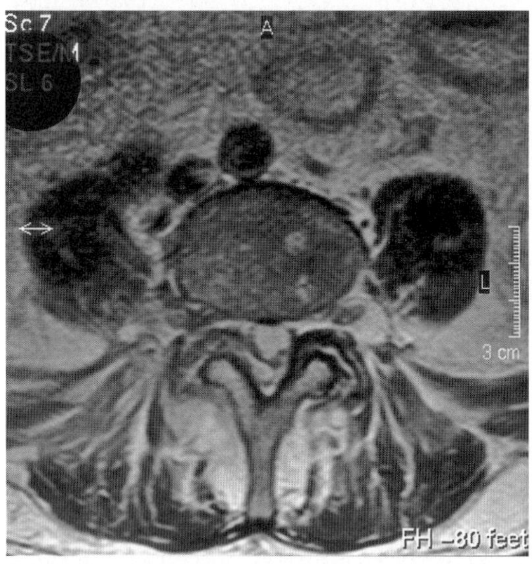

Fig. 5.17. Axial T2-weighted image through the L4-5 level with expansion and partial destruction of the right facet joint. Increased fluid with blurring of surrounding soft tissue structures and of the ligamentum flavum. Appearance consistent with spondylitis on the right

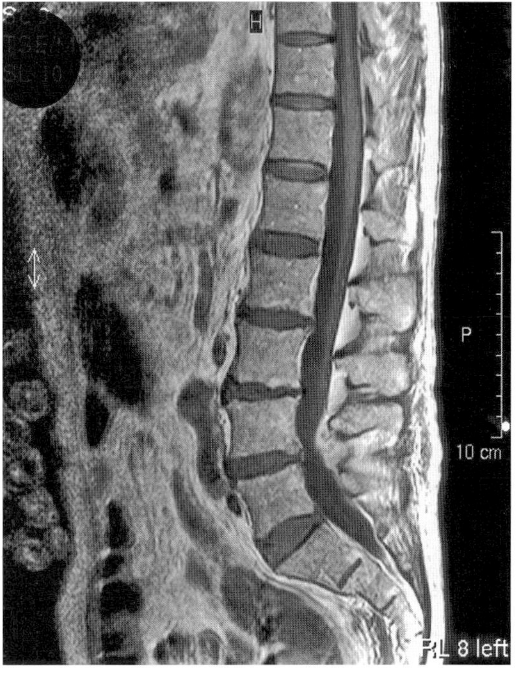

Fig. 5.18. Same patient. Sagittal T1-weighted image of the lumbar region showing abnormal contrast enhancement of the posterior portions at the L4-5 level. Spondylitis with slight posterior narrowing of the spinal canal

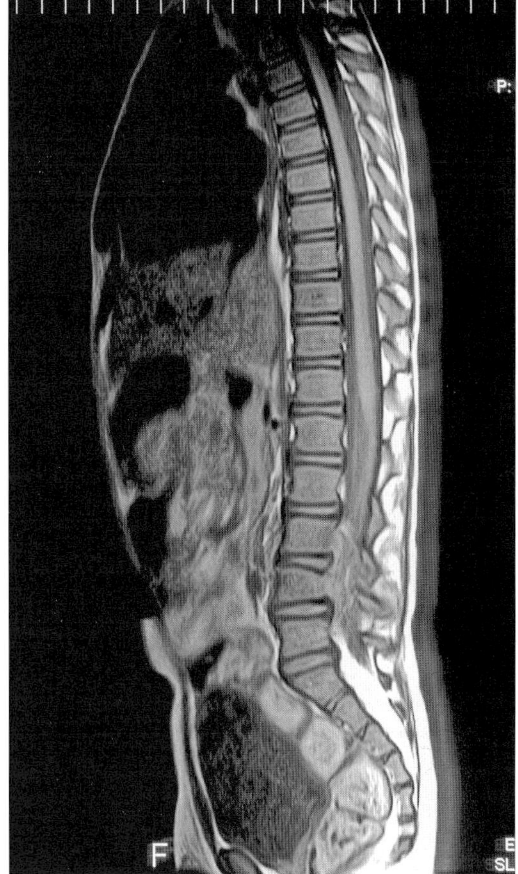

Fig. 5.19. Sagittal T1-weighted image of the thoracic and lumbar regions depicting the soft-tissue-signal mass posterior to the L3 and L4 vertebral bodies with extension to the L4/5 disc space

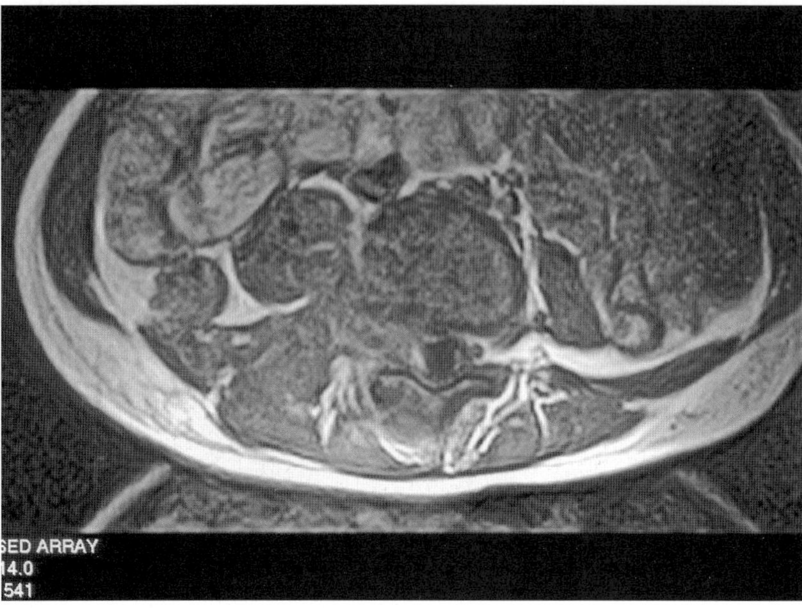

Fig. 5.20. Same patient as in preceding figures. Axial T1-weighted image through the L3-4 level depicting a large soft tissue-signal mass posterior and to the right of the vertebra, which is blurred. The appearance is consistent with tuberculous spondylitis with partial vertebral destruction

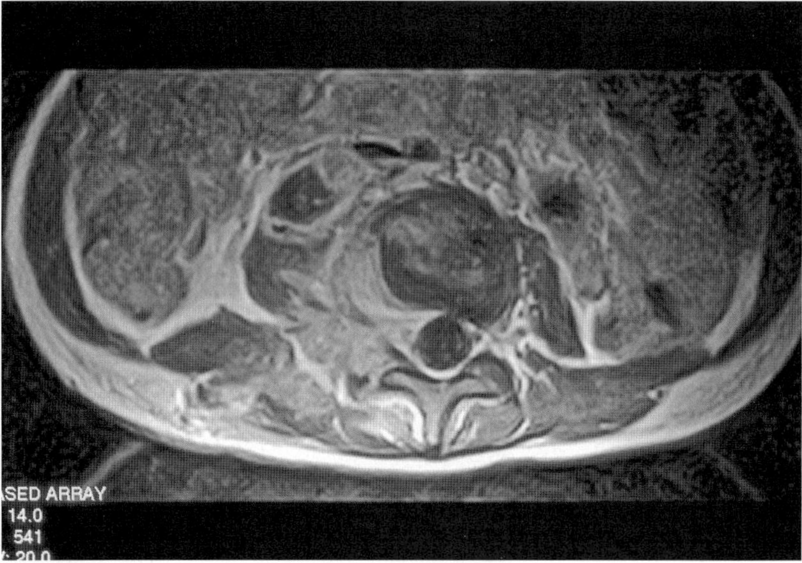

Fig. 5.21. Contrast-enhanced axial T1-weighted image through the L3-4 level showing marked abnormal enhancement of the extensive soft-tissue-signal-intensity structures to the right and posterior to L3-4 with extension into the spinal canal. Appearance consistent with tuberculous spondylitis

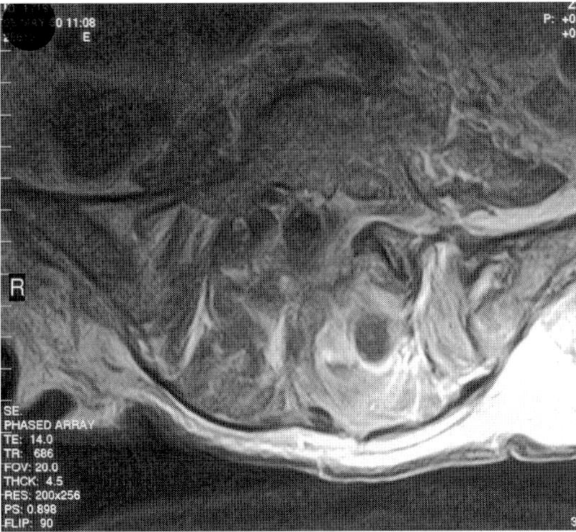

Fig. 5.22. Same patient. Contrast-enhanced axial T1-weighted image through the L4-5 level. The large paravertebral inflammatory process/abscess extends into the spinal canal. In addition, a small area of liquefaction is depicted in the posterior soft tissue

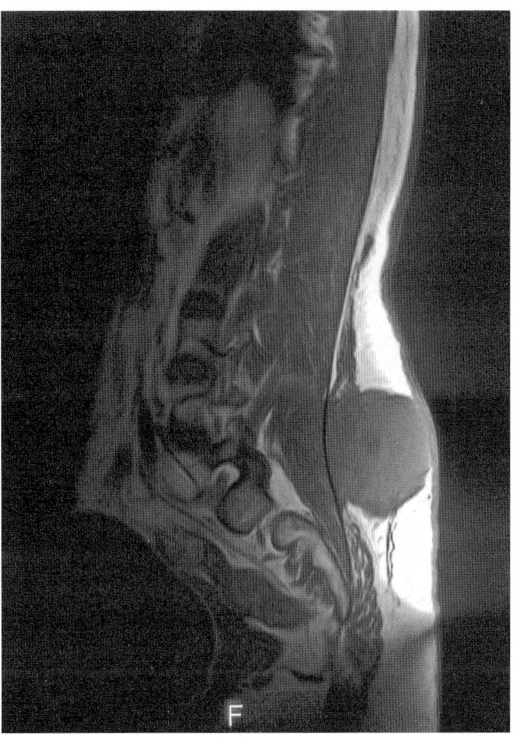

Fig. 5.23. Sagittal T1-weighted image of the lumbar region. Round mass of low signal intensity in the epifascial subcutaneous soft tissue structures at the levels of L4 and L5 with an epifascial extension up to the L2 level

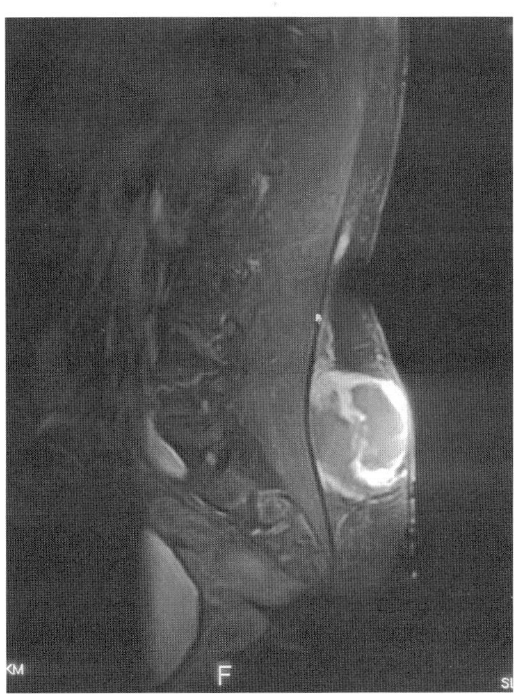

Fig. 5.24. Sagittal T1-weighted image with fat saturation after contrast administration. Wide margin of enhancement around the large subcutaneous abscess at the L4-5 level with a tongue-shaped extension up to L2

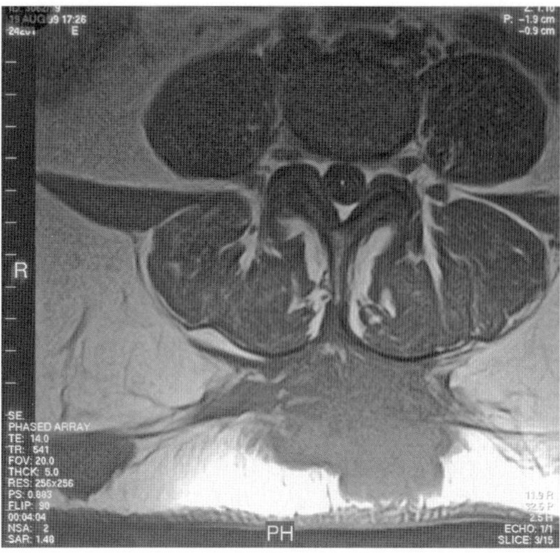

Fig. 5.25. Same patient. Axial T1-weighted image at the L4-5 level depicting the abscess in the posterior soft tissue as a well-defined mass of low signal intensity

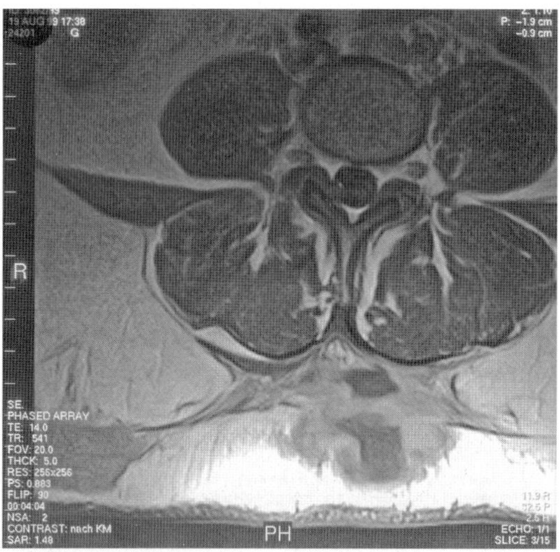

Fig. 5.26. Axial T1-weighted image after contrast administration showing clear abnormal peripheral enhancement of the abscess with foci of liquefaction located centrally in the subcutaneous fatty tissue posterior to L4-5

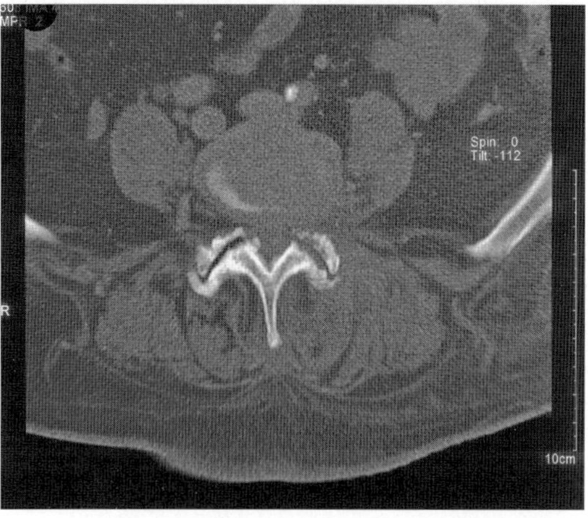

Fig. 5.27. 62-year-old woman with low back pain, predominantly on the left. Axial CT scan at L4-5. Suspected spondylitis with blurring of the left L4-5 facet joint, increased periarticular fluid, and partial destruction of bony structures

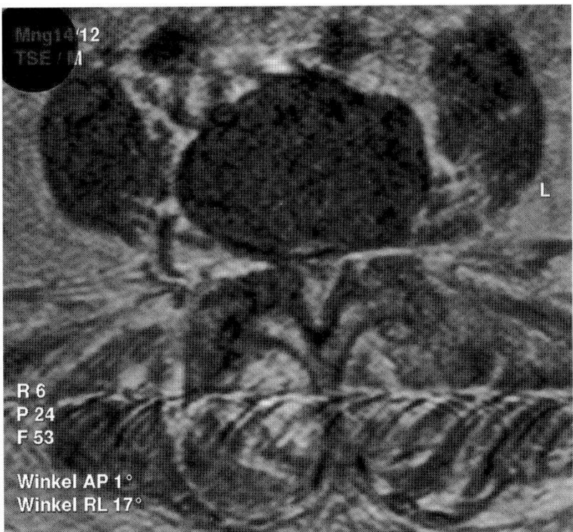

Fig. 5.28. Same patient as Fig. 5.27. Axial T1-weighted image through L4-5 with irregular appearance of the left facet joint. Bony destruction cannot be excluded

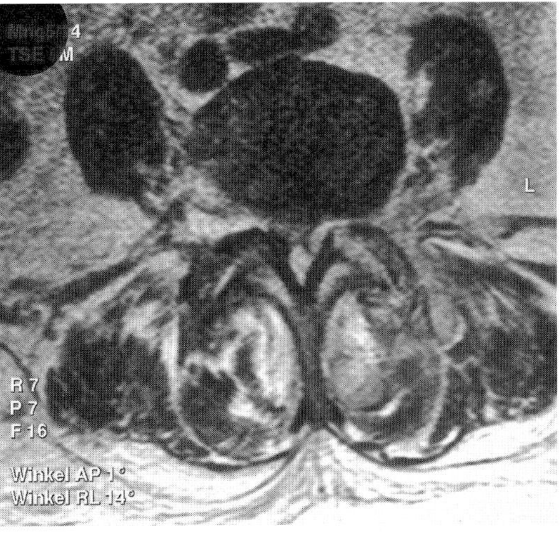

Fig. 5.29. Contrast-enhanced axial T1-weighted image through L4-5. There is pronounced abnormal enhancement around the left facet joint with demonstration of bony destruction and irregular appearance of the joint

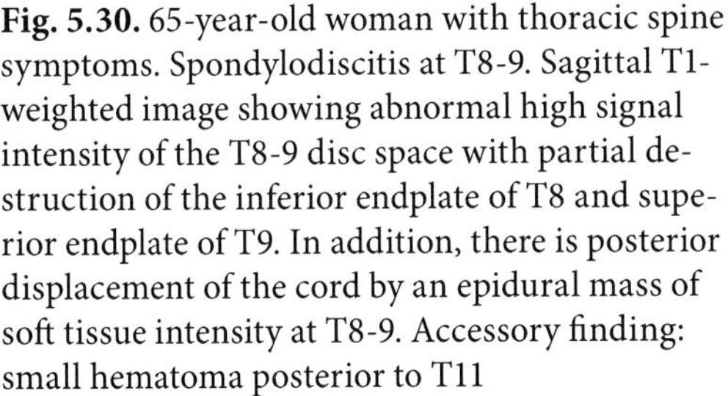

Fig. 5.30. 65-year-old woman with thoracic spine symptoms. Spondylodiscitis at T8-9. Sagittal T1-weighted image showing abnormal high signal intensity of the T8-9 disc space with partial destruction of the inferior endplate of T8 and superior endplate of T9. In addition, there is posterior displacement of the cord by an epidural mass of soft tissue intensity at T8-9. Accessory finding: small hematoma posterior to T11

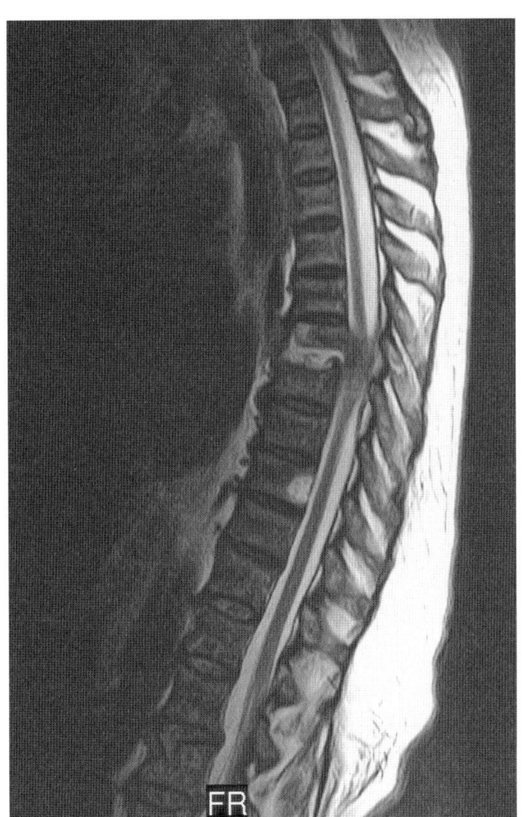

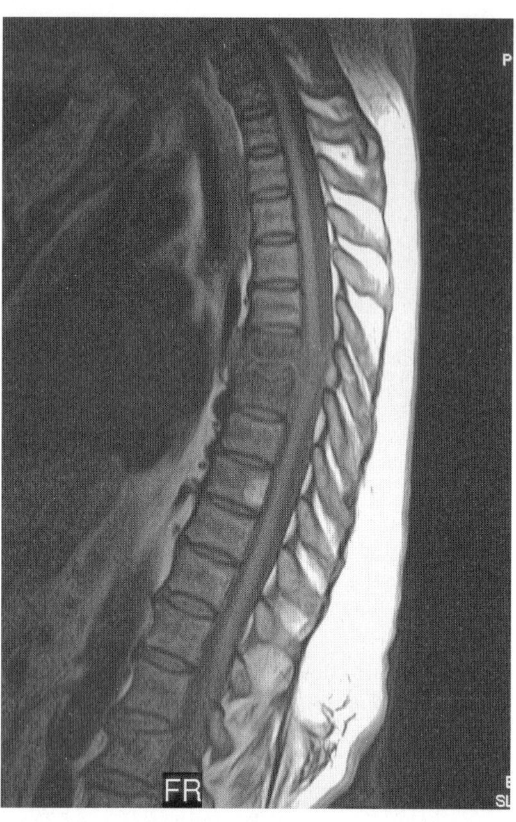

Fig. 5.31. Same patient as Fig. 5.30. Sagittal T1-weighted image with low signal intensity of the T8 and 9 vertebral bodies. The posterior epidural abscess is just barely discernible

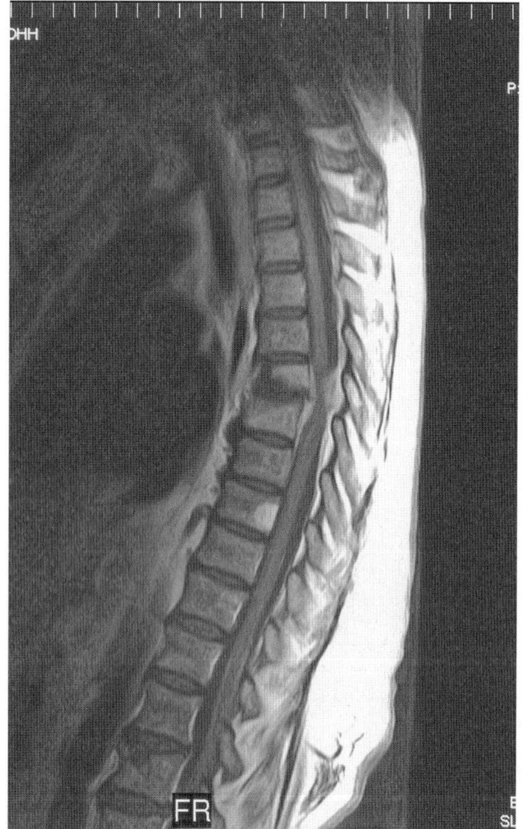

Fig. 5.32. Sagittal T1-weighted image of the thoracic spine with clear epidural contrast enhancement at the T8-9 level, consistent with abscess formation in spondylodiscites. The extent of bony destruction of the anteroinferior portion of T8 and at the superior endplate of T9 is outlined by the enhancement of the remainder of the vertebral bodies. Slight displacement of T8 over T9 with tilting of the upper vertebral body

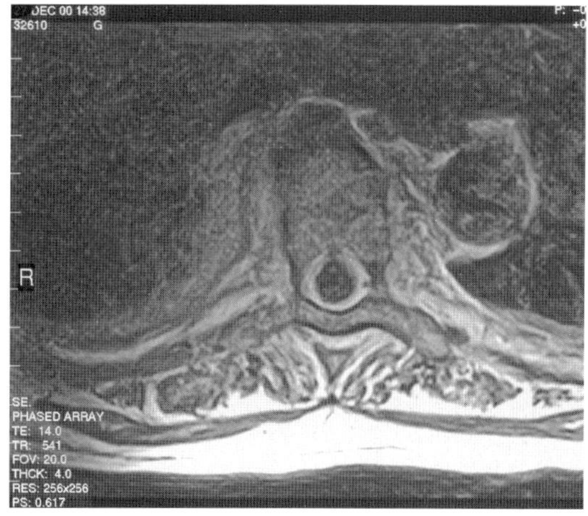

Fig. 5.33. Same patient. Axial T1-weighted image of the T8-9 level showing bilateral paravertebral abscess extending to the descending aorta. There is no definitive spinal stenosis and the spinal cord appears unremarkable

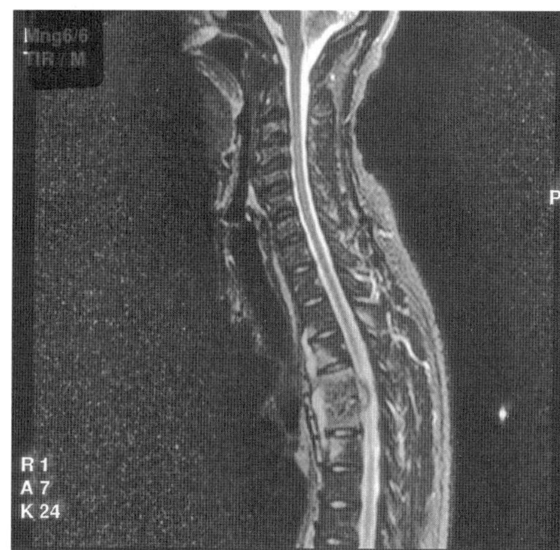

Fig. 5.34. 26-year-old man presenting with spinal symptoms at the cervicothoracic junction. Spondylodiscitis at T5-6. Sagittal T2-weighted image with fat saturation of the cervical spine and cervicothoracic junction down to the T9 level. Altered signal of the T5 and T6 vertebral bodies and anterior portions of T4 and T7 with a prevertebral mass of fluid intensity extending from T4 to T6. Smaller epidural mass posteriorly

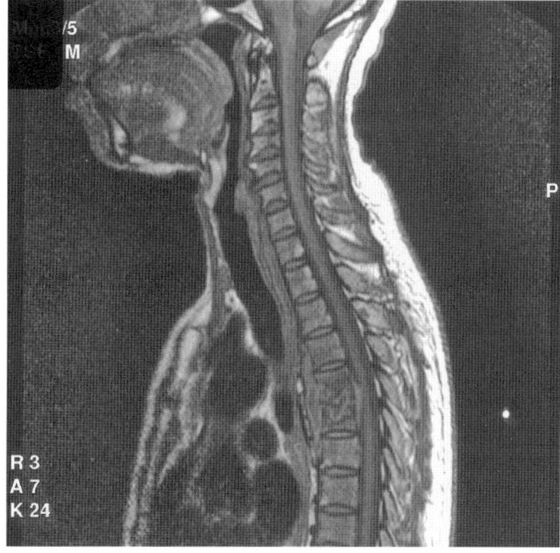

Fig. 5.35. Sagittal T1-weighted image of the cervical and upper thoracic spine showing reduced signal intensity of the T5 and T6 vertebral bodies with a slightly inhomogeneous appearance of the posterior epidural and anterior abscess formations

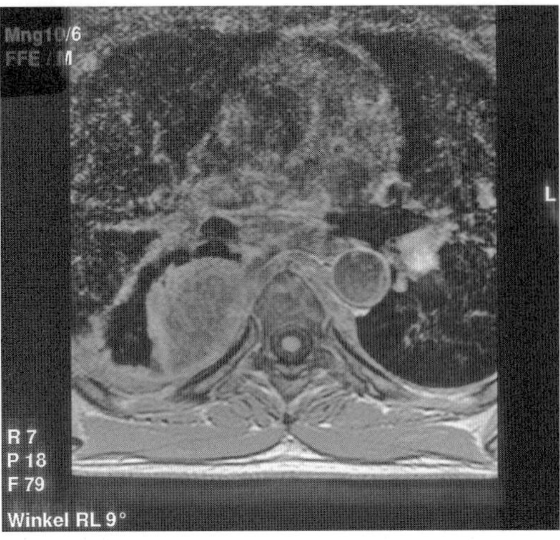

Fig. 5.36. Same patient as in preceding figures. Axial T1-weighted image through the T5-6 level showing large soft-tissue-signal-intensity mass to the right of the spine and smaller lesions anteriorly and on the left. Normal appearance of the spinal canal

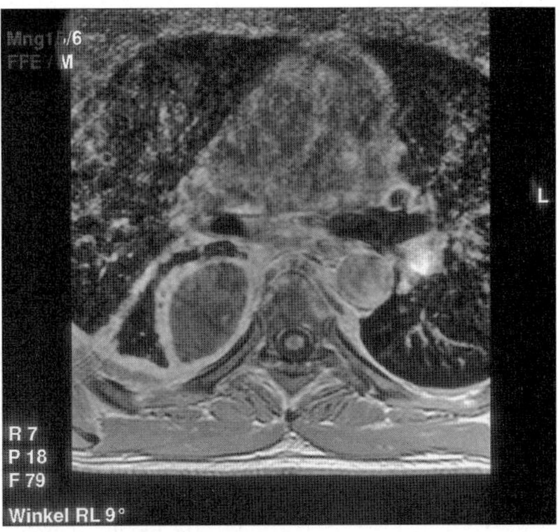

Fig. 5.37. Contrast-enhanced axial T1-weighted image through the T5-6 level showing the large abscess with central liquefaction to the right of the spine as well as more inhomogeneous abscess structures anteriorly and to the left of the vertebra. Abnormal contrast enhancement of T5 vertebra confined to anterior portion. Appearance consistent with T5-6 spondylodiscitis. Suggestion of minimal epidural contrast enhancement anteriorly on the left

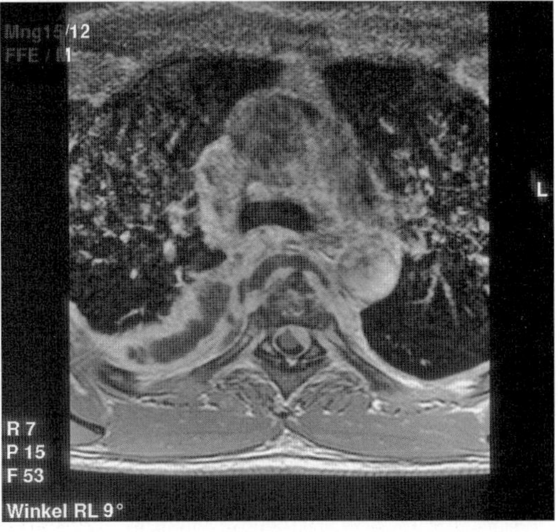

Fig. 5.38. Contrast-enhanced axial T1-weighted image through the T6 level showing the larger vertebral defect at the superior endplate of T6 and the smaller right anterolateral abscess. Larger anterior epidural abscess on the left with narrowing of the spinal canal and displacement of the cord

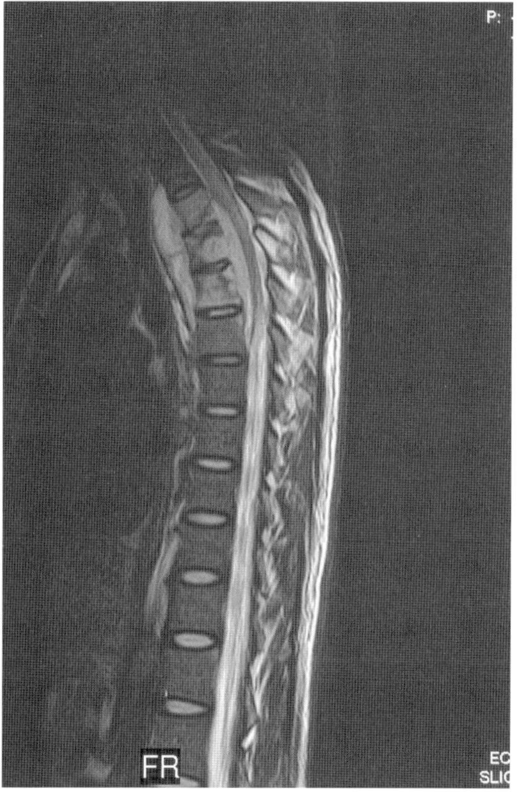

Fig. 5.39. 40-year-old patient with symptoms around the cervicothoracic junction. Paravertebral abscess from T3 through T5. Sagittal T2-weighted image of the thoracic region with signal alteration of the T3 to T5 vertebral bodies and posterior epidural mass nearly isointense to fluid. Additional anterior abscess of similar signal intensity

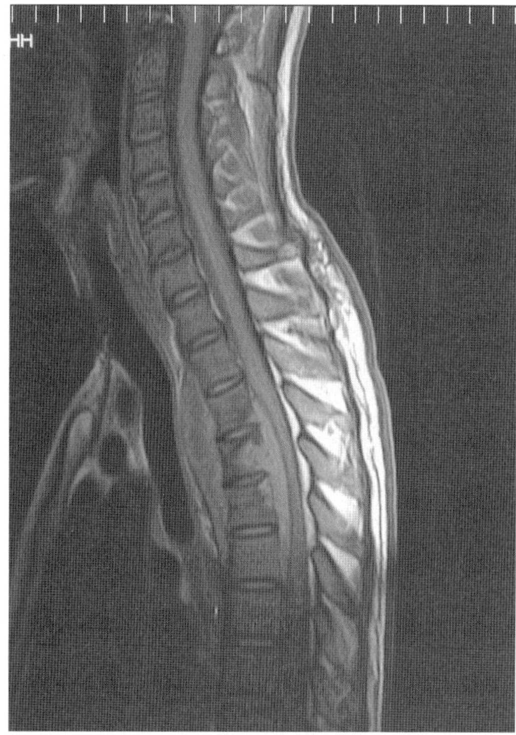

Fig. 5.40. Sagittal T1-weighted image of the cervical and upper thoracic spine showing the paravertebral abscess formation with soft tissue intensity extending from T2 through T6 anteriorly and from T3 through T6 posteriorly. There is disruption of the posterior surface of T4 and less extensive disruption also of the T5 posterior surface. No major signal changes of the intervertebral discs

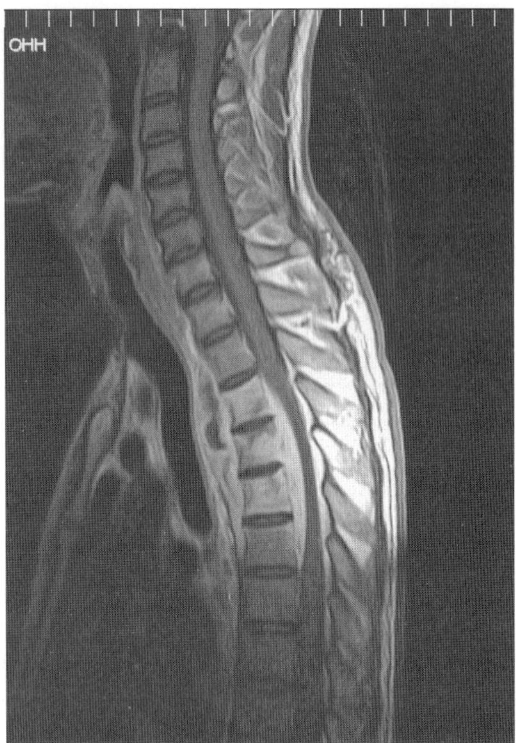

Fig. 5.41. Same patient as Figs. 5.39 and 5.40. Contrast-enhanced sagittal T1-weighted image of the cervical and upper thoracic spine showing marked abnormal enhancement of the abscess structures from T2 through T6 and pronounced narrowing of the spinal canal as well as abnormal enhancement of the T3 to T5 vertebral bodies

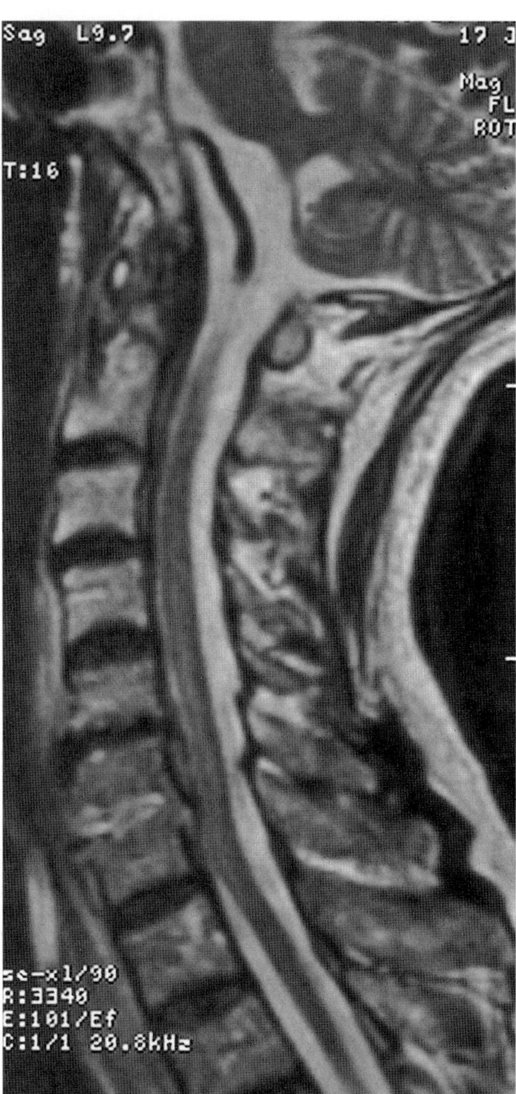

Fig. 5.43. Spondylitis. Sagittal T2-weighted image showing high signal intensity of the C6-7 disc space

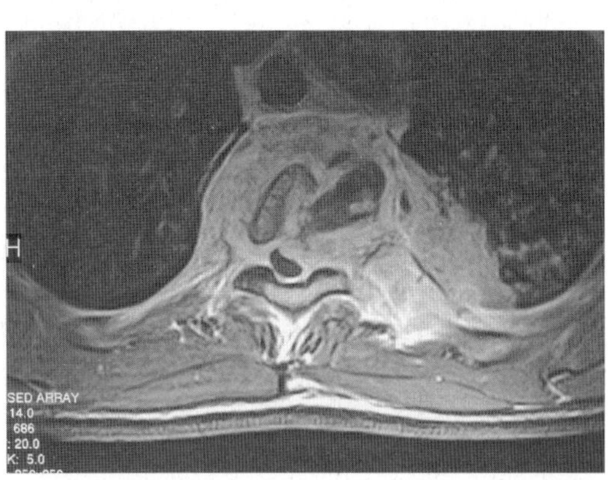

Fig. 5.42. Contrast-enhanced axial T1-weighted image through the T4 level. Pronounced contrast enhancement of the slightly inhomogeneous abscess structures paravertebrally and intraspinally. There is marked displacement and deformity of the spinal cord with partial destruction of the T4 vertebral body and early erosive changes of the left T5 costotransverse joint

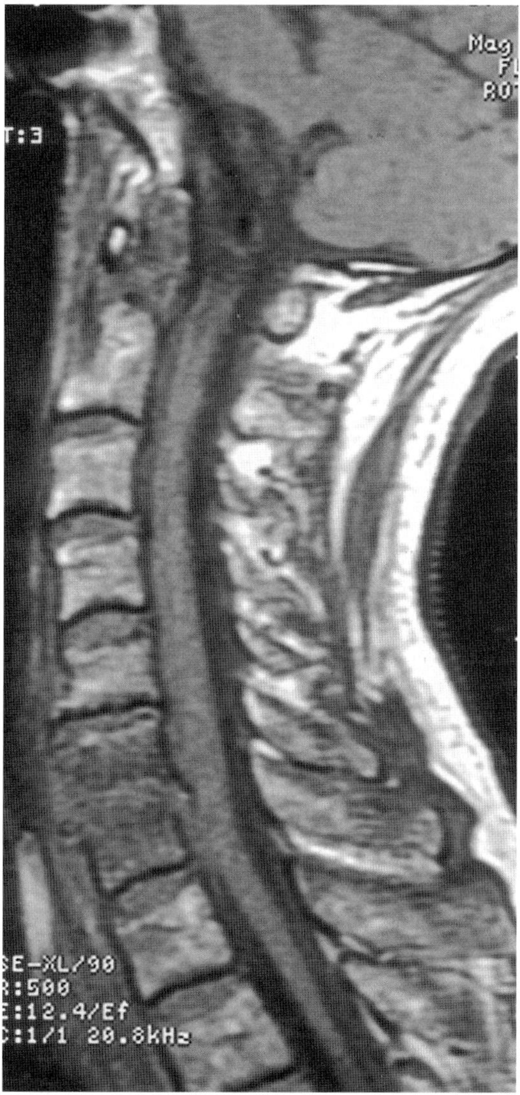

Fig. 5.44. Same patient. Sagittal T1-weighted image (unenhanced) depicting the interspace with normal disc signal. There is thickening of the prevertebral soft tissue layer and edematous signal reduction of the affected vertebral bodies

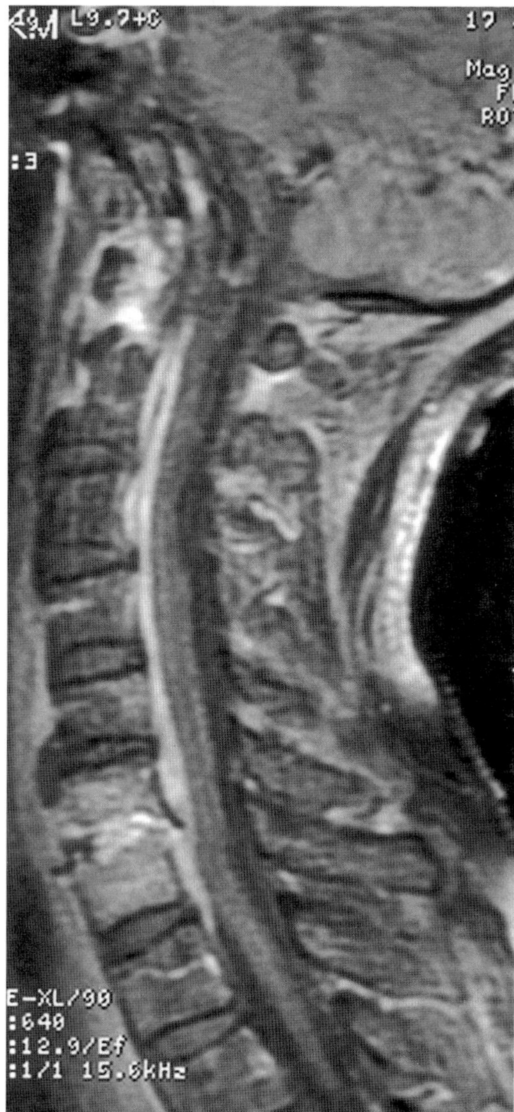

Fig. 5.45. Sagittal T1-weighted image with fat suppression after IV contrast administration. Inflammatory signal increase in the C6-7 disc space and affected vertebral bodies; epidural inflammatory reaction, and inflammatory thickening of the prevertebral soft tissue layer

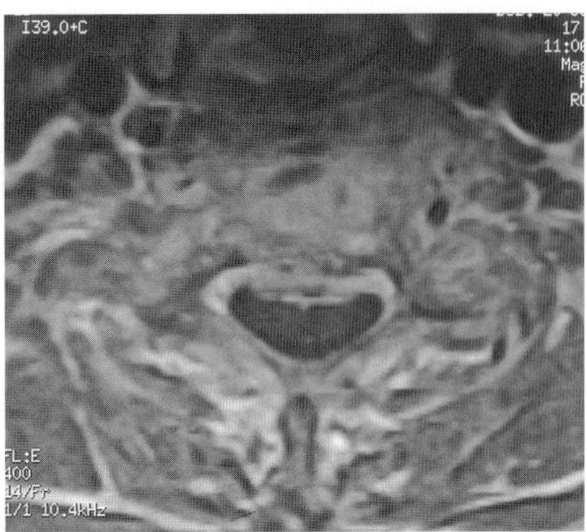

Fig. 5.46. Same patient as in preceding figures. Transverse T1-weighted image after IV contrast administration: increased signal of the inflammatory process at the disc level with colliquation at the 11 to 12 o'clock position and inflammatory infiltration of paravertebral tissue

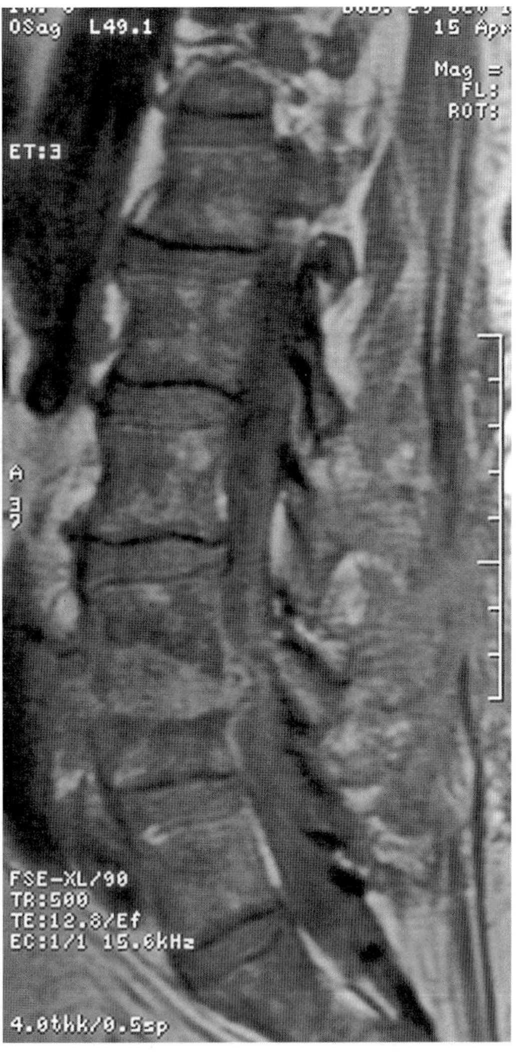

Fig. 5.47. Unenhanced sagittal T1-weighted image showing melting of the vertebral endplates of L3 and L4. The interspace appears to be widened and the process extends into the spinal canal

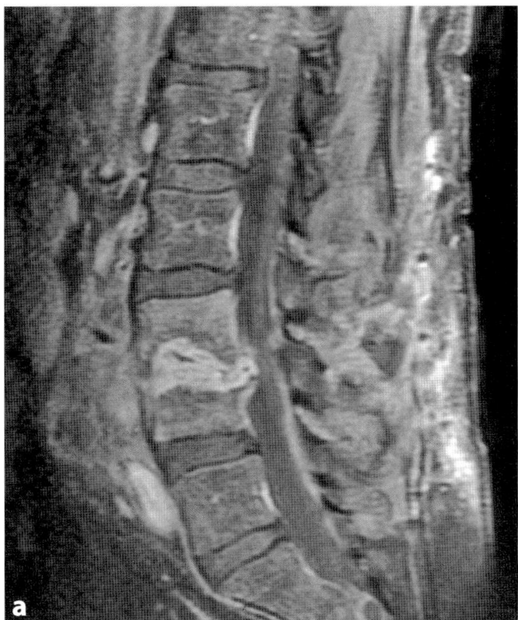

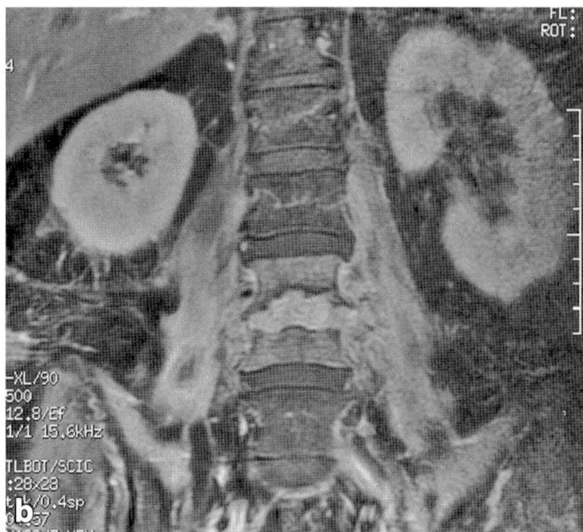

Fig. 5.48a, b. Same patient. Sagittal T1-weighted image with fat suppression (**a**) and coronal T1-weighted image with fat suppression (**b**), both after contrast administration: inflammatory signal increase in the L3-4 disc space and inflammatory involvement of the adjacent vertebral bodies. There is paravertebral extension of the inflammatory process (gravitation abscess in right psoas muscle) with a small epidural abscess component

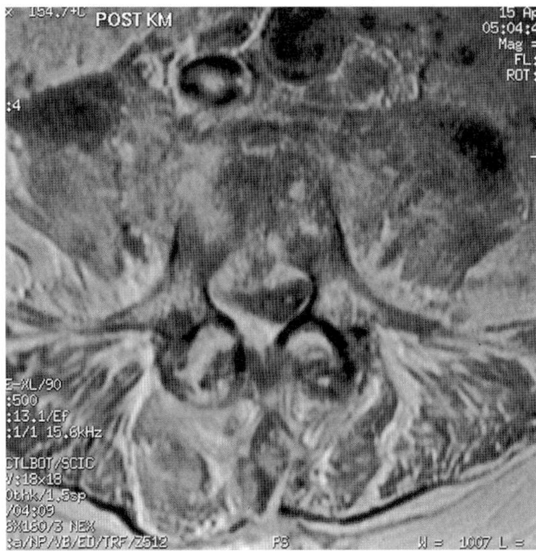

Fig. 5.49. Transverse T1-weighted image after contrast administration providing a good overview of the extent of spondylodiscitis: there is involvement of the right psoas muscle, an epidural component with dural tube deformity, and extension of the inflammatory process to the right extensor muscle

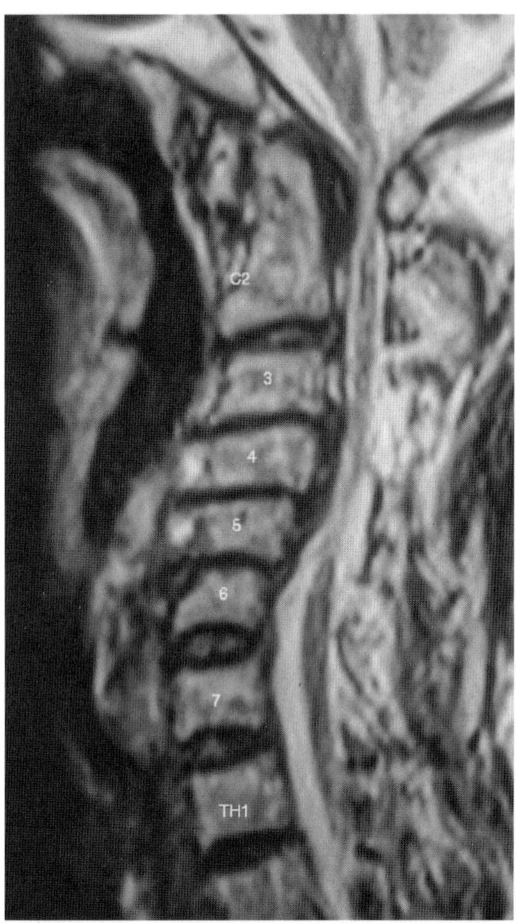

Fig. 5.50. Sagittal T2-weighted image. Low-signal-intensity pannus posterior to the dens, marked narrowing of the upper cervical canal

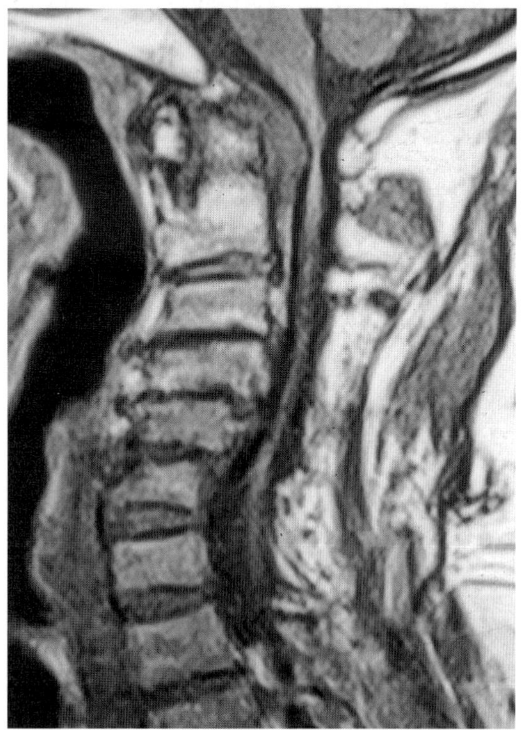

Fig. 5.51. Sagittal T1-weighted image showing severe pannus at the atlantoaxial junction with narrowing of the spinal cord and advanced spinal cord atrophy

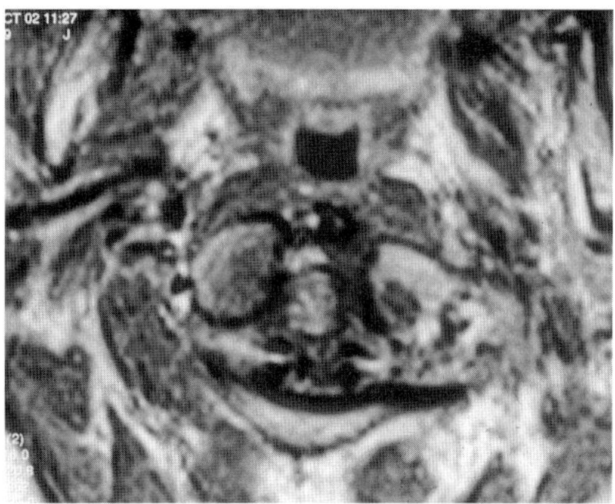

Fig. 5.52. Same patient. Transverse T1-weighted image after contrast administration: spinal cord reduced to a line by atrophy, inflammatory signal increase of pannus, asymmetric position of the tip of the dens with erosive changes

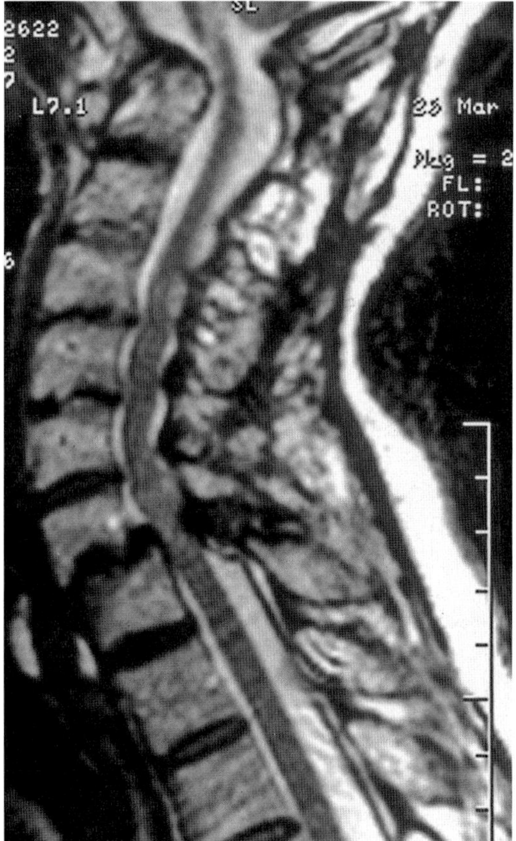

Fig. 5.53. Sagittal T2-weighted image: subluxation of C7 on T1 with involvement of the posterior portions of the vertebral arch and ligamenta flava; spinal cord compression

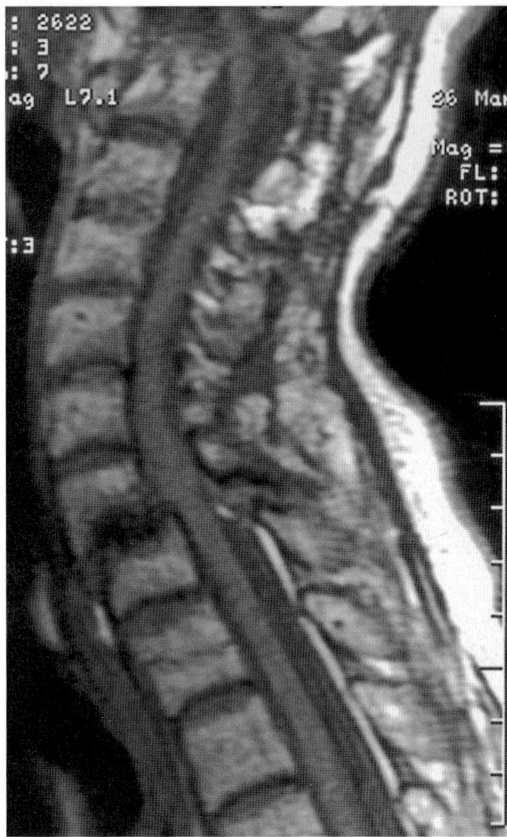

Fig. 5.54. Same patient as in preceding figures. Sagittal T1-weighted image: inflammatory erosions and destruction of the vertebral endplates. Inflammatory pannus in posterior space of spinal canal

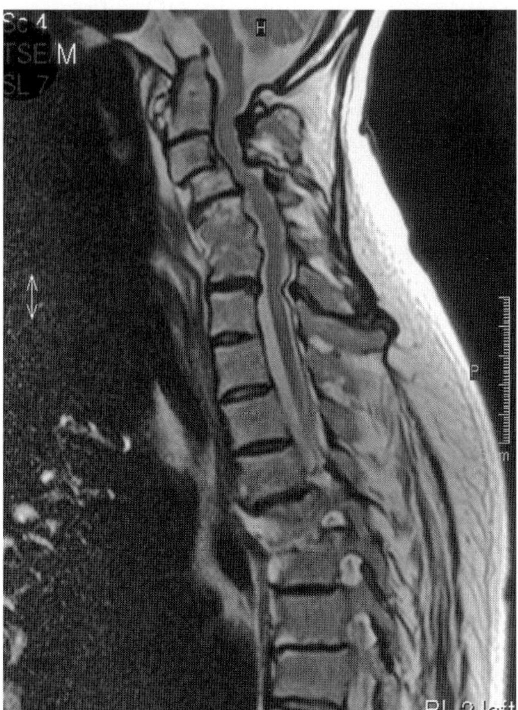

Fig. 5.56. 65-year-old patient with known chronic polyarthritis. Sagittal T2-weighted image of the cervical region including the craniocervical and cervicothoracic junctions. Subluxation of the atlantoaxial joint with pseudobulbar displacement of the dens axis into the foramen magnum. The spinal cord is markedly displaced with slight spinal stenosis at the level of the foramen magnum. Subluxation of the C3-4 joint with anterior displacement of C3. Synostoses of C5, C6, and C7 with destruction of intervening disc spaces and postural kyphosis. Additional synostosis at the T5-6 level with complete loss of the disc

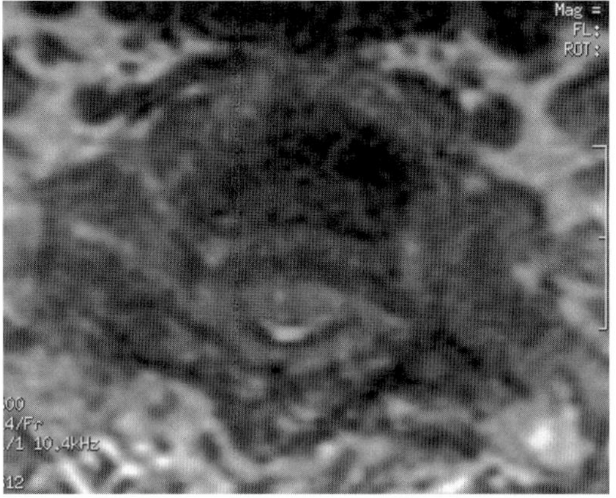

Fig. 5.55. Transverse T1-weighted image. Step formation at C7-T1. Expansion of the facet joints and thickening of the ligamentum flavum

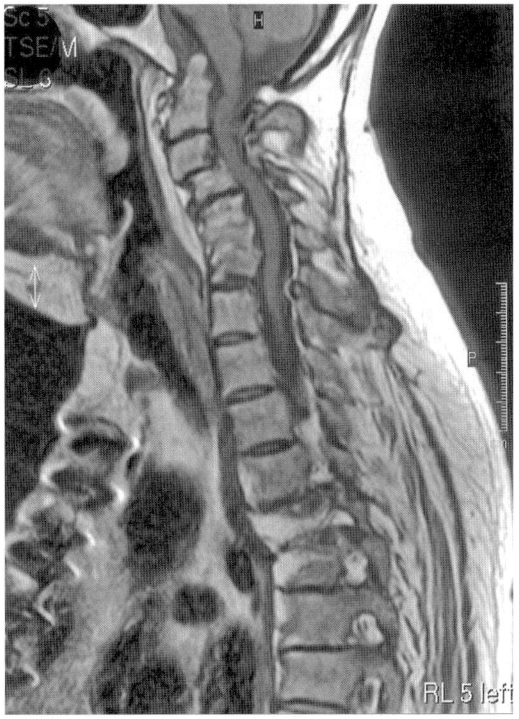

Fig. 5.57. Same patient. Sagittal T1-weighted image showing dislocation of the atlantoaxial joint with synostoses from C5 through C7 and less clear depiction of the T5-6 synosthosis

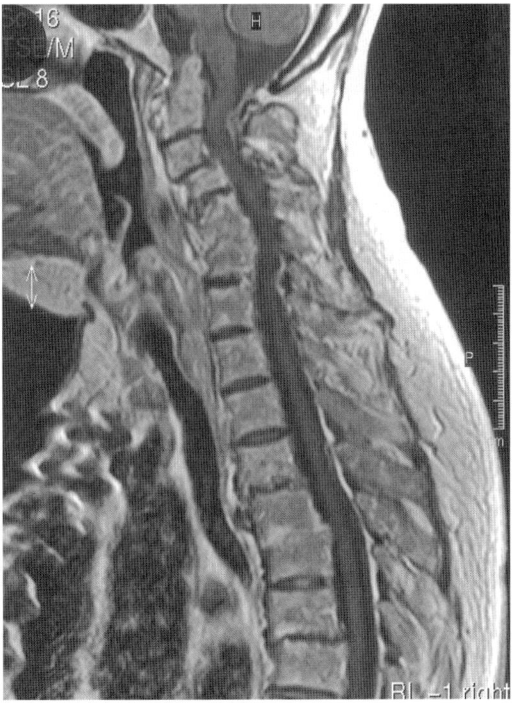

Fig. 5.58. Sagittal T1-weighted image after contrast administration showing relatively homogeneous contrast enhancement of the marrow spaces. No evidence of abscess formation. The consolidated T5-6 disc is slightly more conspicuous

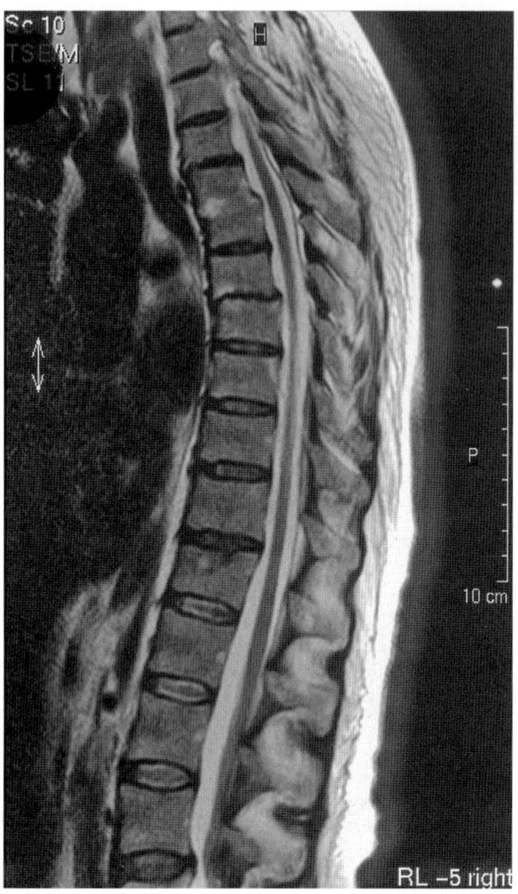

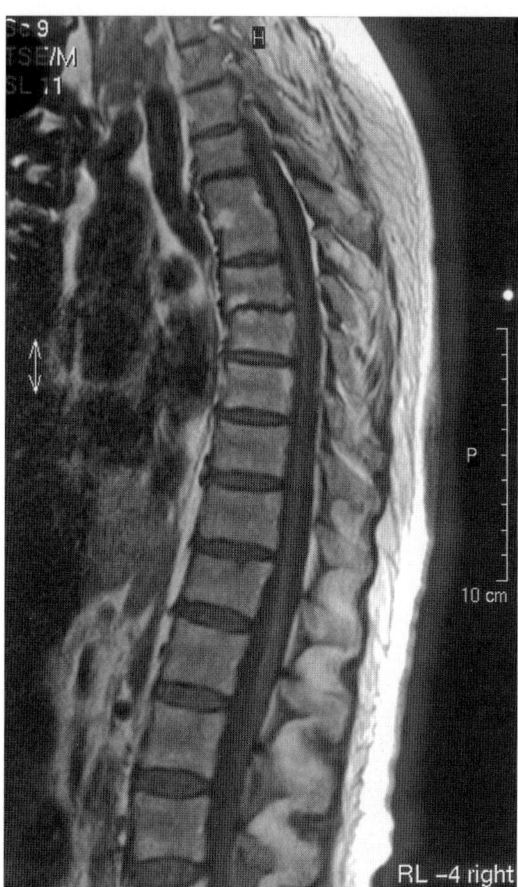

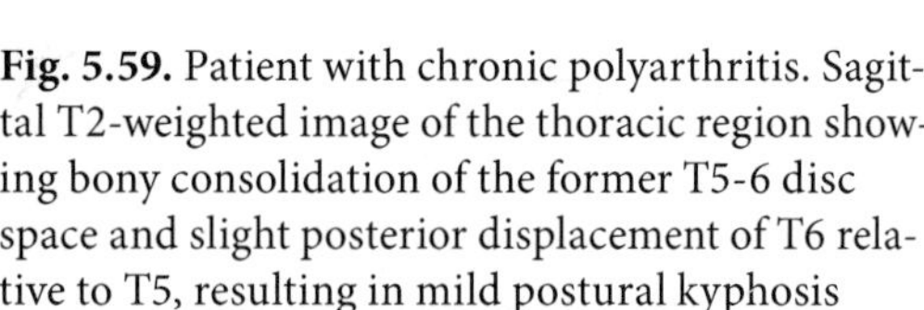
Fig. 5.59. Patient with chronic polyarthritis. Sagittal T2-weighted image of the thoracic region showing bony consolidation of the former T5-6 disc space and slight posterior displacement of T6 relative to T5, resulting in mild postural kyphosis

Fig. 5.60. Sagittal T1-weighted image of the T5-6 synostosis in chronic polyarthritis

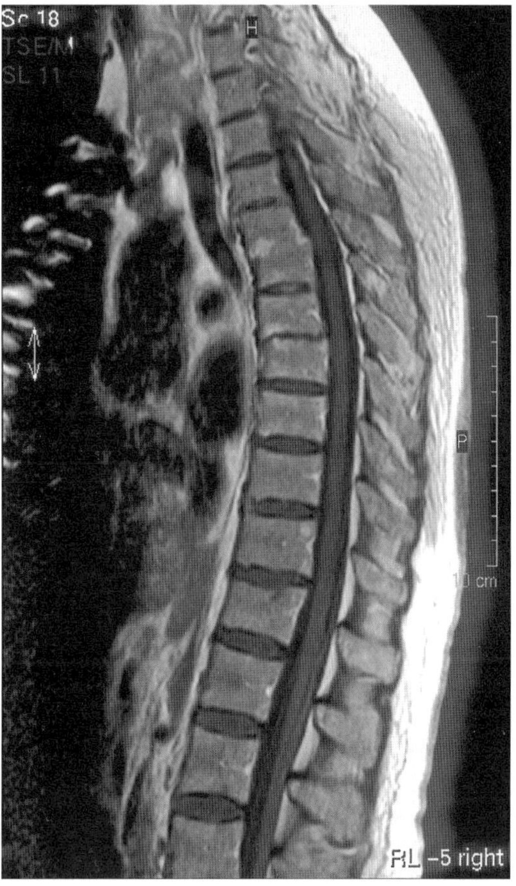

Fig. 5.61. Same patient (chronic polyarthritis). Contrast-enhanced sagittal T1-weighted image of the cervical region. No abnormal contrast enhancement in the area of synostosis or the other vertebrae depicted. The image shows additional narrowing of the T6-7 disc space without signs of acute erosion or abnormal contrast enhancement

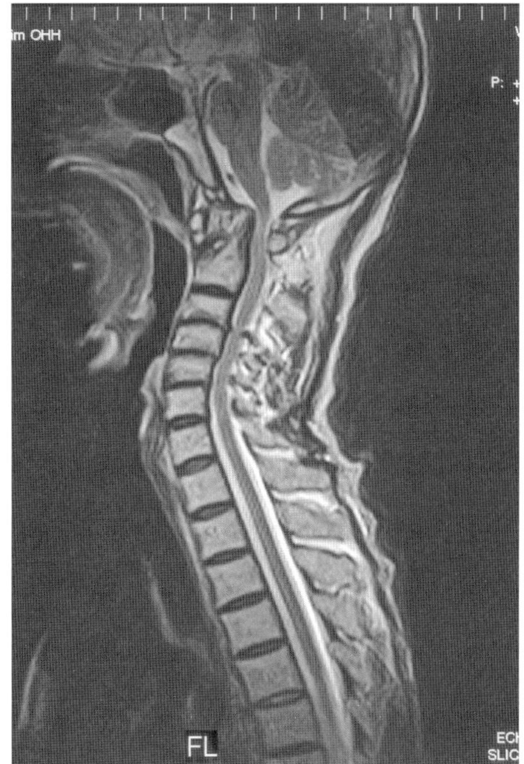

Fig. 5.62. 46-year-old man with pain around the craniocervical junction. Sagittal T2-weighted image of the cervical region and craniocervical junction showing abnormal posterior position of the mutilated and rarefied dens axis. Soft tissue structures are depicted in the atlantoaxial joint and there is marked posterior displacement and compression of the proximal cervical spinal cord. Degenerative changes of upper cervical spine with narrowing of the C3-4, C4-5, and C5-6 disc spaces

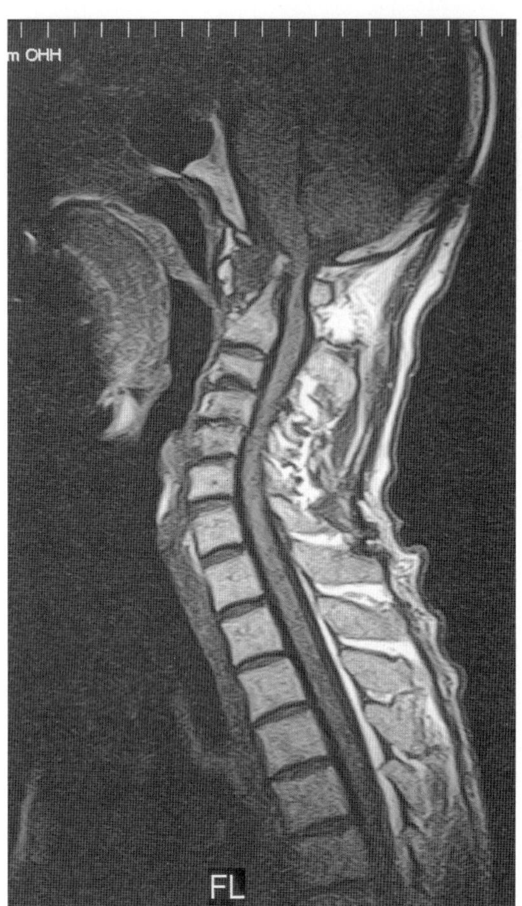

Fig. 5.63. Same patient as Fig. 5.62 (atlantoaxial arthritis). Sagittal T1-weighted image showing mutilation and bony destruction of the dens axis, which is displaced posteriorly. Depiction of soft tissue structures anterior to the dens and pronounced compression of the spinal cord

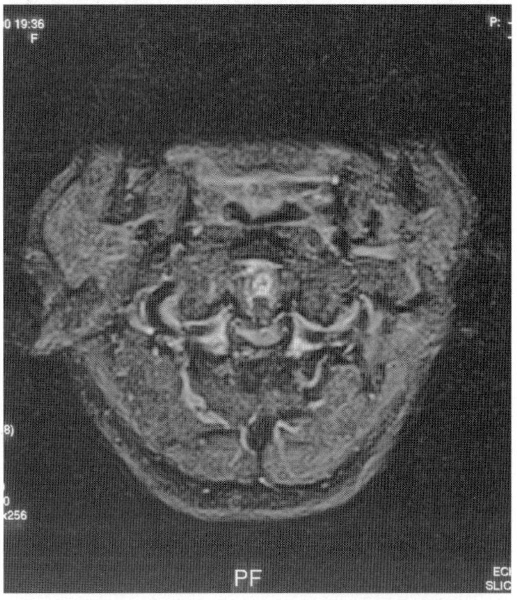

Fig. 5.64. Axial T2-weighted image at the level of the atlantoaxial joint showing posterior displacement of the residual dens relative to the atlas with marked deformity of the spinal cord

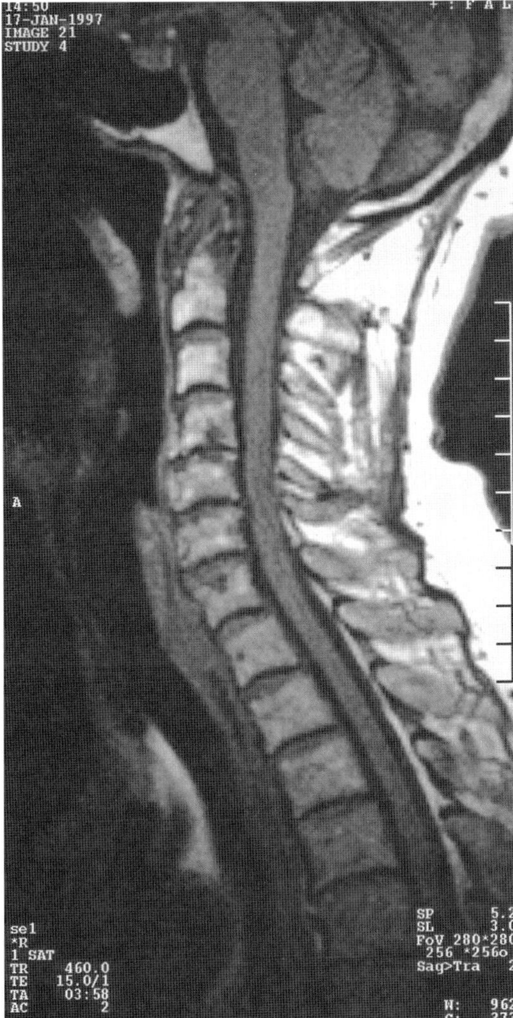

Fig. 5.65. Sagittal T1-weighted image of the cervical region including the craniocervical junction in a 75-year-old patient. There is partial destruction and posterior displacement of the dens with slight deformity of the medulla oblongata at the level of the foramen magnum

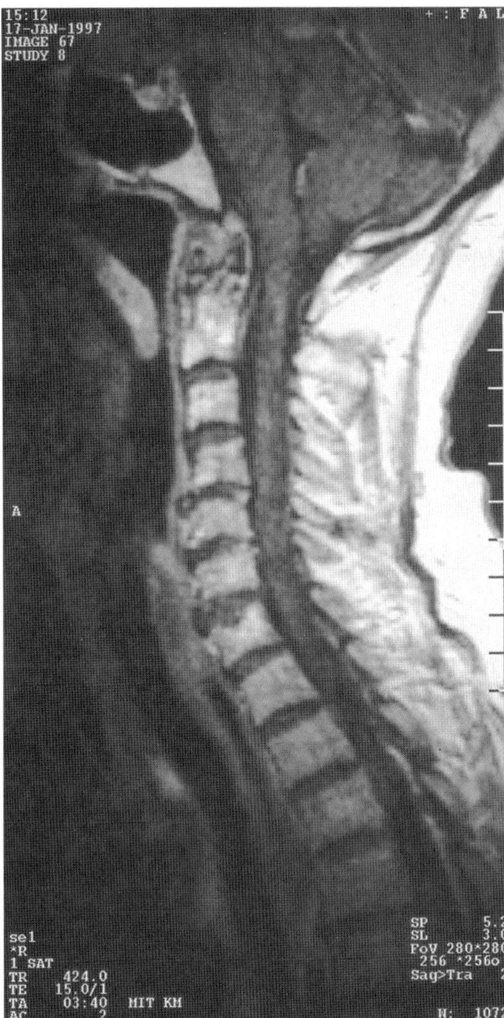

Fig. 5.66. Sagittal T1-weighted image after contrast administration. The image shows extensive and pronounced enhancement of the soft tissue anterior to the destroyed dens in atlantoaxial arthritis

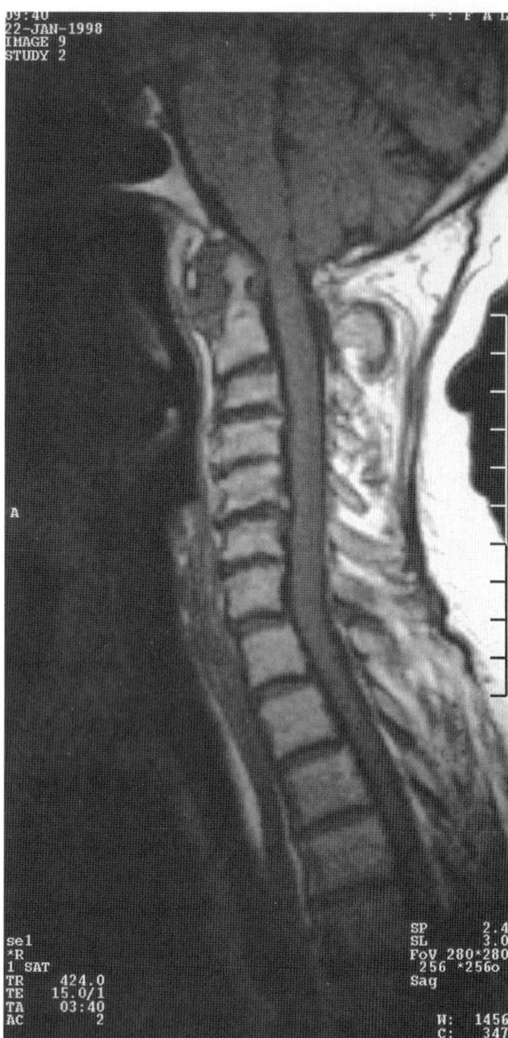

Fig. 5.67. Same patient as Figs. 5.65 and 5.66. Sagittal T1-weighted image of the cervical region showing partial destruction of the dens axis with luxation of the atlantoaxial joint and soft tissue in the joint. Slight deformity of the medulla oblongata at the level of the foramen magnum

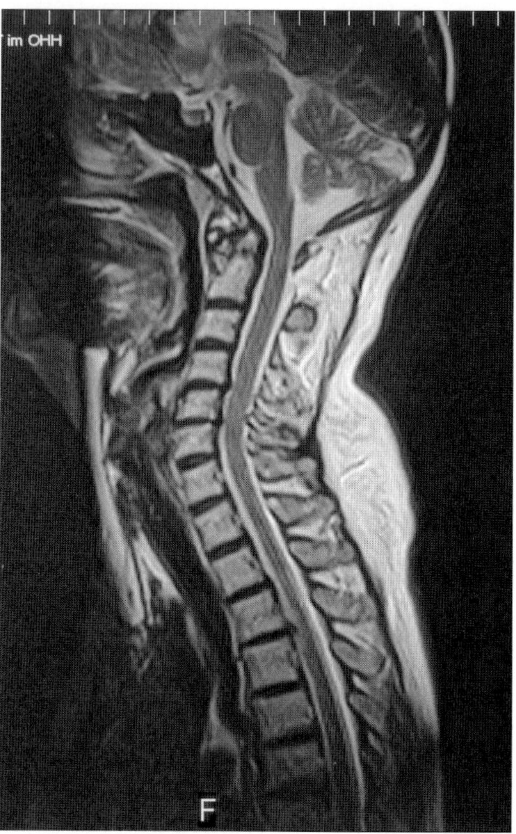

Fig. 5.68. Sagittal T2-weighted image of the cervical region in a 60-year-old patient with luxation of the atlantoaxial joint and partial destruction of the dens axis. The distance between the anterior arch of atlas and dens is increased. Soft tissue signal intensity in the former joint space. Slight posterior displacement of the spinal cord at the level of the foramen magnum

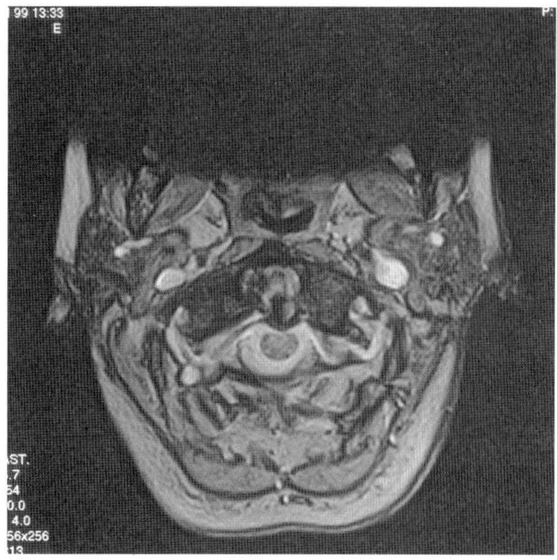

Fig. 5.69. Same patient. Axial T2-weighted image through the level of the atlantoaxial joint showing posterior subluxation of the dens axis with slight deformity of the cervical spinal cord and obstruction of the anterior subarachnoid space

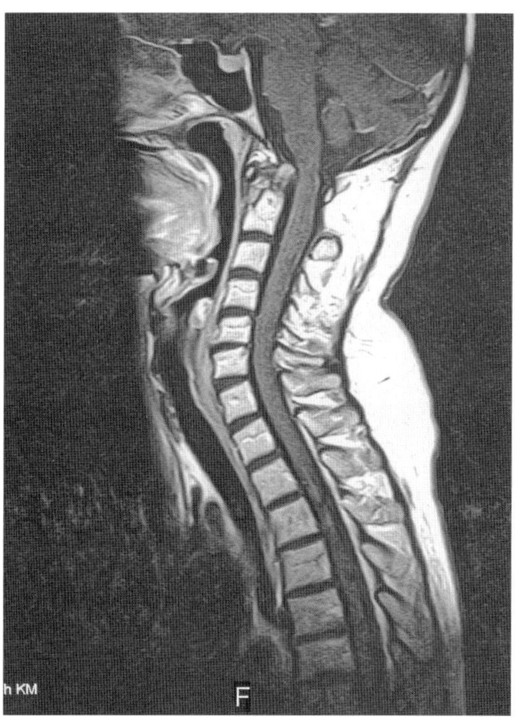

Fig. 5.70. Sagittal T1-weighted image of the cervical region after contrast administration showing moderate contrast enhancement of the soft tissue structures in the atlantoaxial joint. Posterior displacement and subluxation of the dens in atlantoaxial arthritis

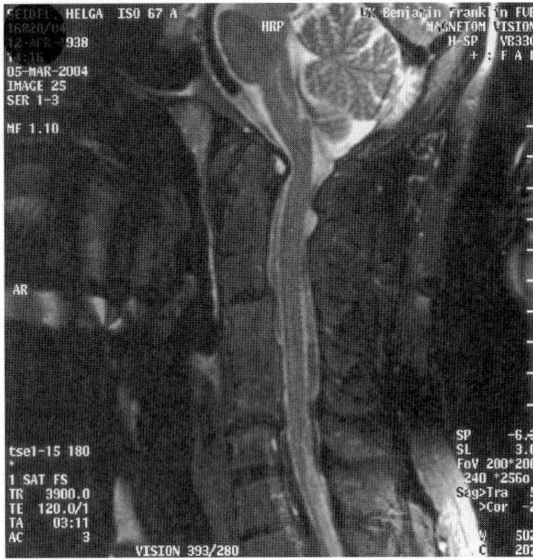

Fig. 5.71. Sagittal T1-weighted image of the cervical spine showing severe atlantoaxial arthrosis with synostoses of C2-C3 and of C4 through C6. Osteophytes at the atlas arch and arthrotic deformity of the dens with narrowing of the joint cleft. Spinal stenosis at the C1-2 level with posterior displacement of the spinal cord and widening of the C1-2 joint

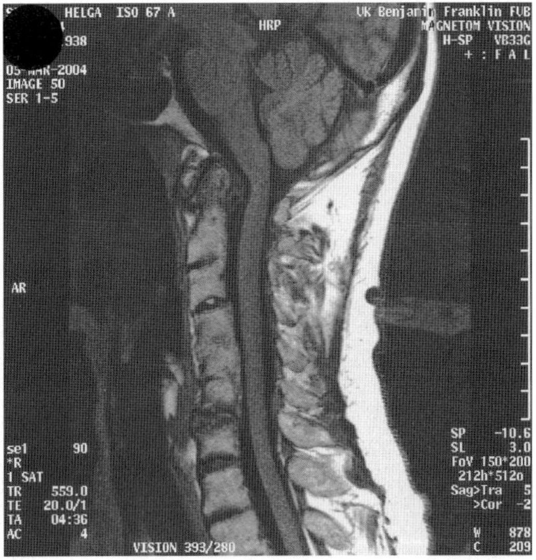

Fig. 5.72. Sagittal T2-weighted image of the upper cervical region. Fluid collection posterior to the dens axis with displacement and compression of the upper end of the spinal cord. The fluid represents joint effusion of the C1-2 joint due to severe arthrosis

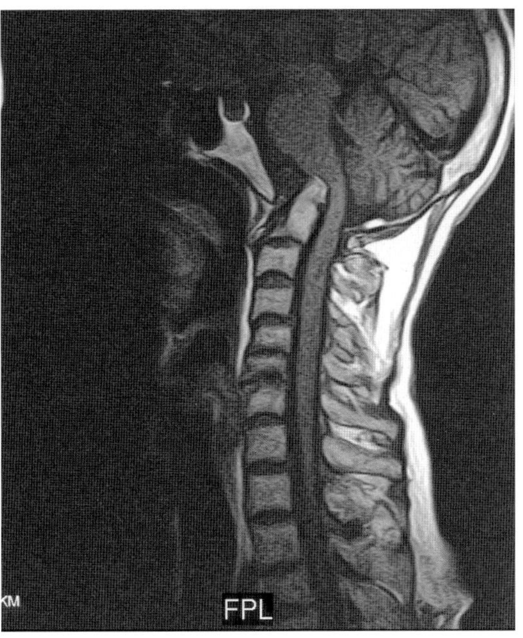

Fig. 5.73. Sagittal T1-weighted image of the craniocervical junction showing marked deformity of the medulla oblongata

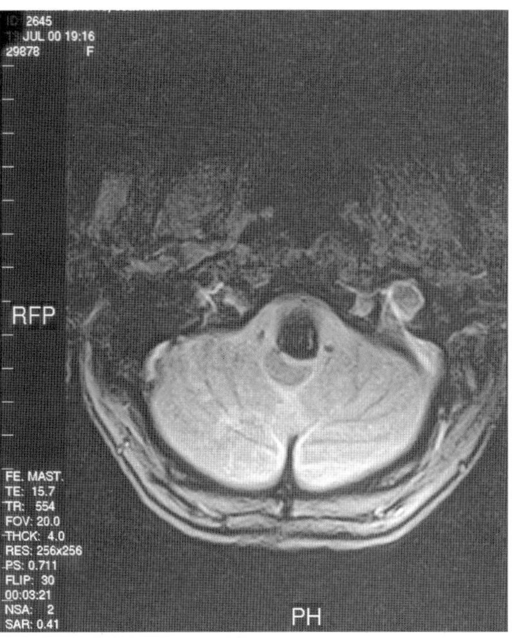

Fig. 5.74. Axial T2-weighted image at the skull base. The dens axis is seen as a circular structure of low signal intensity markedly displacing and indenting the medulla oblongata

Fig. 5.75. Sagittal T2-weighted image of the cervical spine and craniocervical junction in a 35-year-old patient with pseudobulbar basilar impression. The dens is seen at the level of the foramen magnum with partial narrowing of the foramen but without significant displacement of the cervical spinal cord/medulla oblongata

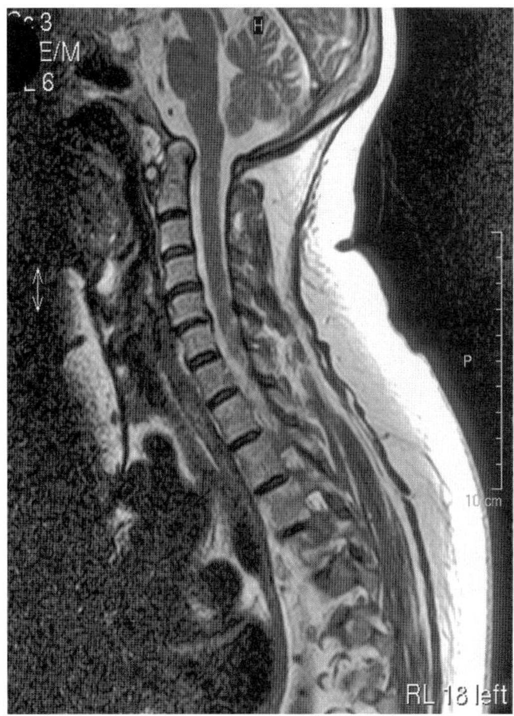

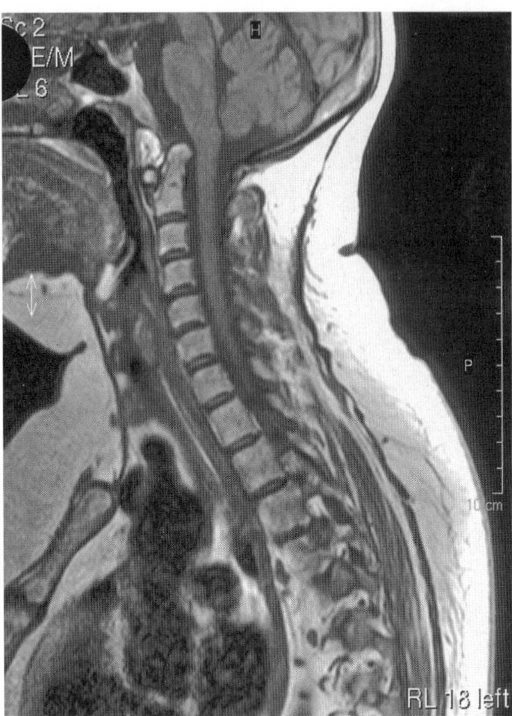

Fig. 5.76. Same patient as Fig. 5.75. Sagittal T1-weighted image of pseudobulbar impression

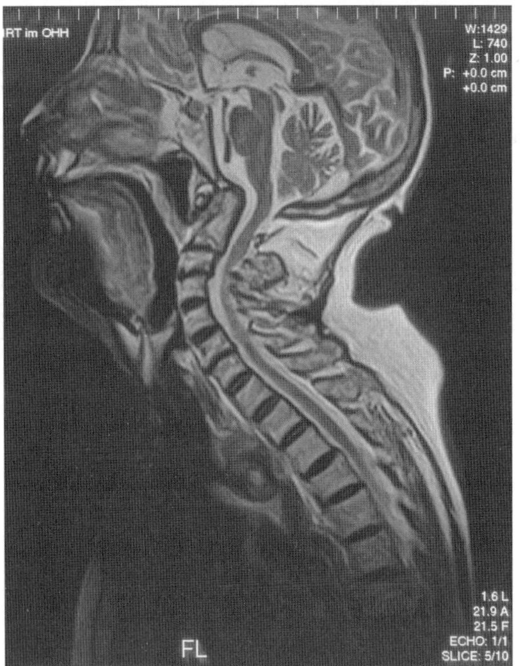

Fig. 5.77. Sagittal T2-weighted image of the cervical spine and craniocervical junction in a 75-year-old patient with pseudobulbar impression. Dens axis displaced upward into the foramen magnum and subluxation of the atlantoaxial joint. Marked deformity and displacement of the cervical spinal cord at the level of the foramen magnum

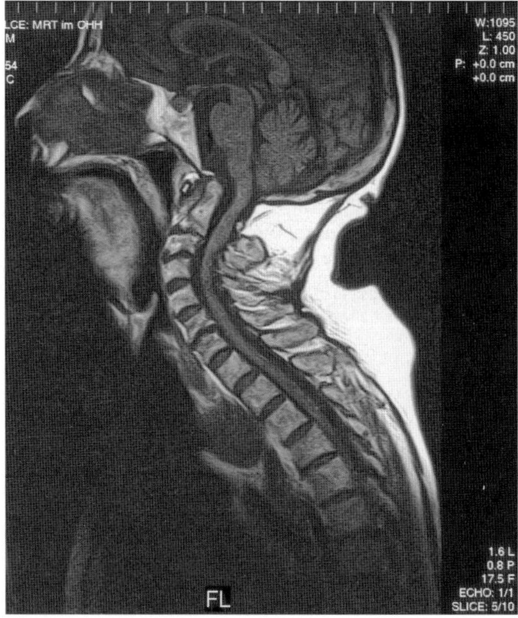

Fig. 5.78. Sagittal T1-weighted image showing pseudobulbar impression with dislocation and cranialization of the dens

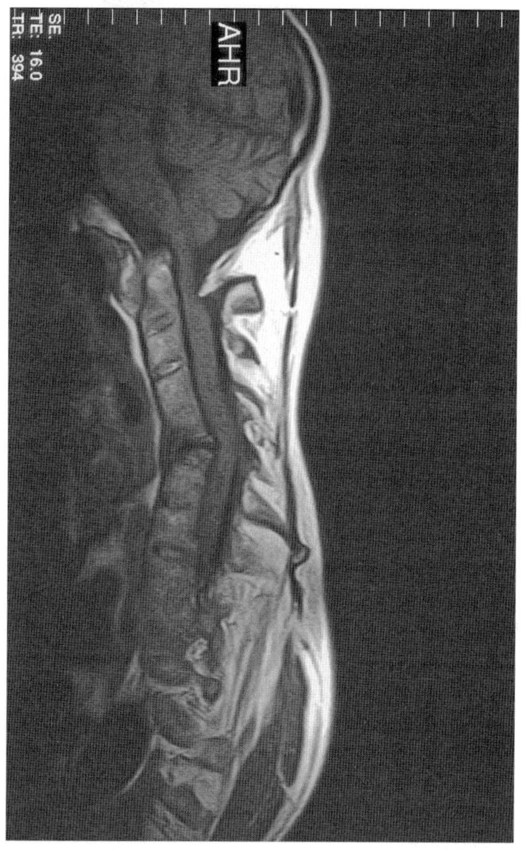

Fig. 5.79. 56-year-old patient with known ankylosing spondylitis. Sagittal T1-weighted image showing basilar impression and the typical changes of ankylosing spondylitis. Fracture and signal alteration at C5-6 and kyphosis with the apex at this level. No irritation of surrounding soft tissue

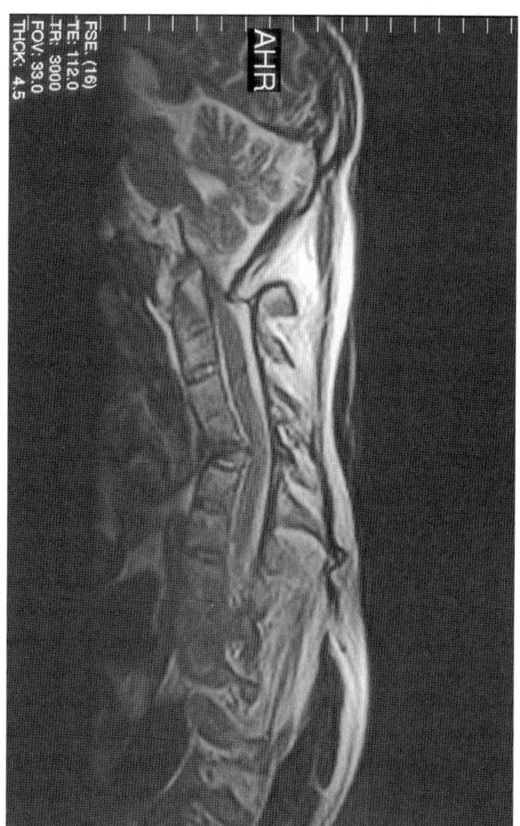

Fig. 5.80. Sagittal T2-weighted image of the cervical region showing the kyphotic curve with posterior displacement of the spinal cord at C5-6. Unaltered signal of the cord. Basilar impression with spinal narrowing at the craniocervical junction

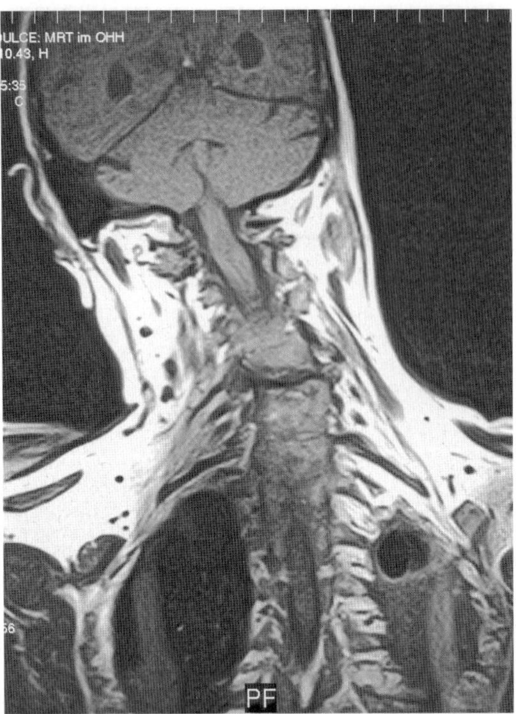

Fig. 5.81. Same patient (ankylosing spondylitis). Coronal T1-weighted image showing the fracture at the C5-6 level with right concave scoliotic curvature

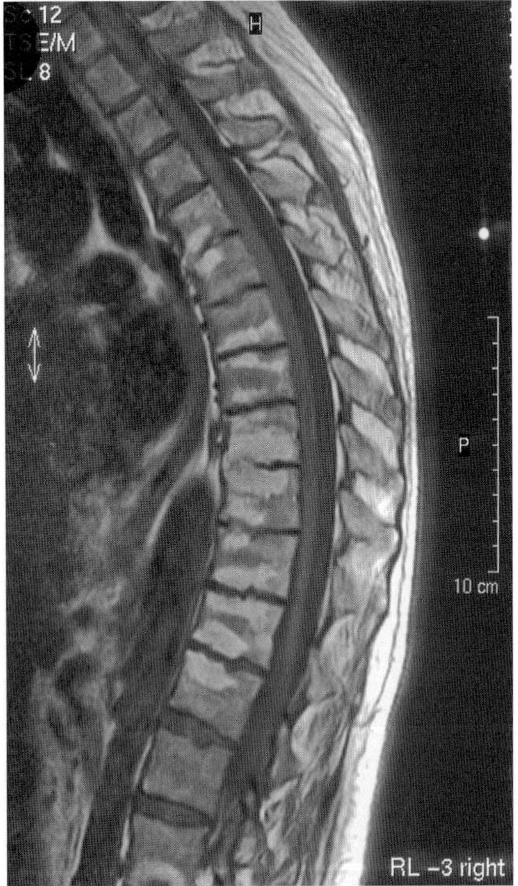

Fig. 5.82. 65-year-old patient with ankylosing spondylitis. Sagittal T1-weighted image of the thoracic region showing the characteristic spinal changes: fatty degeneration at the inferior and superior endplates, mostly anteriorly, in the middle and lower thoracic spine and bony consolidation of the interspaces at T4-5, T8-9, and T9-10; irregular appearance of the intervertebral discs and endplates. No evidence of disc herniation. Postural kyphosis

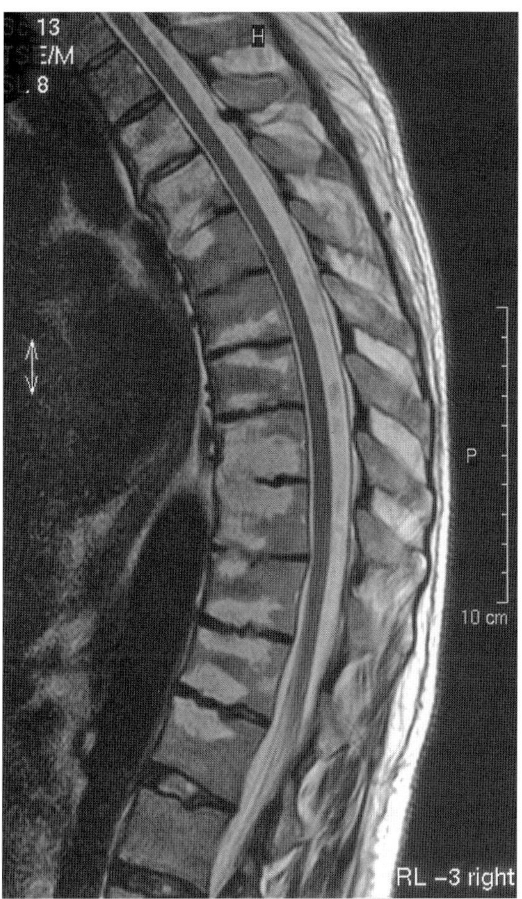

Fig. 5.83. Same patient. Sagittal T2-weighted image. Again, fatty degeneration near the endplates in the middle and lower thoracic spine is indicated by a bright signal. Normal appearance of the thoracic spinal cord and canal

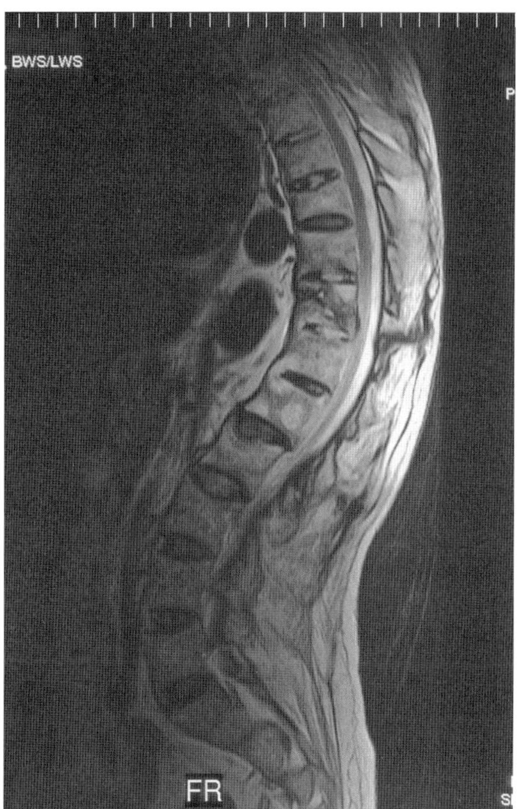

Fig. 5.84. Sagittal T2-weighted image of the lower thoracic region and thoracolumbar junction in a 55-year-old patient with ankylosing spondylitis. Bony consolidation of the anterior portions of T10-11, T11-12, and T12-L1 with postural kyphosis. Transverse fracture of T11 with the characteristic appearance of vertebral fracture associated with ankylosing spondylitis

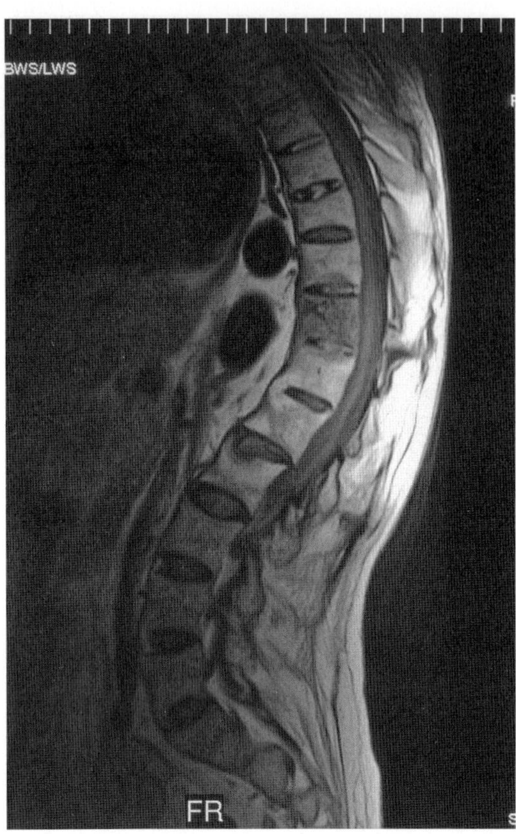

Fig. 5.85. Same patient as Fig. 5.84 (ankylosing spondylitis). Sagittal T1-weighted image before contrast administration. Reduced signal intensity of the T11 vertebral body with irregular transverse fracture cleft of low signal intensity

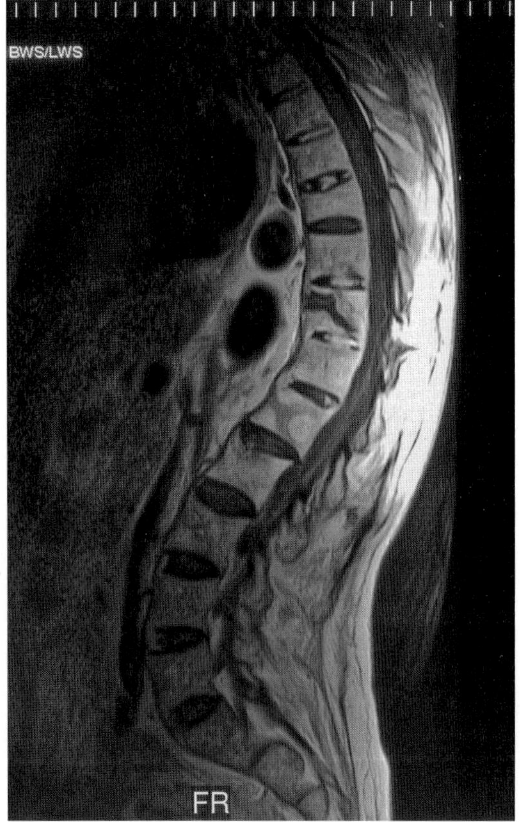

Fig. 5.86. Sagittal T1-weighted image of the lower thoracic region showing the T11 vertebral fracture outlined by contrast enhancement of the surrounding vertebra. There is good visualization of the anterior synostoses from T10 through L1 due to postural kyphosis

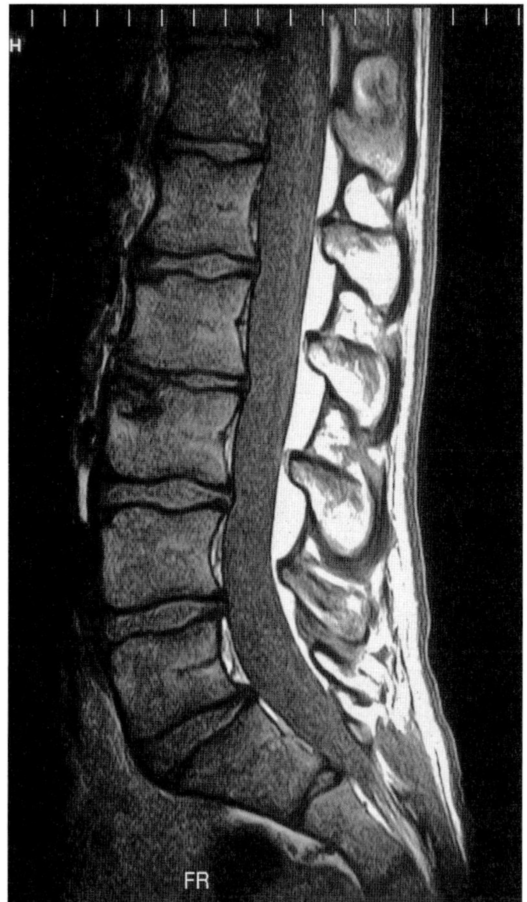

Fig. 5.87. Sagittal T1-weighted image of a 15-year-old patient with known ankylosing spondylitis showing typical Andersson lesion of the upper anterior corner of the L3 vertebra and less obvious lesion of L2

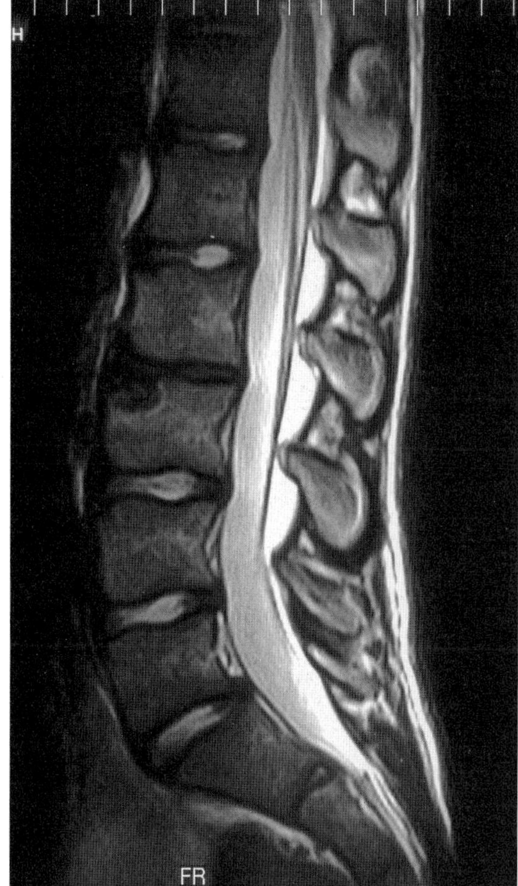

Fig. 5.88. Sagittal T2-weighted image of the L3 and L2 Andersson lesions with focal signal loss and deformity of the anterior upper endplate

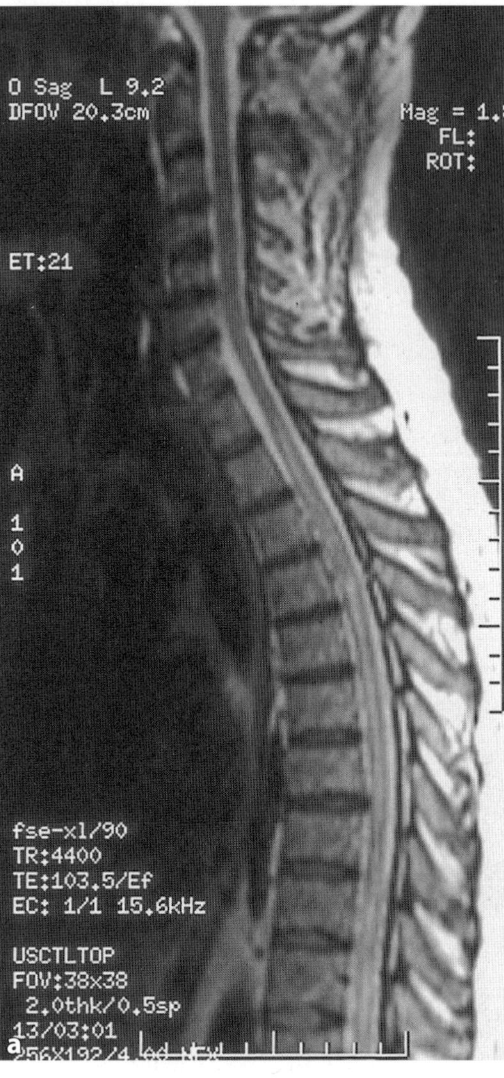

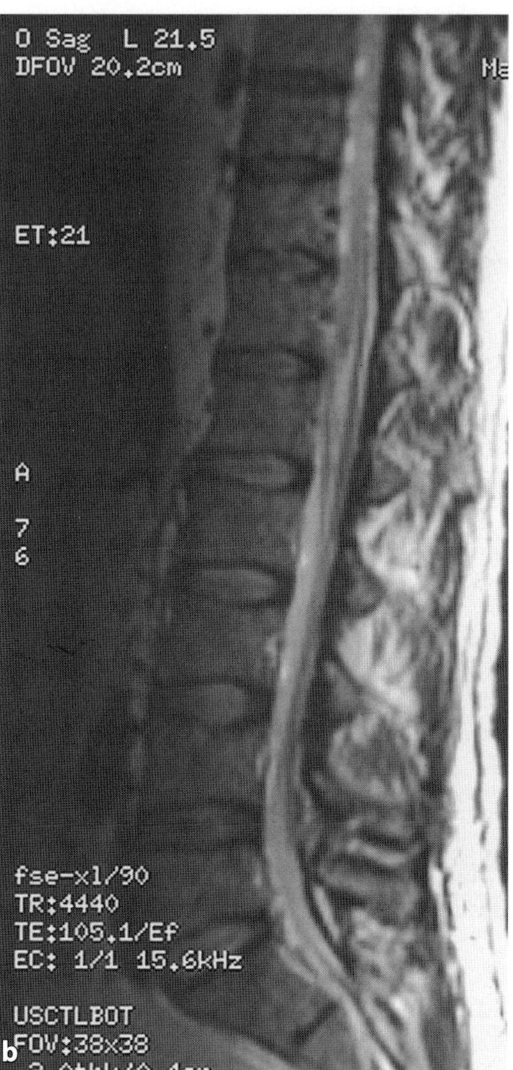

Fig. 5.89a, b. Sagittal T2-weighted images of the cervical and lumbar regions. Myelitic lesion extending from T4 through L1 (conus medullaris)

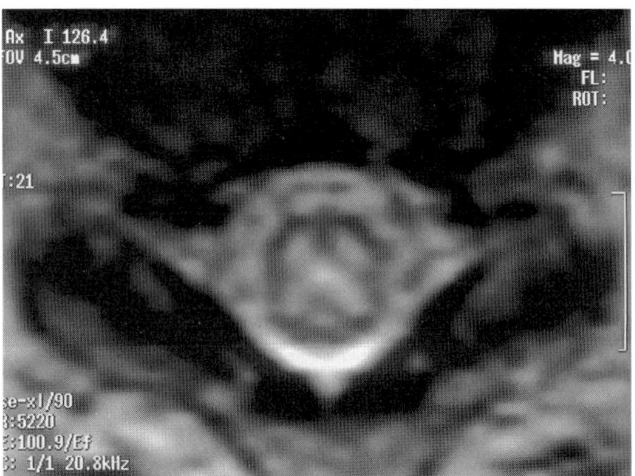

Fig. 5.90. Transverse T2-weighted image: central high-signal-intensity myelitic lesion

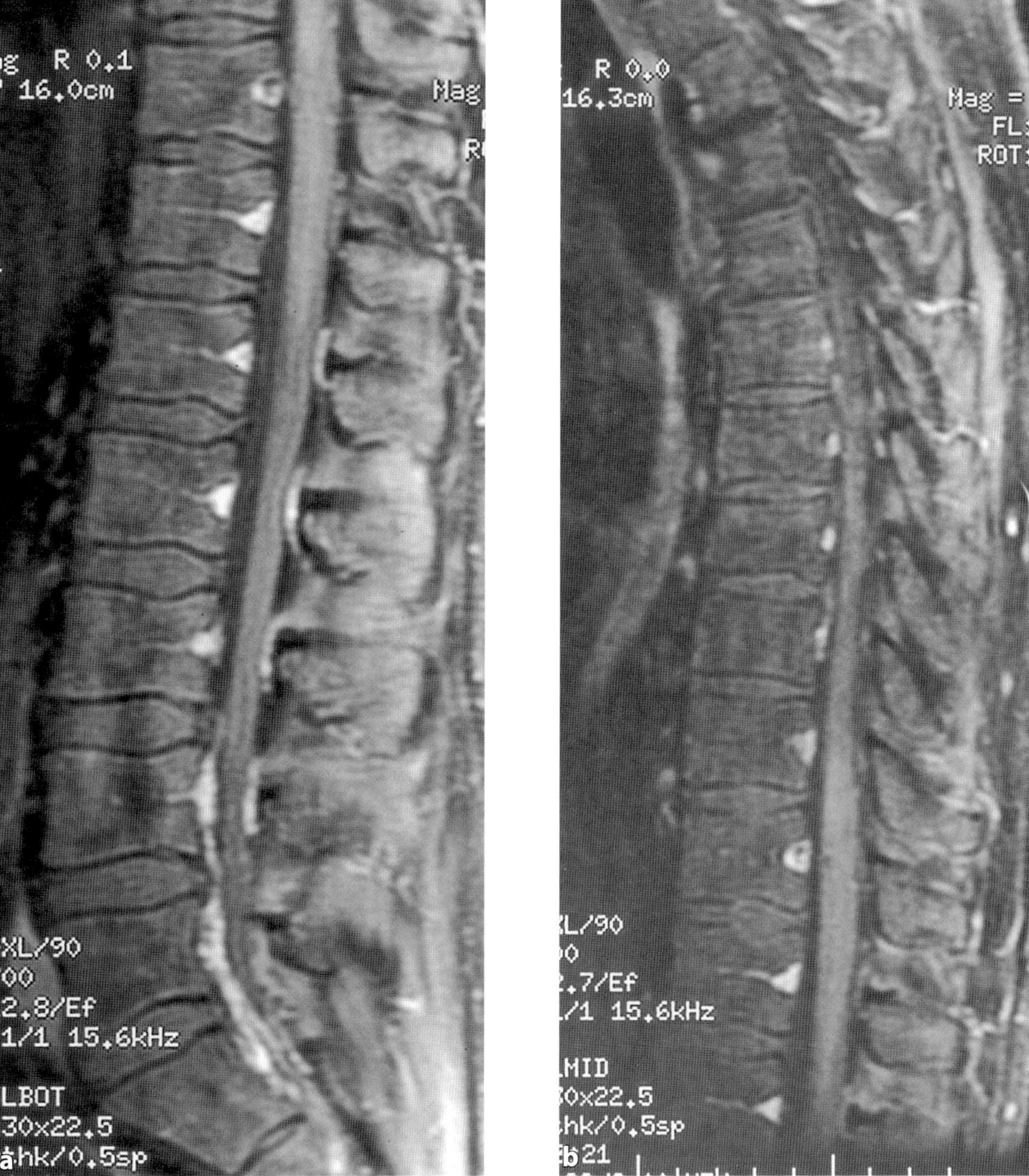

Fig. 5.91a, b. Same patient. Sagittal T1-weighted sequence with fat suppression after contrast administration. Only very weak contrast enhancement of the myelitic lesion in the center of the lower thoracic spinal cord just above the conus medullaris

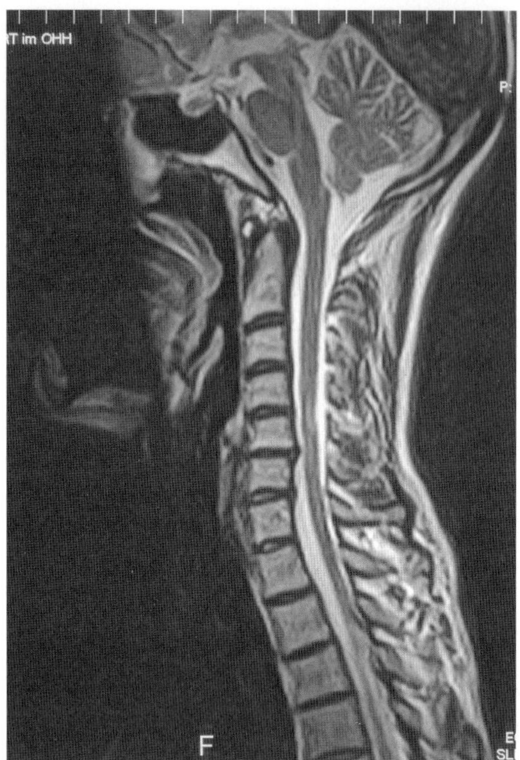

Fig. 5.92. Sagittal T2-weighted image of the cervical region and craniocervical junction in an 88-year-old patient with known multiple sclerosis. Band-like signal increase of the spinal cord at the level of C4-5 with mild kyphosis with the apex at C5-6 and posterior disc protrusion at C5-6 and C6-7

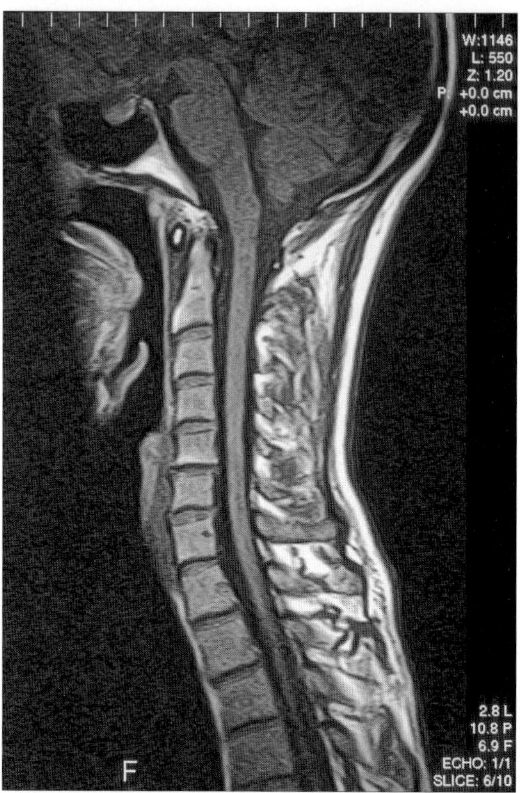

Fig. 5.93. Sagittal T1-weighted image showing normal appearance of the cervical spinal cord in multiple sclerosis

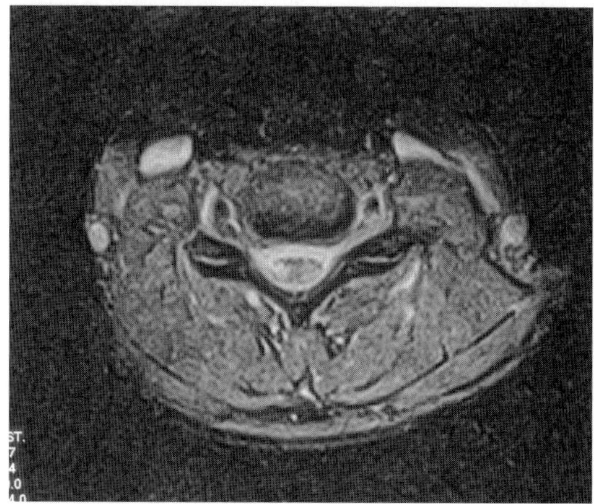

Fig. 5.94. Axial T2-weighted image at the C4-5 level showing a high-signal-intensity intraspinal MS lesion in the right aspect of the cord. Normal size and shape of the cord

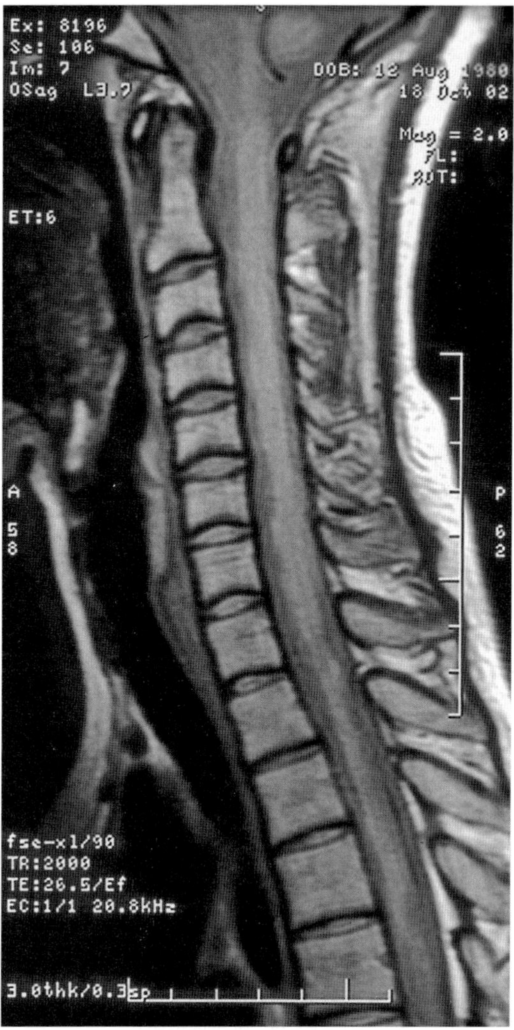

Fig. 5.95. Sagittal proton-density-weighted image. Large confluent signal alterations of the cervical spinal cord from C3 through C6-7 in a patient with acute disseminated encephalomyelitis

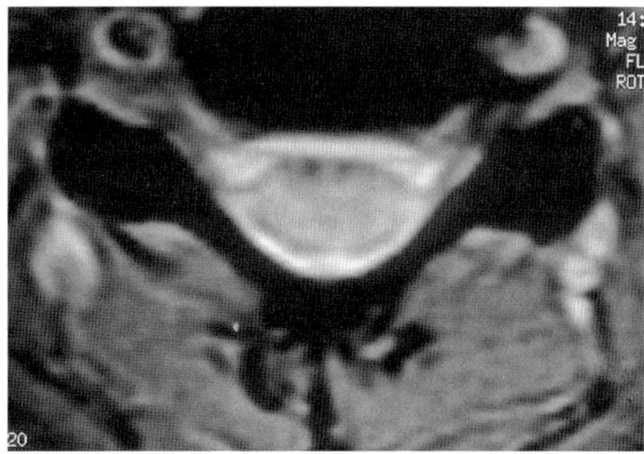

Fig. 5.96. Transverse T2-weighted image. Extensive inflammatory signal alteration of the cervical cord

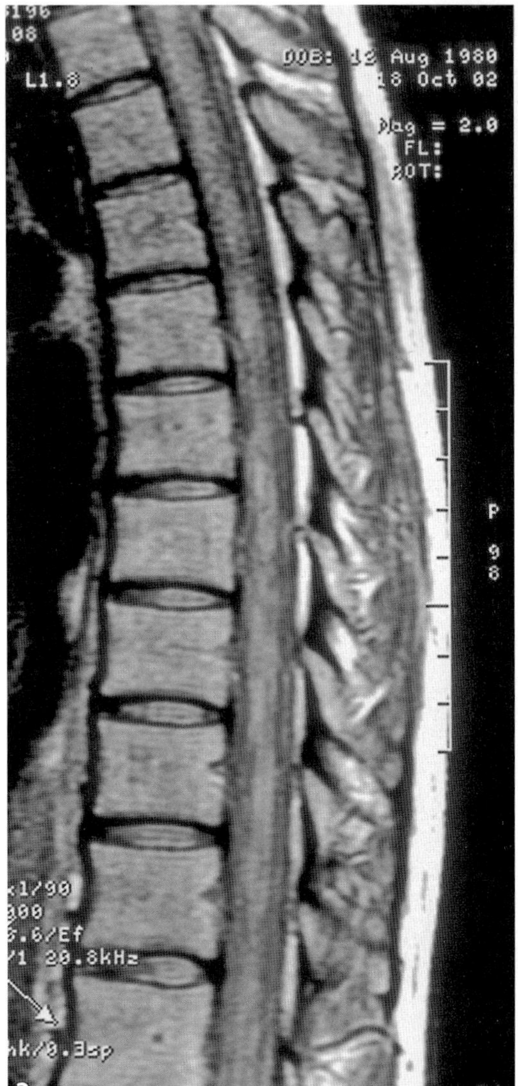

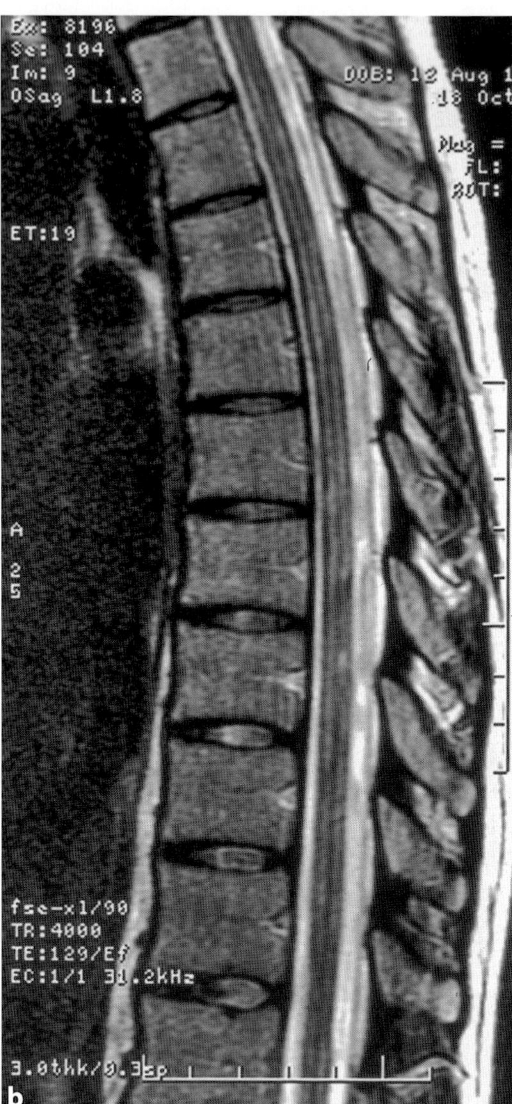

Fig. 5.97a, b. Proton-density- and T2-weighted sagittal images. Multisegmental manifestations of disseminated encephalomyelitis in the thoracic cord and prominent central canal

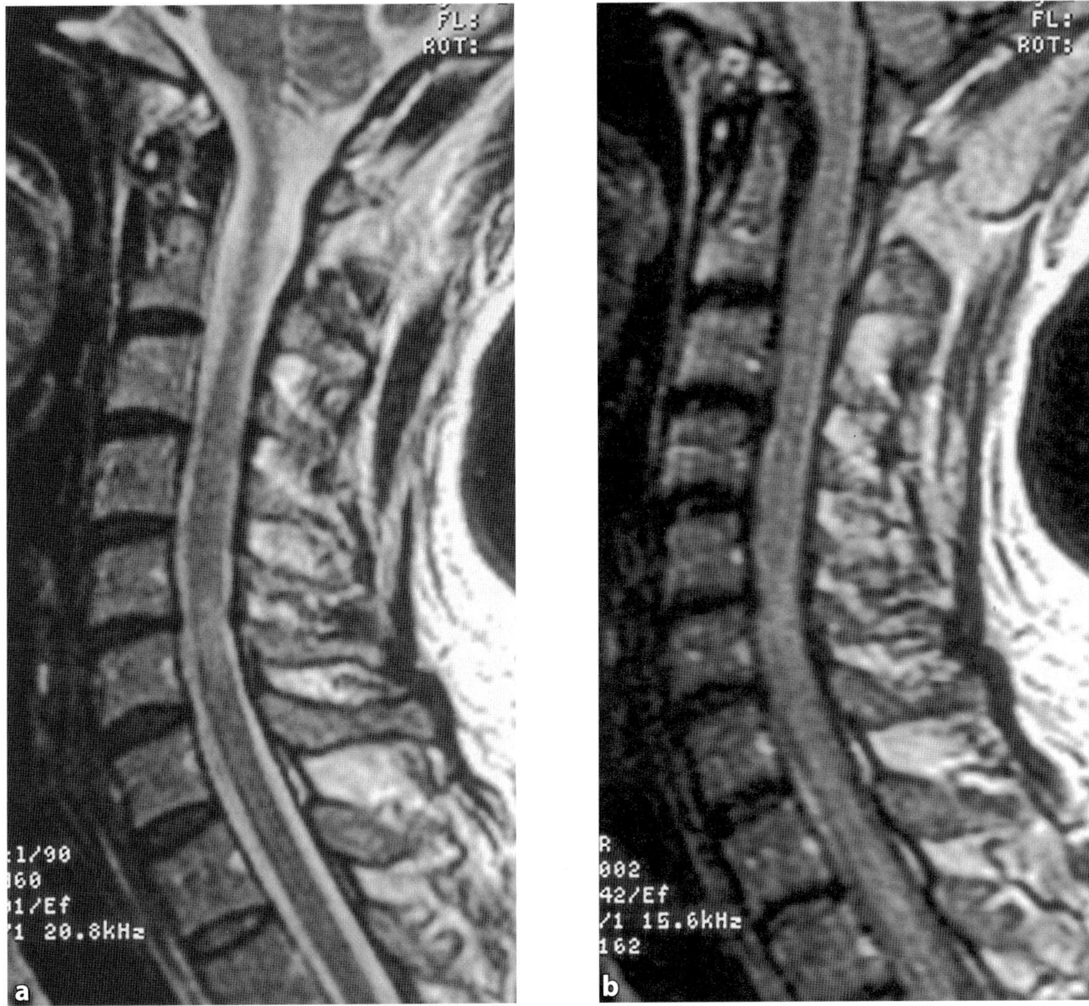

Fig. 5.98. a, b Sagittal T2-weighted image (**a**) and FLAIR image (**b**): manifestation of disseminated encephalomyelitis at C5-6

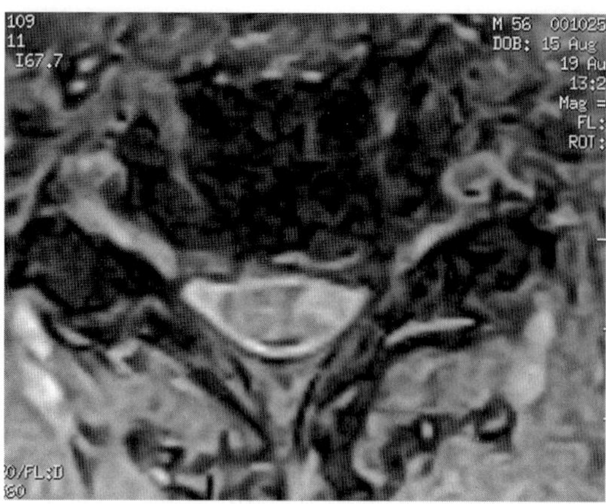

Fig. 5.99. Transverse T2*-weighted image showing eccentric lesion of disseminated encephalomyelitis in the cervical cord

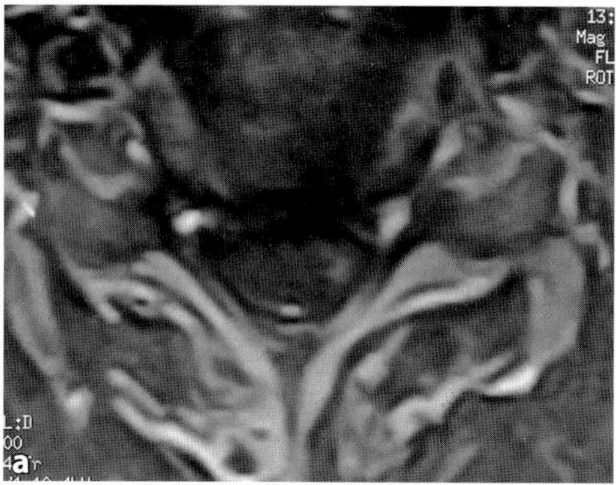

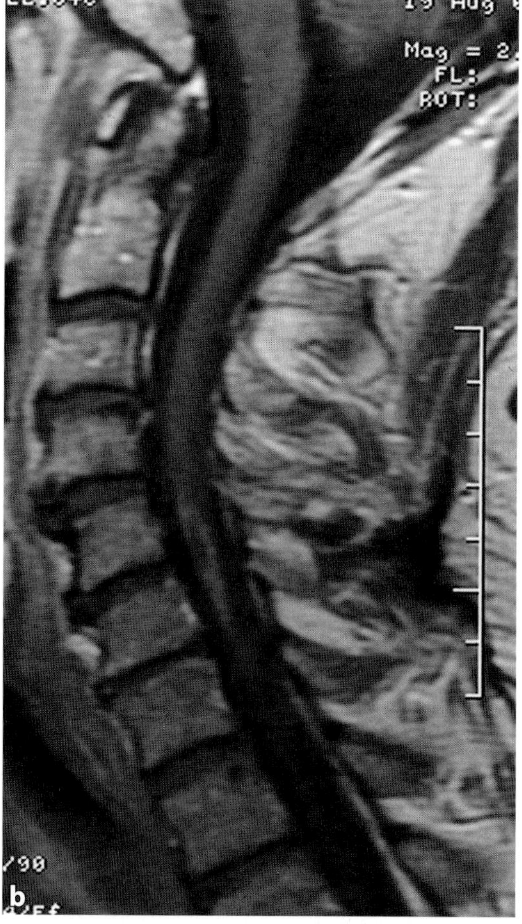

Fig. 5.100a, b. Transverse and sagittal T1-weighted images after contrast administration. Sagittal image showing pronounced peripheral enhancement of the florid disseminated encephalomyelitis lesion

6 Tumors and Tumor-like Lesions

6.1 Neurinoma, Schwannoma, Neurofibroma, and Meningioma

Pathoanatomy and Pathophysiology

Nerve sheaths tumors and meningiomas are tumors of the intradural extramedullary compartment and are relatively uncommon in the general neurosurgical or orthopedic patient population. About 10% to 20% of all primary tumors of the CNS arise in the spinal cord and about 50% of these are extramedullary in location. These tumors are typically seen as well-circumscribed lesions, rarely invade the neural axis, and are benign in over 90% of cases.

Two main types of nerve sheath tumors are distinguished: neurofibromas and neurinomas/schwannomas. Spinal neurinomas are intra-arachnoid tumors while meningiomas are extra-arachnoid in location. Anterior location of a neurinoma is extremely rare, while meningiomas are typically found laterally or anterolaterally in the canal, as they are thought to arise anterior to the denticulate ligament.

Neurofibromas are associated with neurofibromatosis type I (NF-I, also known as von Recklinghausen's or peripheral neurofibromatosis). NF-I is an autosomal dominant disorder related to the long arm of chromosome 17 and is characterized by the presence of cutaneous neurofibromas, café-au-lait spots, iris hamartomas (Lisch nodules), and skeletal changes such as scoliosis or lytic defects (e.g. of the skull).

Multiple peripheral neurofibromas may occur but are often asymptomatic. Peripheral spinal neurofibromas originate among the dorsal sensory nerve roots in close vicinity to the dorsal nerve root ganglia with secondary penetration of the spinal canal.

Other associated tumors of the CNS are gliomas of the optical nerve and hypothalamus, ependymomas, peripheral neuroectodermal tumors (PNETs), meningiomas, and hamartomas.

Neurofibromatosis type II (NF-II, central neurofibromatosis) is also an autosomal dominant disorder with complex genetic defects. It is characterized by bilateral acoustic neurinomas of the statoacoustic nerve, and there is an association with meningiomas. NF-II patients sporadically develop spinal schwannomas or ependymomas.

Malignant degeneration of nerve sheath tumors (neurofibrosarcoma, malignant schwannoma) is uncommon (2-4%) and occurs in adults. De novo malignant spinal schwannomas and neurofibrosarcomas have also been observed after local radiotherapy.

Neurinomas and schwannomas are usually easier to delineate than neurofibromas, which are typically fusiform. They also arise from the dorsal nerve root, more specifically, from one of its components (root cells or fascicle). Neurofibromas and schwannomas differ in their histologic appearance and biologic features although they may originate from the same class of stem cells.

Meningiomas arise from clusters of arachnoid cells at the exit sites of nerve roots or entry sites of segmental arteries. This also seems to explain the typical lateral and anterolateral localization of meningiomas as compared with neurinomas.

Intradural meningiomas are twice as common in women than in men and are typically diagnosed in women between 50 and 70 years. Multiple intradural meningiomas are found in 1% to 2% of cases. Some meningiomas have intradural and extradural components. Hormonal and genetic factors are involved in the pathogenesis of meningiomas, as there is an association with pregnancy and an increased incidence in women with breast cancer. An association between meningioma development and prior trauma or irradiation is known for intracranial tumors but has not been confirmed for spinal meningioma. Most spinal meningiomas are of the psammomatous type, while younger patients may occasionally present with a more aggressive angioblastic meningioma.

MR Technique

MR imaging is the modality of choice for the diagnostic assessment of intradural extramedullary tumors. The standard protocol comprises sagittal and axial T1- and T2-weighted sequences including T1-weighted imaging after Gd-DTPA administration. Slice orientation and coil selection depend on the site of the tumor.

MR Findings

Neurinomas and neurofibromas are typically isointense to neural structures on T1-weighted images with a very high signal on T2-weighted images. Both tumors show strong enhancement after contrast administration, occasionally the appearance is heterogeneous with areas of less pronounced enhancement. These two tumors must be differentiated from other extramedullary lesions, in particular meningiomas. The following features help differentiate neurinomas and meningiomas on MRI:

- Localization:
  Neurinoma – mainly cervical and lumbar regions,
  Meningioma – mainly thoracic region;
- T2-weighted images:
  Neurinoma – pronounced hyperintensity,
  Meningioma – slight or no hyperintensity;
- T1-weighted images after Gd-DTPA:
  Neurinoma – high signal intensity, heterogeneous, small cysts,
  Meningioma – moderately high signal, homogeneous;
- Dura:
  Neurinoma – normal appearance,
  Meningioma – prominent enhancement of adjacent dura (meningeal tail sign).

On T1-weighted images, the tumors are isointense or slightly hypointense.

When MRI demonstrates a meningioma at the craniocervical junction or a dumbbell neurinoma in the cervical region, MR angiography should be performed to identify possible displacement or encasement of the vertebral arteries by the tumor (Figs. 6.1–6.55).

MR Pitfalls

The diagnosis of a neurinoma with a typical growth pattern (extramedullary intradural tumor with extradural extension through the intervertebral foramina [dumbbell neurinoma]) is usually straightforward. An occasional tumor may be difficult or impossible to differentiate from a purely extradural meningioma.

Clinical Significance

MR imaging of the entire CNS and genetic testing are mandatory in patients with clinically suspected neurofibromatosis.

Patients in whom radiography or a CT scan demonstrates marked widening of an intervertebral foramen or smooth bone erosions should undergo an MRI examination for further diagnostic evaluation even when they have no symptoms.

While neurinomas typically present with initial radicular symptoms, meningiomas are more commonly associated with symptoms of spinal cord compression. Characteristically, these tumors are associated with slow progression of symptoms. As the tumors grow slowly, the spinal cord can adjust to increasing compression, which enables almost complete recovery of function after surgery even in patients with severe neurologic deficits. Even very large dumbbell-shaped neurinomas at the craniocervical junction or in the throacolumbar region may be asymptomatic or cause only unspecific symptoms for months or years. Hence, there are no specific clinical symptoms that would enable the differentiation of intraspinal extramedullary tumors from other spinal conditions such as syringomyelia, spondylotic radiculomyelopathy, spinal arteriovenous malformation, multiple sclerosis, or a granulomatous inflammatory process.

Careful evaluation of the relationship of the tumor to the spinal cord is important for choosing the most appropriate surgical access. Purely anterior approaches are rarely necessary. Surgical removal of a meningioma at the foramen magnum may occasionally require a far lateral access with condylectomy and the need for subsequent stabilization. Most tumors can be accessed by laminotomy, possibly in conjunction with unilateral facetectomy.

6.2 Astrocytoma

MR Technique

Typical T2- and T1-weighted sequences in sagittal and transverse planes, supplemented by coronal images as needed. Contrast-enhanced T1-weighted images to identify hemorrhage/calcification. T2-weighted gradient echo sequences.

MR Findings

Spinal astrocytomas are characterized by an increased signal intensity on T2-weighted images and may appear homogeneous or inhomogeneous (hemorrhage, necrosis, cysts). Perifocal edema is typical. On T1-weighted images, they are isointense or slightly hypointense relative to the spinal cord. Nearly all spinal astrocytomas show enhancement on postcontrast images (and, in contrast to cerebral astrocytomas, enhancement is independent of the tumor grade). See Figs. 6.56–6.62.

MR Pitfalls

It is often not possible to differentiate a spinal astrocytoma from ependymoma (astrocytoma tends to be eccentric in location, while ependymoma is more commonly found centrally and is more likely to show hemorrhage).

6.3 Ependymoma

Pathoanatomy and Pathophysiology

Intraspinal ependymomas can be found in the intramedullary or extramedullary compartment with extramedullary tumors occurring exclusively in the cauda equina. They arise from residual ependymal cells in the central canal of the spinal cord or in the filum terminale. Intramedullary ependymomas with an extramedullary, exophytic component are extremely rare. Large intramedullary ependymomas may extend throughout the cervical or thoracic spinal cord, but cervical tumors involving 2 to 3 segments are the most common form.

Ependymomas are slow-growing tumors that may become very large but cause only mild clinical symptoms such as unspecific back pain or radicular pain and paresthesia. Three histologic subtypes - cellular, papillary, and myopapillary - are distinguished with the myxopapillary type being the most common. Anaplastic spinal ependymoma is rare and the only form with secondary intraspinal spread.

Ependymal tumors are well-defined lesions that are easily distinguished from the normal spinal cord or cauda equina and are characterized by expansive growth. In contrast, an intraspinal astrocytoma may be difficult to differentiate from the normal cord. Hemorrhage or infarction of an ependymoma in the cauda equina can cause an acute cauda equina syndrome.

Cauda equina ependymoma may be associated with a syndrome of increased intracranial pressure with headaches and papillary edema via a mechanism (increased protein?) that is not yet fully understood.

MR Findings

An early ependymoma may present as a small mass of the same signal intensity as the surrounding cord on T1-weighted images with slight contrast enhancement, making it difficult to differentiate from other entities. With further growth, the MR appearance becomes more characteristic with the intramedullary tumor assuming a sausage-like shape and typically showing heterogeneous enhancement after Gd-DTPA administration. The residual spinal cord around the tumor is reduced to a thin line. There may be cysts at the upper and lower poles of the solid tumor, which are most clearly visualized on T2-weighted images. The MR appearance does not allow differentiation of an intramedullary ependymoma from an astrocytoma (Figs. 6.63–6.66).

Clinical Significance

The good demarcation of an intramedullary ependymoma from the normal cord makes the tumor amenable to complete resection by myelotomy and microsurgical resection. In contrast to intracranial ependymomas, spinal tumors rarely recur when complete resection is achieved of a cauda equina or intramedullary ependymoma histologically classified as grade I or II.

Early surgical removal is desirable even if slight neurologic deficits occur after the intervention (e.g. impaired proprioception). No neurologic improvement can be achieved in patients with paresis or muscular atrophy. Radiotherapy is not indicated and biopsy with decompression and radiotherapy have been abandoned. Only highly malignant intraspinal tumors such as glioblastoma or anaplastic astrocytoma are treated by irradiation.

6.4 Hemangioblastoma

Pathoanatomy and Pathophysiology

Although hemangioblastomas are the most common tumors of the posterior cranial fossa in adults, they rarely occur in the spinal column, constituting only about 3% of intramedullary tumors. Multiple spinal hemangioblastomas, which are frequently asymptomatic, may occur in patients with von Hippel-Lindau syndrome (cerebellar hemangioblastoma, retinal angiomatosis, renal cell carcinoma). A hemangioblastoma is a highly vascularized tumor that is pial or subpial in location but may also occur extradurally. More than half of the tumors are associated with cysts. The cyst fluid has a high protein content from transudation of fluid by the tumor. The cysts may become very large relative to the tumor size and are not part of the tumor.

MR Findings

Hemangioblastomas are characterized by vigorous contrast enhancement. The signal from the cyst cavity varies with the protein content of the fluid. Large edema is another common finding. The diagnosis of hemangioblastoma is further corroborated by the demonstration of vessels, which are depicted as signal voids.

MR angiography may be useful when evaluating a solid tumor (Figs. 6.67–6.69). Angiography may be indicated for embolization of feeding vessels.

MR Pitfalls

Hemangioblastoma must be distinguished from intramedullary metastasis, which is associated with edema.

Clinical Significance

Small multiple hemangioblastomas should be followed up by MRI. Symptomatic lesions in the spinal canal are operated on, especially when they have a cystic component.

6.5 Epidermoids and Dermoids

Pathoanatomy and Pathophysiology

Epidermoid and dermoid cysts arise from displaced ectoderm at the time of closure of the neural tube at three to for weeks of gestation. An epidermoid cyst is lined with squamous epithelium and contains soft, bead-like masses of keratin, which increase with the age of the cyst. Dermoid cysts have the same lining but contain complete cutaneous appendages such as hair follicles. The fluid has an oily consistency.

MR Findings

MRI allows evaluation of the relationship of an epidermoid or dermoid cyst to the spinal cord or cauda equina. The lesions may be isointense to CSF on T2-weighted sequences. Differentiation is possible with diffusion-weighted imaging (DWI), which will depict epidermoids with a bright signal (Figs. 6.70–6.72).

MR Pitfalls

Problems may arise in differentiating epidermoid or dermoid cysts from tumor cysts. This is why contrast-enhanced sequences are mandatory to exclude a neoplasm. Tarlov cysts can be distinguished from other cysts by their location at the sacral roots. Epithelial cysts (neurenteric cysts) developing from an abnormal, persisting canal between ectoderm and endoderm are commonly but not exclusively located anteriorly and may be associated with other anomalies (diastematomyelia, cleft vertebra).

Clinical Significance

Epidermoid und dermoid cysts are characterized by slow growth. A congenital dermal sinus should be excised together with the epidermoid.

Intradural epidermoid cysts occur secondary to the introduction of epithelial cells, e.g. through lumbar puncture. This type of cyst is rare.

6.6 Vascular Lesions

Pathoanatomy and Pathophysiology

The spinal cord is supplied by three arteries extending from the medulla oblongata to the conus medullaris: a single anterior spinal artery and paired posterior spinal arteries.

The anterior spinal artery originates from the distal branches of the vertebral arteries and courses through the anterior sulcus where it is joined by the radiculomedullary arteries arising from the vertebral, ascending cervical, segmental intercostal, and lumbar arteries. The radiculomedullary arteries penetrate the dura at the nerve root sleeves where they give off a regular dural branch to supply the dura and the nerve root. Medullary branches, which are not consistently present, interconnect the anterior spinal artery and the posterior spinal arteries. The radiculomedullary arteries run intradurally and have an ascending course. The largest medullary feeder is the artery of Adamkiewicz, which arises from the intercostal branches of the lower thoracic aorta, typically at the T9 level. It occurs on the left side in 80% of subjects. In a similar manner, the cervical portion of the spinal cord is supplied by the artery of Lazorthes, the large radiculomedullary artery of the C5 or C6 segment.

The anterior spinal artery gives off radial branches that supply the anterior two thirds of the spinal cord. The posterior spinal arteries supply the posterior portion. Venous drainage is through radial veins opening into the coronal venous plexus.

Four types of spinal arteriovenous malformations (AVMs) are distinguished:

- dural arteriovenous fistula (type I AVM),
- intramedullary arteriovenous malformations (types II and III, so-called glomus AVM and juvenile AVM),
- extramedullary and perimedullary AVMs (type IV).

Type I AVMs are located at a neural foramen and are supplied by dural branches of the radicular arteries. The intradural component of such a fistula consists of a convolution of tortuous arterialized veins on the posterior surface of the spinal cord. Dural fistulas are the most common type and are regarded as acquired malformations. They typically present with slowly progressive myelopathy in the second half of life.

Intramedullary type II AVMs consist of a compact intramedullary nidus fed from the anterior spinal artery and draining into the coronal plexus. The juvenile type (type III) is extremely rare. The malformation has a very complex architecture and is supplied by radiculomedullary branches from different levels. It may be large with extramedullary and even extraspinal extension.

Type IV AVMs are extramedullary in location, typically on the anterior surface of the spinal cord and rarely on the posterior surface. The draining veins are extremely dilated.

AVMs damage the spinal cord by various mechanisms. These include venous congestion with subsequent ischemia and myelopathy (e.g. dural AV fistula and peridural AVM), intramedullary bleeding with direct damage to the cord (e.g. glomus AVM), thrombosis, compression by the convoluted varicose vessels, and concomitant aneurysm.

MR Findings

An intramedullary AVM (types II and III) is seen as a low-signal-intensity area with flow voids on T1-weighted sequences. The surrounding spinal cord may appear heterogeneous. Focal areas of high signal intensity indicate earlier hemorrhage. MRI is currently the method of choice for evaluating both the intramedullary and the extramedullary components of such malformations.

The absence of spinal cord enlargement and the presence of flow voids representing the tortuous vessels on the posterior surface of the cord are characteristic of spinal dural AV fistulas on MRI.

A high signal within the cord on T2-weighted images indicates edema due to vascular congestion. These intramedullary changes are reversible if closure of the fistula is achieved before the patient develops myelomalacia (Fig. 6.73–6.79).

MR Pitfalls

MR angiography is indicated in patients with suspected spinal AVM but does not allow accurate evaluation of feeding and draining vessels. Great care must be taken not to mistake pulsation artifacts for flow voids. Inconclusive cases may be resolved using gradient echo sequences.

Conventional, selective, and superselective angiography continues to be the gold standard and is indicated for selecting the most suitable therapeutic approach in patients with strong MR evidence of spinal AVM.

Clinical Significance

MRI enables early diagnosis of a spinal vascular malformation, which would otherwise require invasive diagnostic tests such as myelography or angiography. Type I spinal AVMs can be operated on with a very low risk, while the other types are usually treated by (repeated) endovascular embolization or a combination of embolization and surgery.

6.7 Sarcoidosis

Pathoanatomy and Pathophysiology

Sarcoidosis may affect the peripheral or central nervous system. Involvement of the spinal cord is less common than sarcoidosis of the meninges or intracranial nerves, hypothalamus, or pituitary gland.

MR Findings

Sarcoidosis is characterized by a patchy or diffuse signal increase of the spinal cord on T2-weighted images. T1-weighted sequences show thickening of the cord and occasionally a decreased signal intensity. Linear meningeal contrast enhancement is more common than focal or diffuse enhancement of the spinal cord (Fig. 6.80).

MR Pitfalls

MRI does not allow differentiation of sarcoidosis lesions from small intraspinal neoplasms, since both types of lesions expand the spinal cord. Unspecific myelitis and disseminated encephalomyelitis are other entities to be considered in the differential diagnosis, especially in patients without a history of sarcoidosis.

Clinical Significance

Clinical and radiologic follow-up and the response to corticoid treatment can help corroborate the diagnosis of sarcoidosis. Biopsy of a mass lesion may be considered in cases where the diagnosis cannot be established systemically.

6.8 Bone Tumors

Anatomy and Pathoanatomy

All bone tumors that may affect the bony spine, except for chordoma, also occur elsewhere in the skeleton. While primary bone tumors arising from the spine and sacrum are extremely rare, metastatic spread to the bony spine is common. Data from different bone tumor registries suggests that spinal tumors account for about 3% of all primary bone tumors. These are in decreasing order of frequency:

- aneurysmal bone cysts,
- osteoid osteoma,
- osteoblastoma,
- osteochondroma,
- giant cell tumors.

Among the malignant tumors, chordoma is by far the most common type after tumors not differentiating toward bone tissue (plasmocytoma, malignant lymphoma).

Theoretically, all primary malignant tumors can also occur in the bony spine, although this localization is very rare.

In the vast majority of both benign and malignant bone tumors, the normal vertebral bone is destroyed and replaced by tumor tissue. The tumor may extend beyond the vertebrae and invade paravertebral structures.

The tumor type is suggested by certain localizations within the bony spine (e.g. chordoma in the sacral region or metastasis from hypernephroma at L1) or by the affected part (vertebral arch: osteoid osteoma, osteoblastoma, osteochondroma; vertebral body: hemangioma, giant cell tumor; lesions involving more than one segment: aneurysmal bone cyst).

Pathomechanism

The skeleton is the third most common site of metastatic spread after the lung and liver. Over two thirds of all skeletal metastases are found in the spine. Spread to the spine is hematogenous including rare cases of retrograde venous spread (L1 metastasis from hypernephroma). Some primary nonskeletal malignancies have a conspicuous affinity to bone. These are in decreasing order of frequency: breast cancer, prostate cancer, lung cancer, renal cancer, thyroid cancer, and Hodgkin/non-Hodgkin lymphoma.

Osteoid Osteoma

Questionable neoplasm. Osteoid osteomas are found in children and juveniles in 80% of cases and typically involve the posterior elements. Pain is the leading symptom, which is why painful scoliosis in children or juveniles should alert the physician to the possibility of osteoid osteoma (Figs. 6.81–6.84).

Osteoblastoma

As with osteoid osteomas, osteoblastomas typically affect the posterior elements and can be differentiated from the former by a diameter >1 cm. Histologic differentiation of these two tumors is not possible. Osteoblastoma is the third most common spinal tumor, after aneurysmal bone cysts and osteoid osteoma (Figs. 6.85–6.92).

Aneurysmal Bone Cysts

Aneurysmal bone cysts are expansive osteolytic lesions frequently involving more than one vertebra. The cysts predominantly arise from the posterior elements but also extend to the vertebral bodies. They are highly vascular lesions that may mimic a tumor (Figs. 6.93–6.96).

Chordoma

Chordomas arise from remnants of the embryonic notochord, which normally develop into the nucleus pulposus of the intervertebral disc. The notochord is part of the primitive skeleton between the clivus and sacrum. This is why chordomas can occur anywhere along the spinal axis, but they are typically found in the sacrum (50%) or clivus (35%), less commonly in the cervical and lumbar regions and least often in the thoracic spine. Chordomas invade surrounding structures (soft tissue, vertebral canal) and can metastasize. The macroscopic appearance is that of a lobulated tumor with fibrous septa, which is typically surrounded by a capsule. Based on histologic criteria, chordomas have more features of benign tumors, while their biological behavior makes them malignant tumors, since they are characterized by osteodestructive growth, slow but steady progression, and the ability to metastasize (Figs. 6.97–6.100).

Eosinophilic Granuloma

Eosinophilic granulomas are monostotic or polyostotic tumor-mimicking lesions. Spinal eosinophilic granulomas tend to involve an entire vertebral body, which may collapse as a result (classical vertebra plana) (Figs. 6.101–6.105).

While vertebra plana in children is often due to eosinophilic granuloma, other osteolytic conditions must be considered as well (such as neuroblastoma, malignant lymphoma, leukemia).

Plasmocytoma

See Figs. 6.106–6.115.

Malignant Fibrous Histiocytoma

This highly malignant bone tumor was recognized as a separate tumor entity three decades ago and used to be classified with the group of fibrosarcomas and fibroblastic osteosarcomas. It is a tumor of adulthood. Unlike bone metastases, primary fibroblastic osteolytic tumors show early invasion beyond bony structures and have large extraosseous soft tissue components (Figs. 6.116–6.120). Malignant fibrous histiocytoma is rare and spinal manifestations, like in other primary malignant bone tumors (except for chondrosarcoma and chordoma), are extremely uncommon (only about 1% of the primary malignant bone tumors occur in the spine).

Metastasis

See Figs. 6.121–6.154.

Clinical Significance

MRI has become an indispensable tool in the preoperative diagnostic evaluation of patients with tumors of the bony spine and should be performed before a tissue sample is obtained for histology. It serves to determine extravertebral and intraspinal tumor extension and to evaluate tumor vascularization on contrast-enhanced images (caveat: hypernephroma metastasis, true hemangioma, giant cell tumors, solid aneurysmal bone cysts).

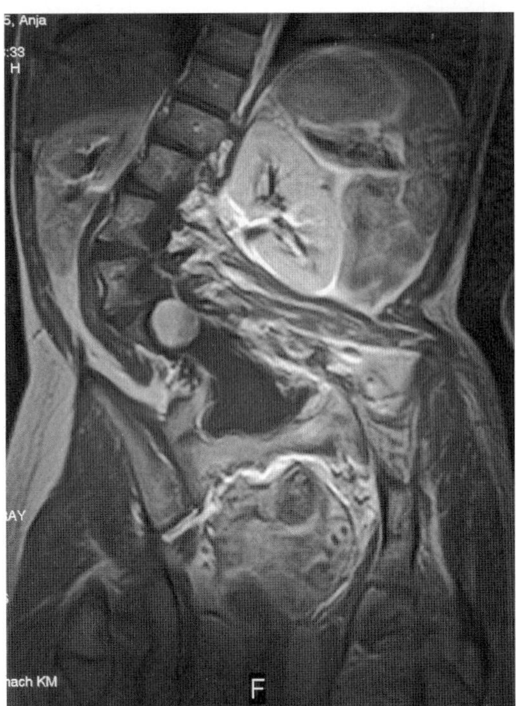

Fig. 6.1. Contrast-enhanced coronal T1-weighted image of the lumbar region in a 16-year-old girl with severe scoliosis. Large neurofibroma at L3-4 with pronounced contrast enhancement in the area of the spinal canal

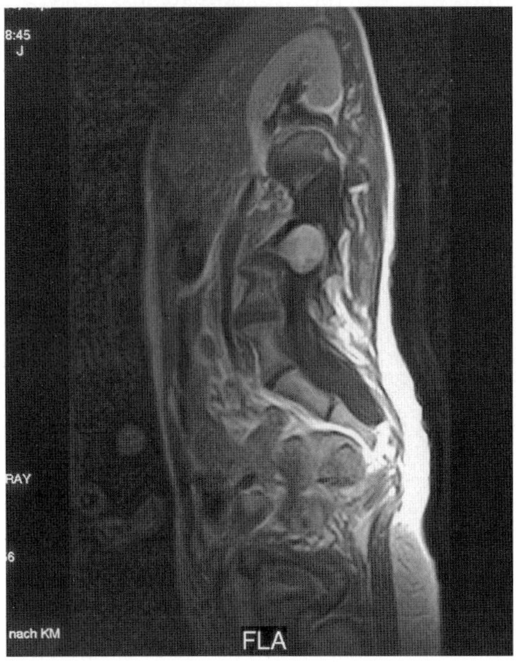

Fig. 6.2. Contrast-enhanced sagittal T1-weighted image of the lumbar region depicting the L3-4 neurofibroma as a large, well-defined, rounded lesion of high signal intensity within the spinal canal

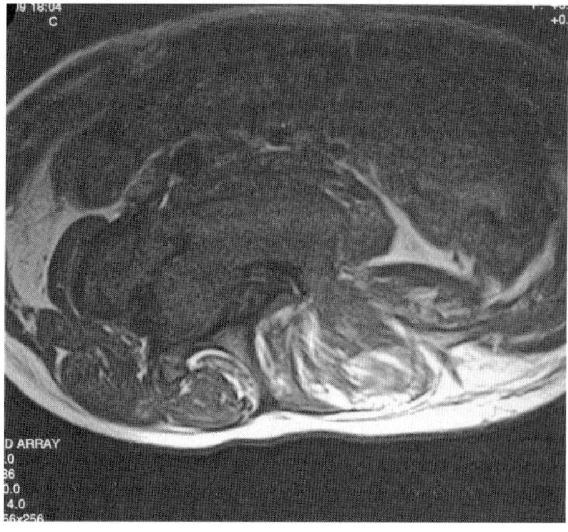

Fig. 6.3. Same patient (L3-4 neurofibroma). Axial T1-weighted image through the L3-4 level depicting the soft-tissue-signal-intensity lesion in the area of the scoliotic curve and paravertebrally on the right side

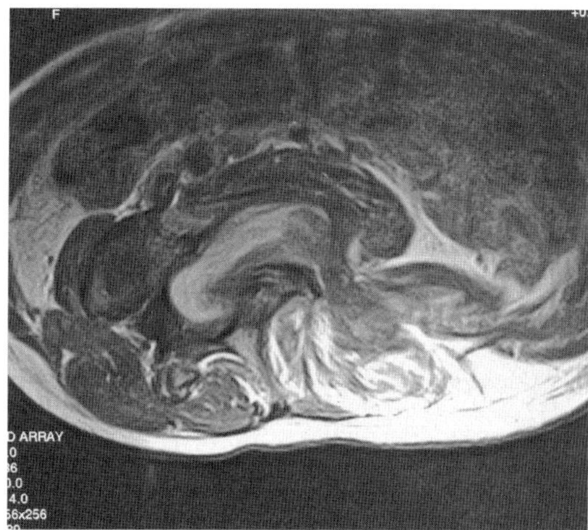

Fig. 6.4. Contrast-enhanced axial T1-weighted image through the L3-4 level showing the markedly enhancing mass intraspinally and to the left of the spinal canal. Neurofibroma with severe left concave scoliosis

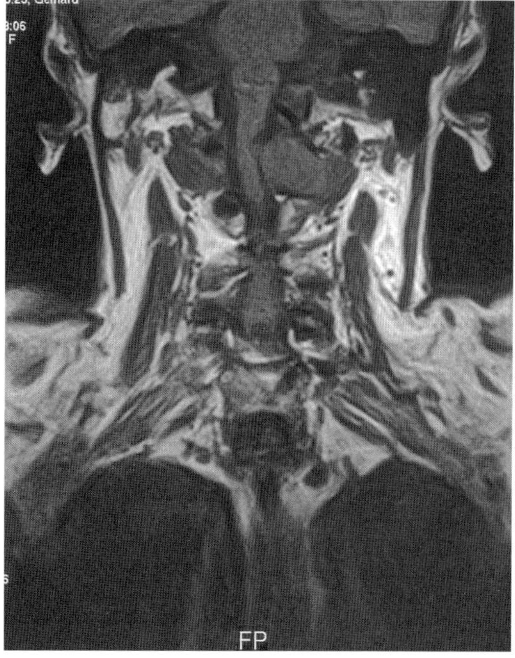

Fig. 6.5. Coronal T1-weighted image in a 76-year-old patient with a large neurinoma at C2-3 on the left. Most of the tumor is located in the left C3 foramen, which is almost completely occupied by tumor tissue and expanded. Deformity and displacement of the proximal cervical spinal cord

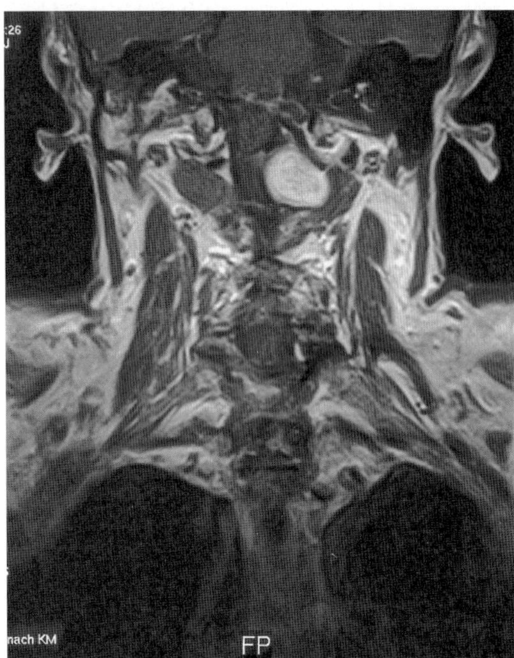

Fig. 6.6. Same patient. Contrast-enhanced coronal T1-weighted image showing clear enhancement of the neurinoma at the C2-3 level on the left

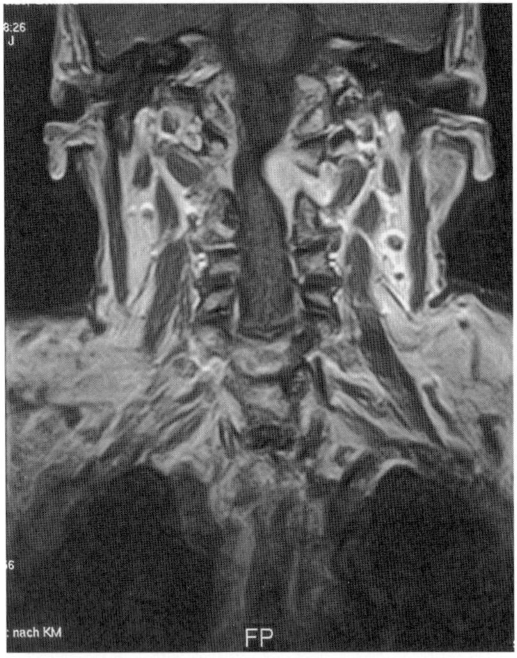

Fig. 6.7. Contrast-enhanced coronal T1-weighted image of the cervical region. Depiction of the intraforaminal portion of the C2-3 neurinoma is improved and the large intraspinal component is also clearly visible

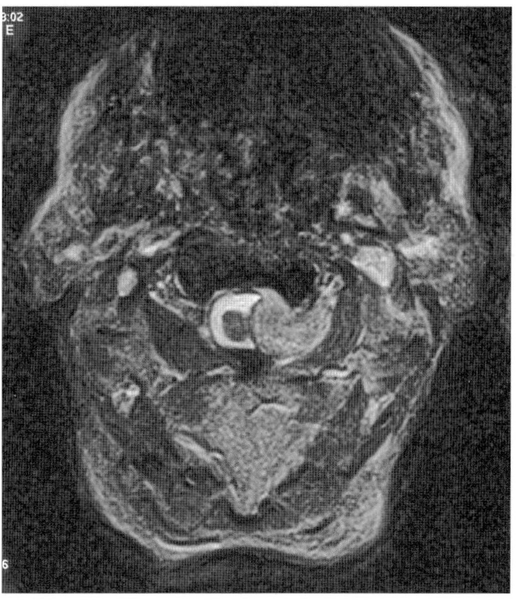

Fig. 6.8. Same patient (C2-3 neurinoma). Axial T2-weighted image showing marked indentation of the dural sac by the neurinoma and slight displacement of the cervical spinal cord to the right. Widening of the left C3 foramen.

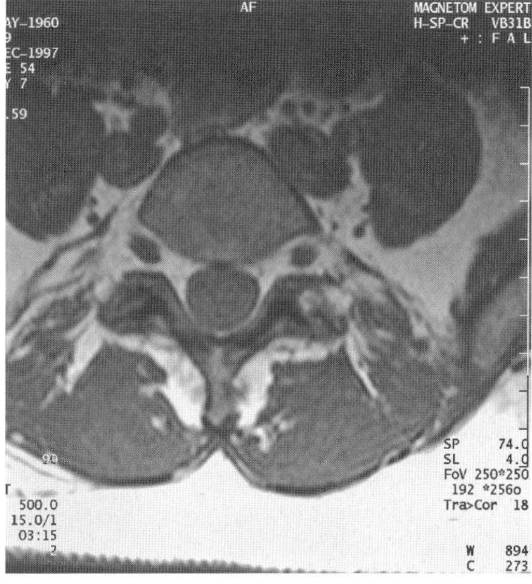

Fig. 6.9. 40-year-old patient with low back symptoms. Axial T1-weighted image of the lumbar spine at the L5-S1 level. Slight signal enhancement of intradural structures without clear evidence of a mass lesion in this patient with schwannoma

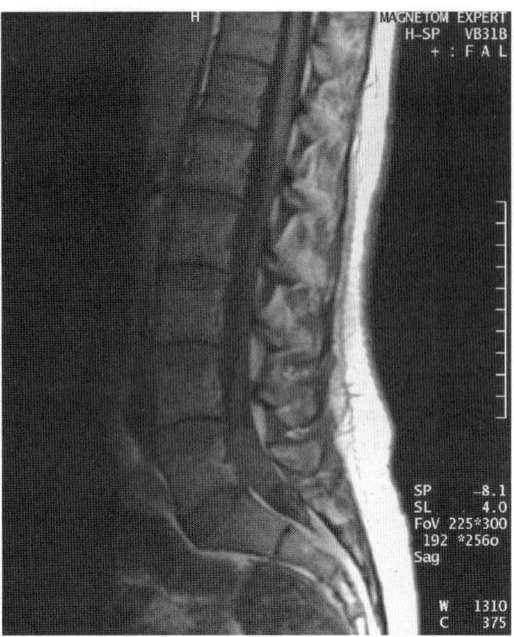

Fig. 6.10. Same patient (schwannoma). Sagittal T1-weighted image showing a poorly demarcated intraspinal tumor extending from L4-5 to L5-S1

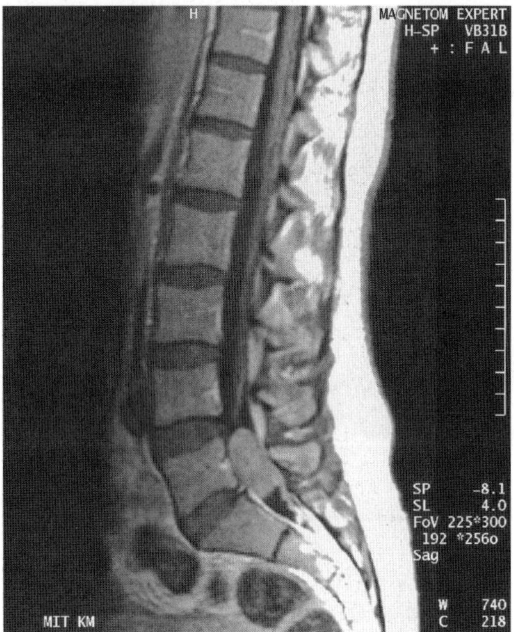

Fig. 6.11. Sagittal T1-weighted image of the lumbar region after contrast administration showing the markedly enhanced intraspinal schwannoma from L4-5 to L5-S1

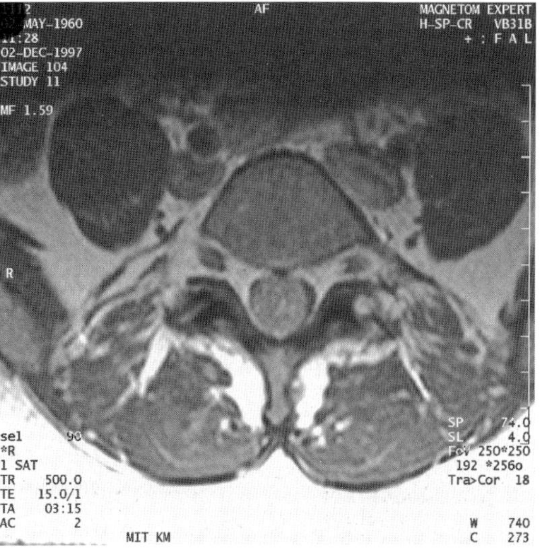

Fig. 6.12. Same patient as in preceding figures. Contrast-enhanced axial T1-weighted image showing the intradural schwannoma as an area of high signal intensity at the L5-S1 level. The tumor is visualized more clearly than on the unenhanced images and nearly completely fills the intradural space. The intraspinal nerve roots are pushed to the side and are seen mostly laterally on the left and anterolaterally on the right

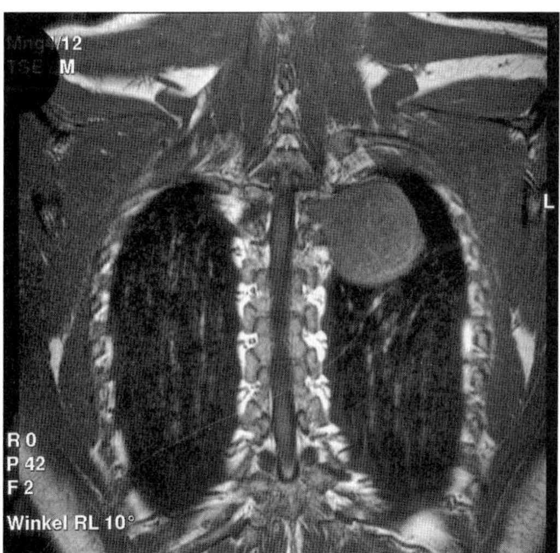

Fig. 6.13. Coronal T1-weighted image of the thoracic spine showing a large paravertebral tumorous lesion on the left at the T3 level. Schwannoma confirmed at surgery

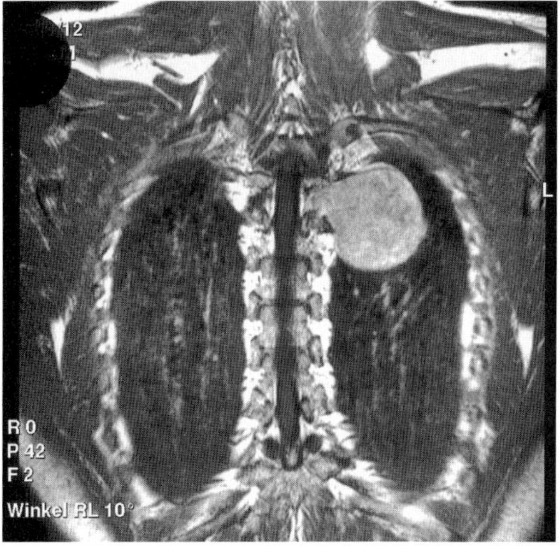

Fig. 6.14. Coronal T1-weighted image after contrast administration showing clear but slightly inhomogeneous enhancement of the left-sided schwannoma, which extends paravertebrally from T3 to T4

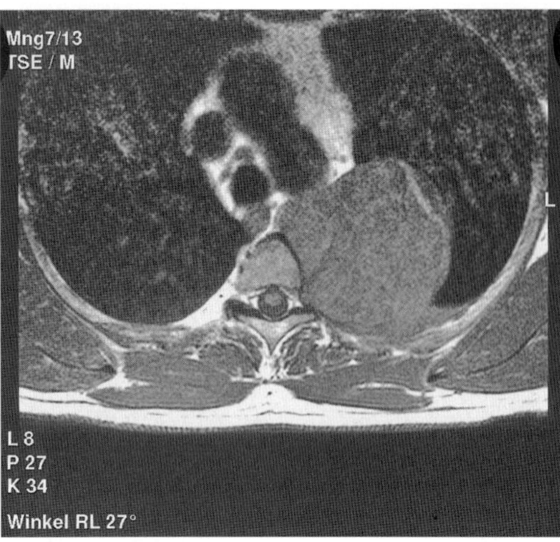

Fig. 6.15. Same patient. Axial T1-weighted image through the T3 level showing the large left paravertebral schwannoma. There is no definitive evidence of extensions into the spinal canal

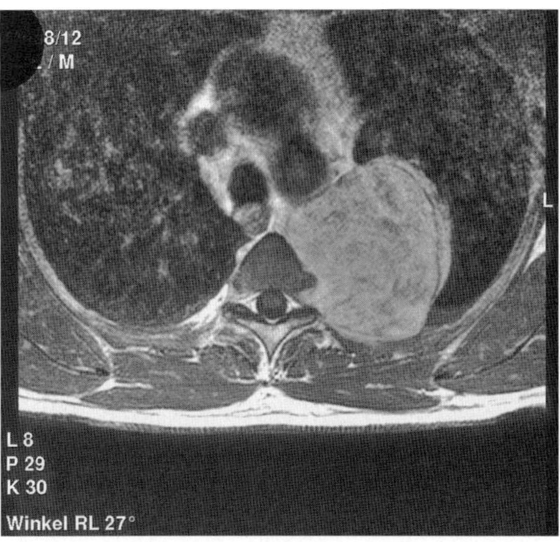

Fig. 6.16. Axial T1-weighted image after contrast administration showing moderate enhancement of the left paravertebral schwannoma and a small extension into the left T3 neural foramen. There is no evidence of bony erosion or destruction of the vertebral body

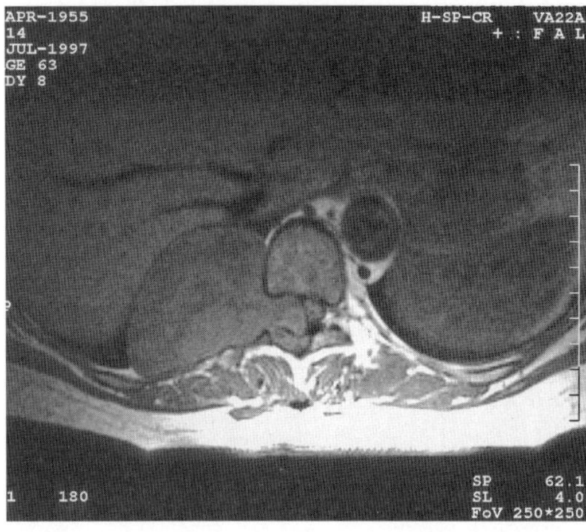

Fig. 6.17. Axial T1-weighted image through the T9 level in a 47-year-old patient with thoracic spine complaints. The image shows a large right paravertebral neurinoma with an intramedullary component. The tumor has low signal intensity, nearly isointense to the liver, and has a size of about 4×5 cm

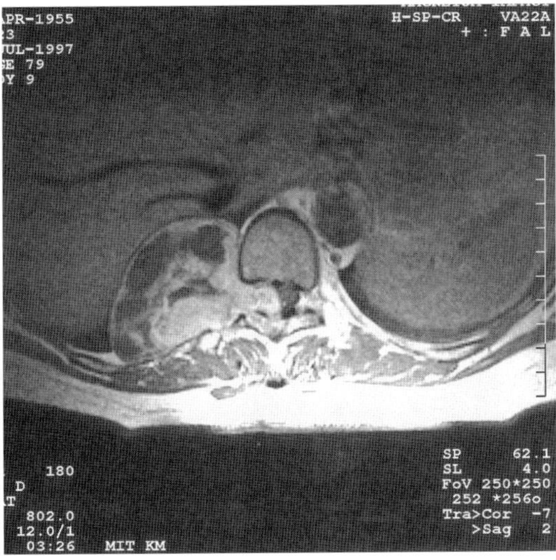

Fig. 6.18. Same patient as Fig. 6.17. Axial T1-weighted image through the T9 level after contrast administration. The neurinoma to the right of T9 and its intramedullary component have high, inhomogeneous signal intensity. The tumor widens the T9 foramen on the right and displaces the thoracic spinal cord

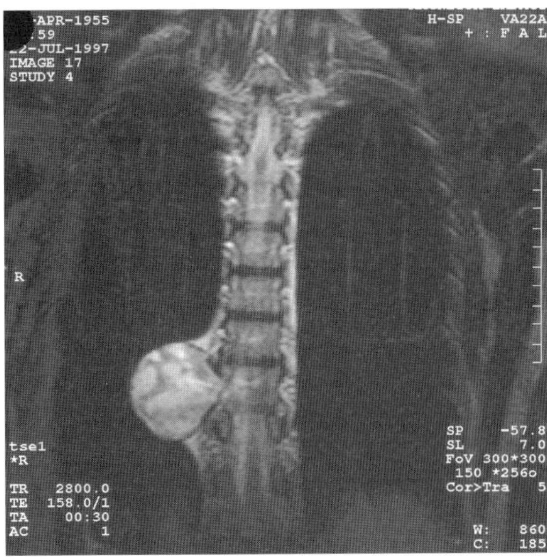

Fig. 6.19. Coronal T2-weighted image of the T9 neurinoma. The image shows an inhomogeneous but mostly high-signal-intensity paravertebral tumor on the right. The tumor is well-defined and appears to be surrounded by a capsule

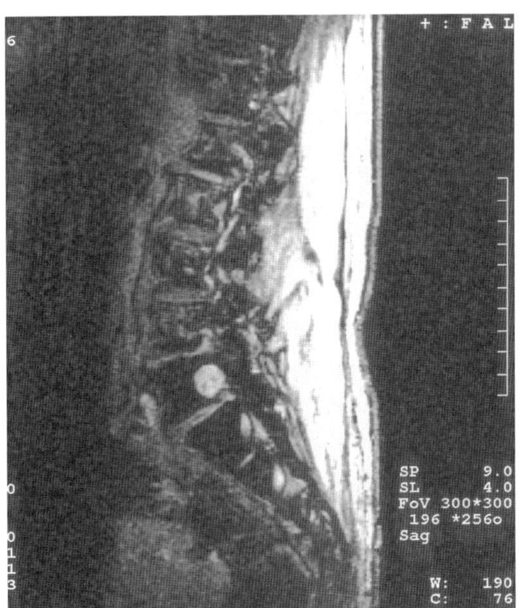

Fig. 6.20. 75-year-old patient with low back symptoms on the left side. Sagittal T2-weighted image with fat saturation of the lower lumbar region showing a sharply demarcated tumor of high signal intensity in the area of the left L5 foramen. Neurinoma with a diameter of about 15 mm

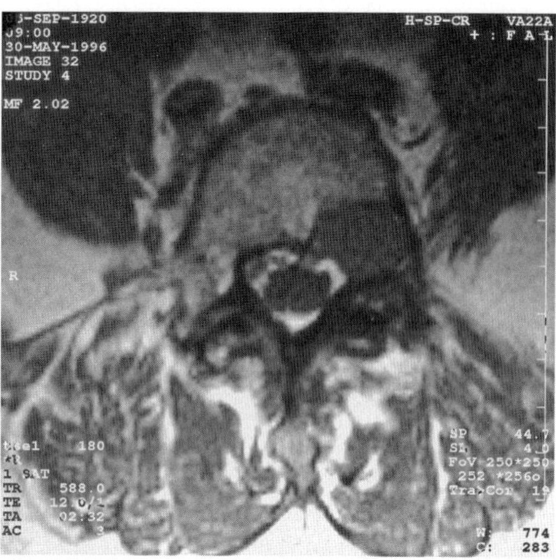

Fig. 6.21. Same patient as Fig. 6.20. Axial T1-weighted image through the L5-S1 level showing the neurinoma in the left neural foramen

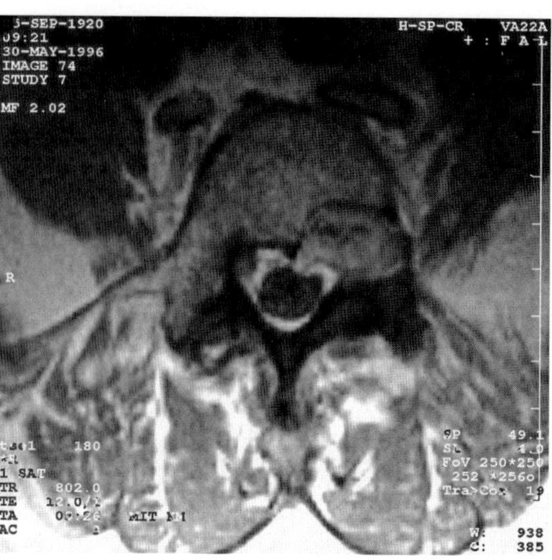

Fig. 6.22. Axial T1-weighted image after contrast administration showing clear but incomplete contrast enhancement of the L5-S1 neurinoma with partial destruction and expansion of the neural foramen and pedicle

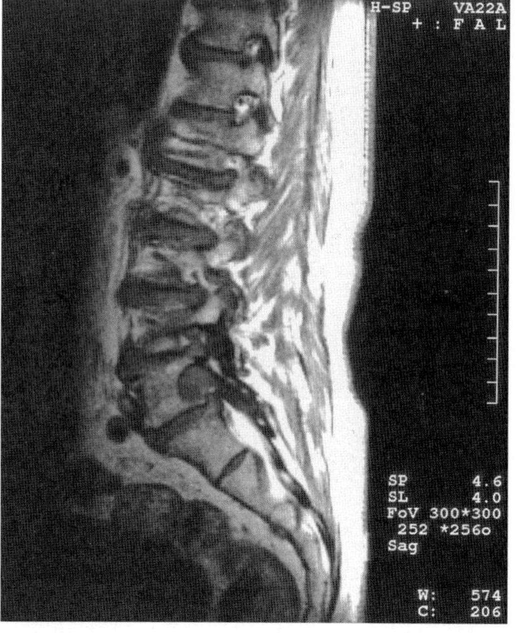

Fig. 6.23. Sagittal T1-weighted image of the lumbar spine showing the L5-S1 neurinoma as a slightly hypointense lesion in the area of the left L5 foramen

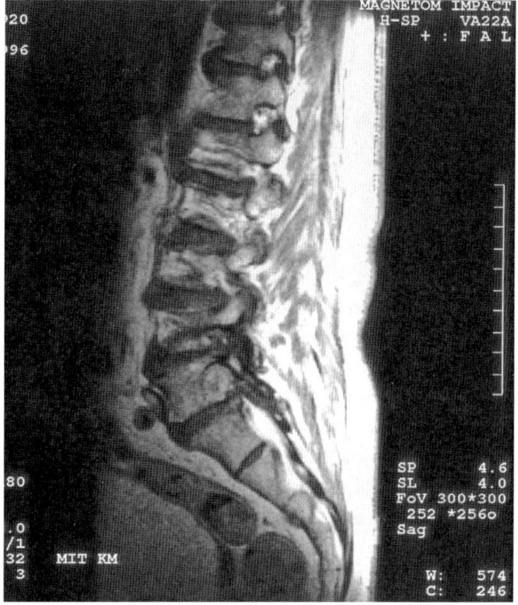

Fig. 6.24. Same patient (L5-S1 neurinoma). Sagittal T1-weighted image after contrast administration. The tumor in the L5-S1 foramen is now nearly isointense to bone marrow

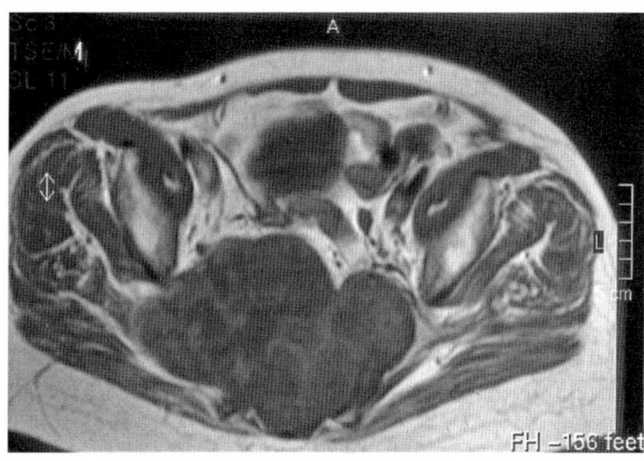

Fig. 6.25. 71-year-old patient with schwannoma. Axial T1-weighted image of the pelvic region depicting a slightly inhomogeneous, low-signal-intensity tumor located posteriorly in the true pelvis. There is partial destruction of the sacrum, which is no longer clearly discernible. The tumor has a size of approximately 8×10 cm

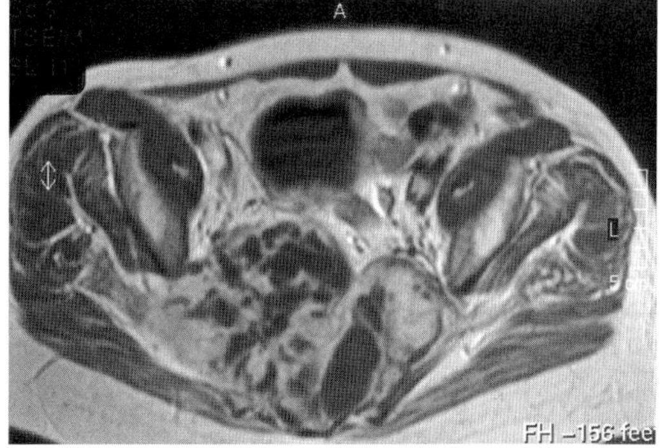

Fig. 6.26. Axial T1-weighted image of the pelvic region after contrast administration showing the well-perfused portions of the schwannoma in the area of the true pelvis/sacrum. The extension of the tumor is as described in the preceding figure. The image shows regressive changes with central liquefaction and necrosis

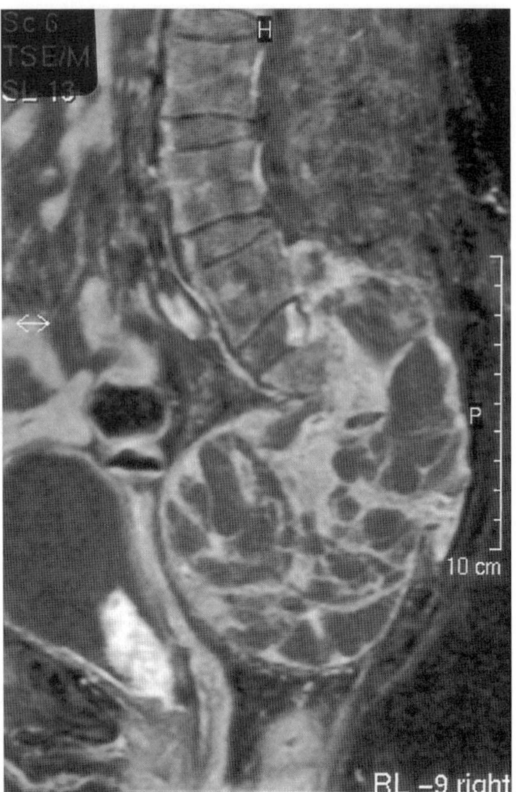

Fig. 6.27. Same patient. Contrast-enhanced sagittal T1-weighted image with fat saturation showing the schwannoma in the sacral region. The total length of the tumor is about 12 cm

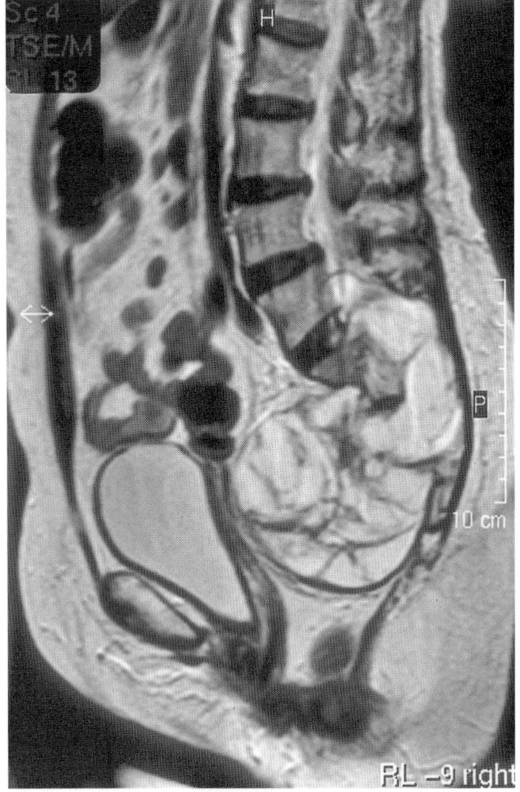

Fig. 6.28. Sagittal T2-weighted image of the large sacral schwannoma. The tumor contains multiple cystic portions and septum-like structures. The spinal canal is completely filled with tumor from L5-S1 downwards

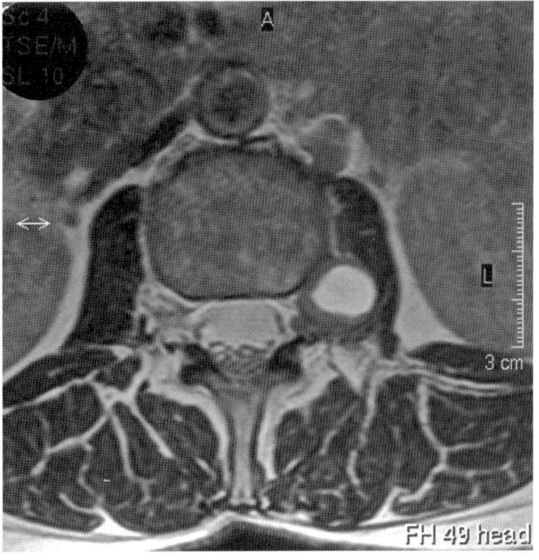

Fig. 6.29. Axial T2-weighted image through the L3-4 level showing a rounded, partially cystic lesion with a parenchymal medial portion surrounding the cyst in a crescent-like manner in the left L3 foramen. The whole tumor has a diameter of about 12 mm. The appearance is consistent with cystic degeneration of a schwannoma

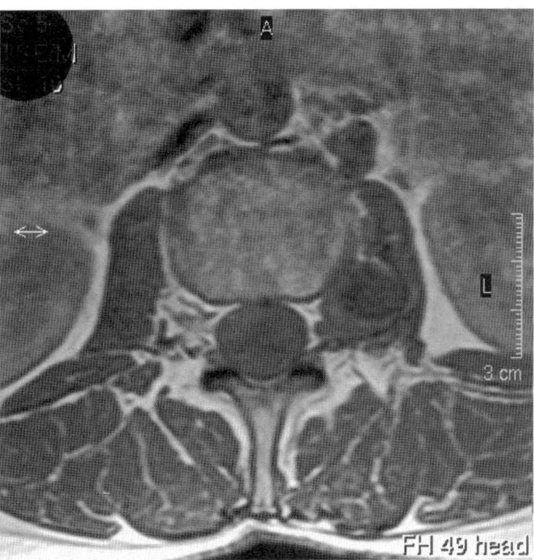

Fig. 6.30. Axial T1-weighted image of the cystic schwannoma at the L3 level

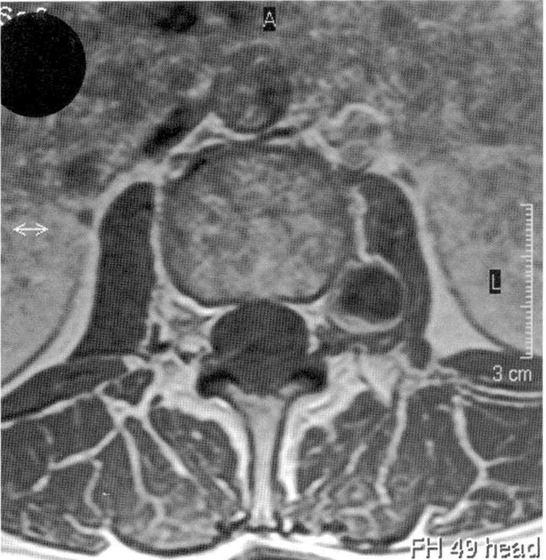

Fig. 6.31. Contrast-enhanced axial T1-weighted image through L3-4 showing enhancement of the parenchymal component of the cystic schwannoma at the L3 level on the left

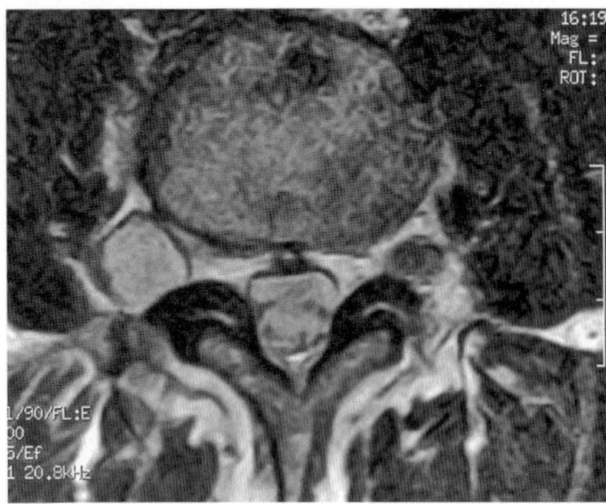

Fig. 6.32. Transverse T2-weighted image depicting an extradural tumor portion in the right neural foramen

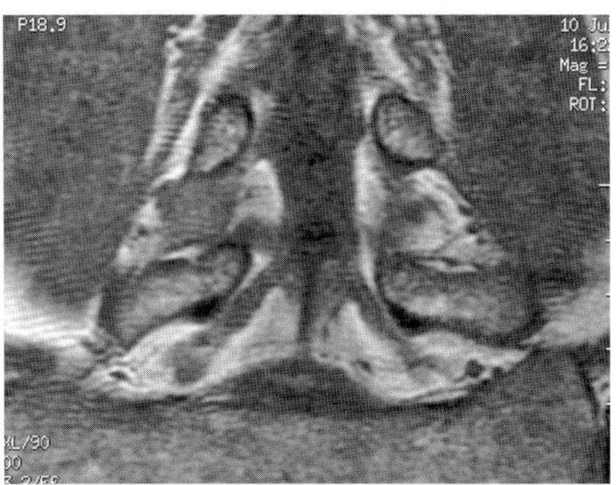

Fig. 6.33. Coronal T1-weighted image of the extradural intraforaminal tumor portion

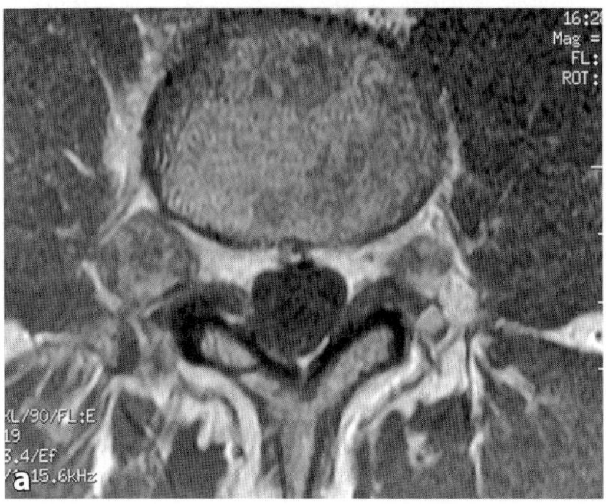

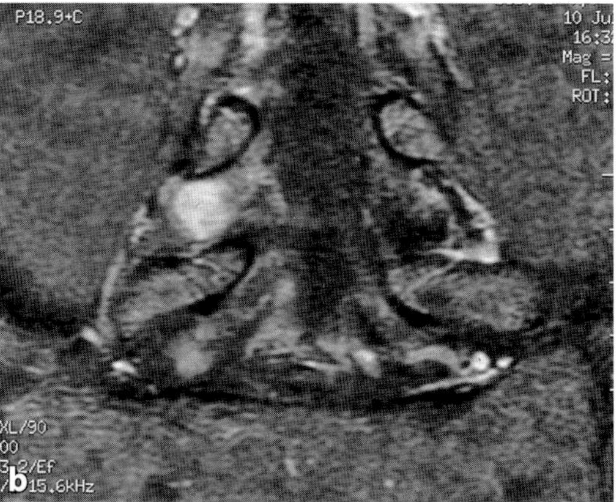

Fig. 6.34a,b. Transverse and coronal T1-weighted images after contrast administration with mostly homogeneous signal enhancement of the tumor

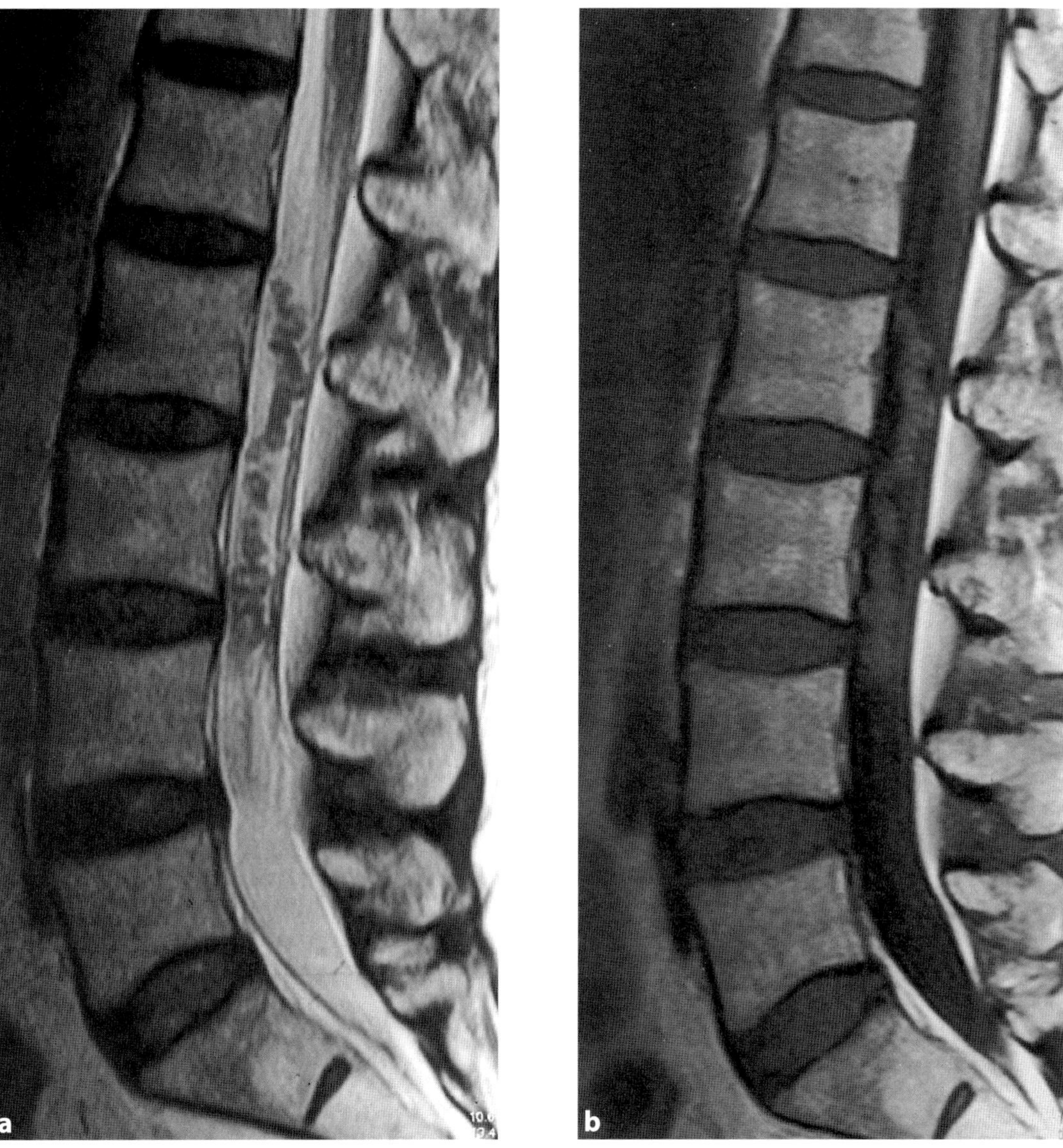

Fig. 6.35a, b. Neurofibromatosis. Sagittal T2- and T1-weighted images showing isointense changes in the dural sac

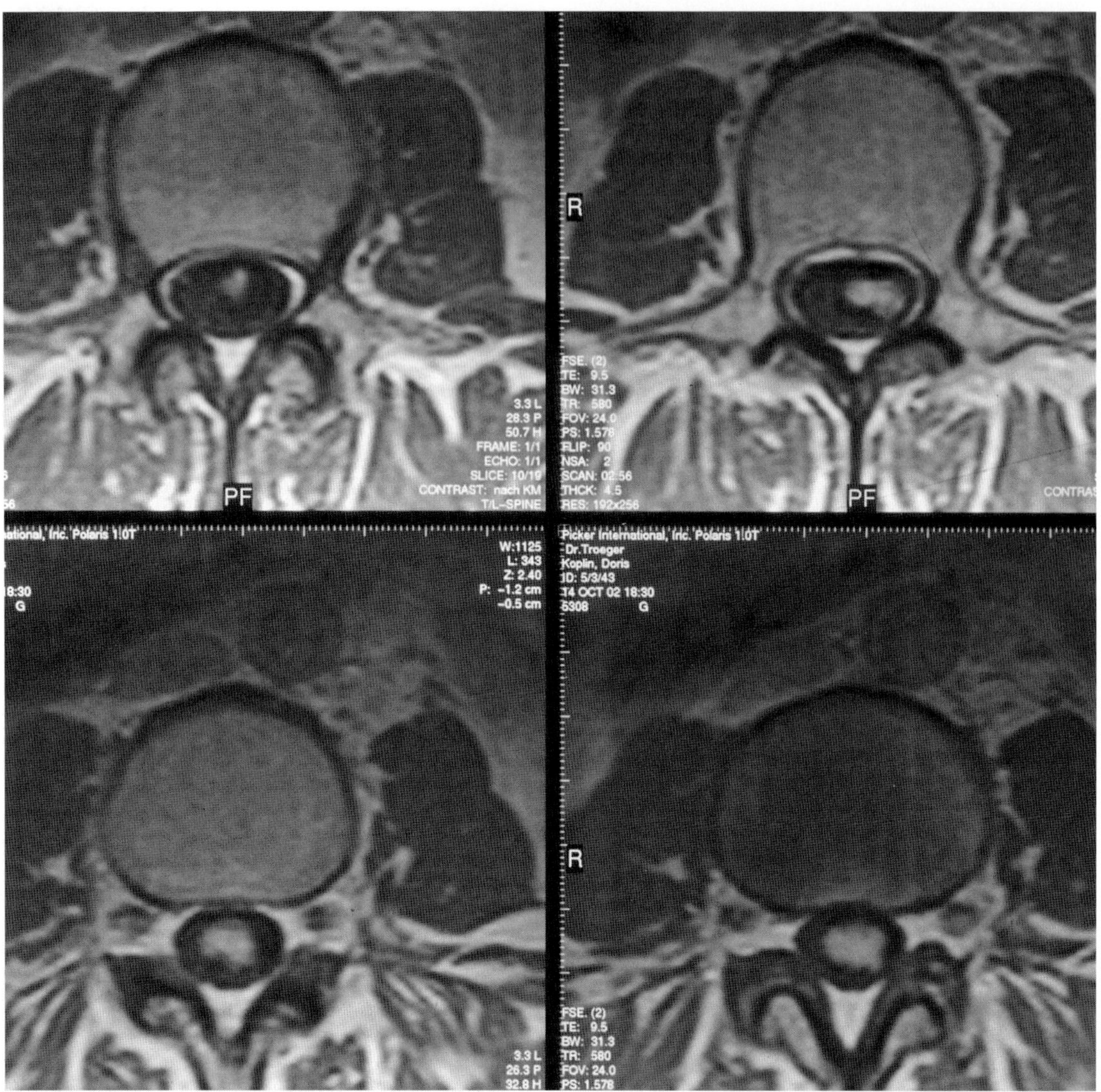

Fig. 6.36. Same patient. Transverse T1-weighted sequence confirming the findings on sagittal images

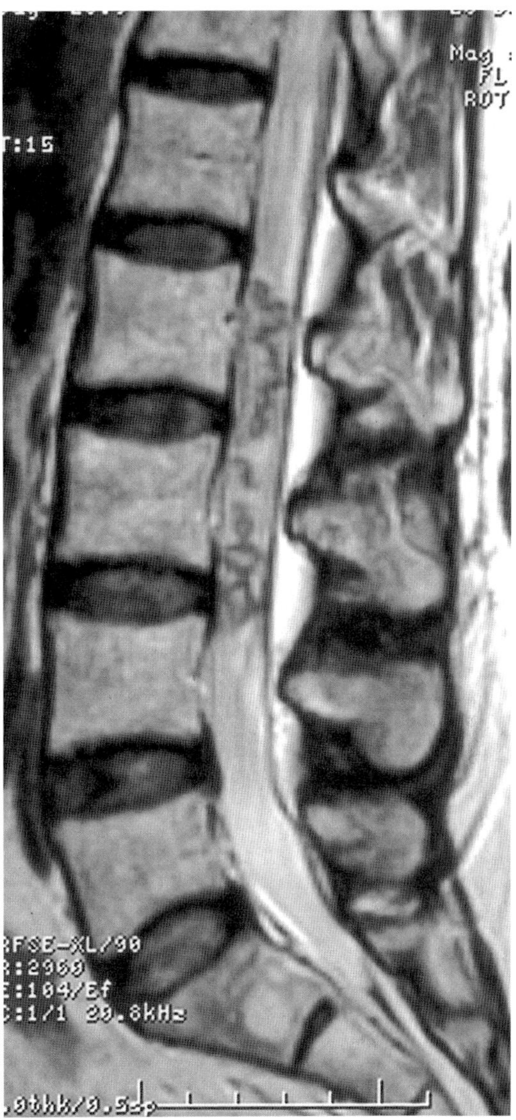

Fig. 6.37. Same patient. Sagittal T2-weighted image confirming the findings seen on preceding images. The appearance suggests ectasia and congestion of intradural veins

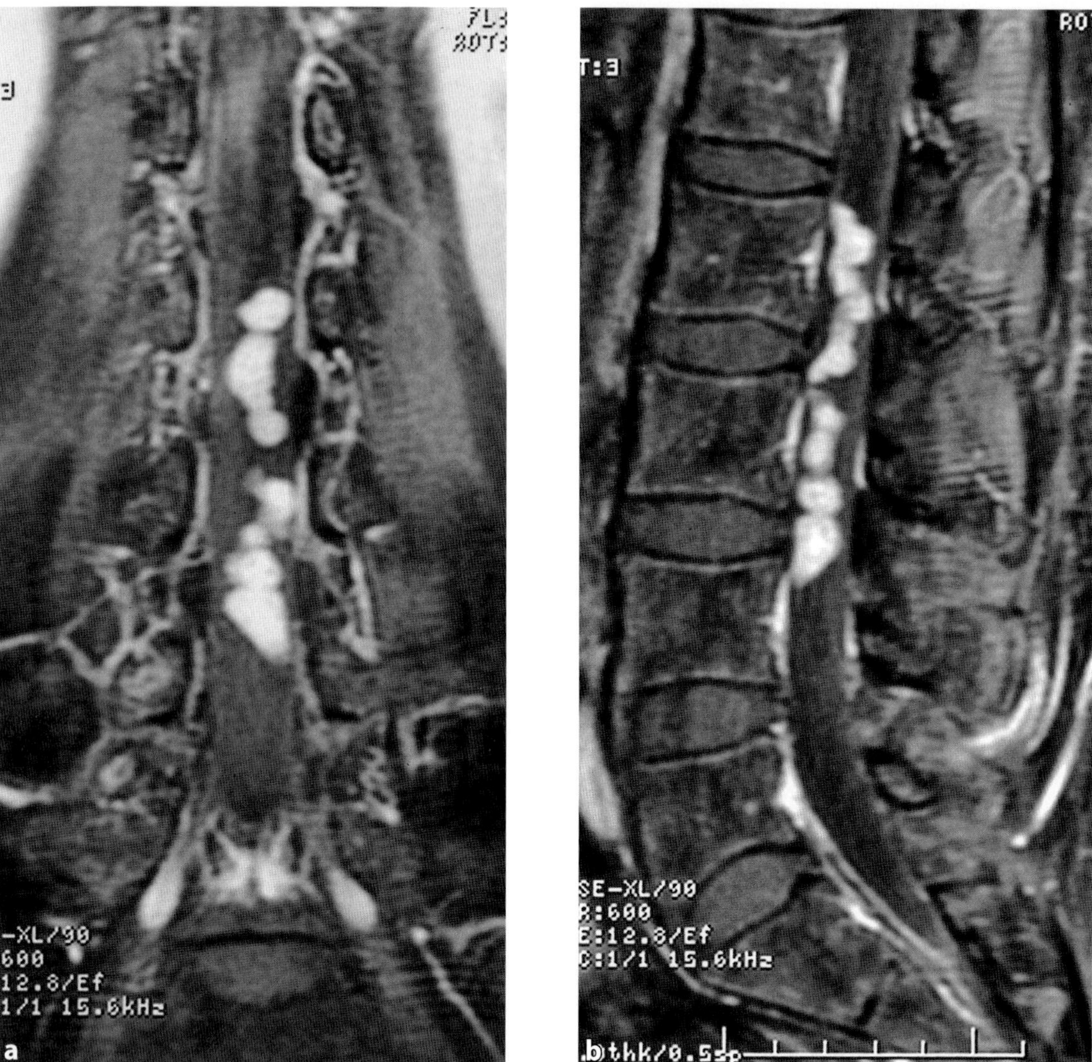

Fig. 6.38a, b. Same patient. Coronal and sagittal T1-weighted images with fat suppression after contrast administration. Strong enhancement of the structures depicted with low intensity on T2

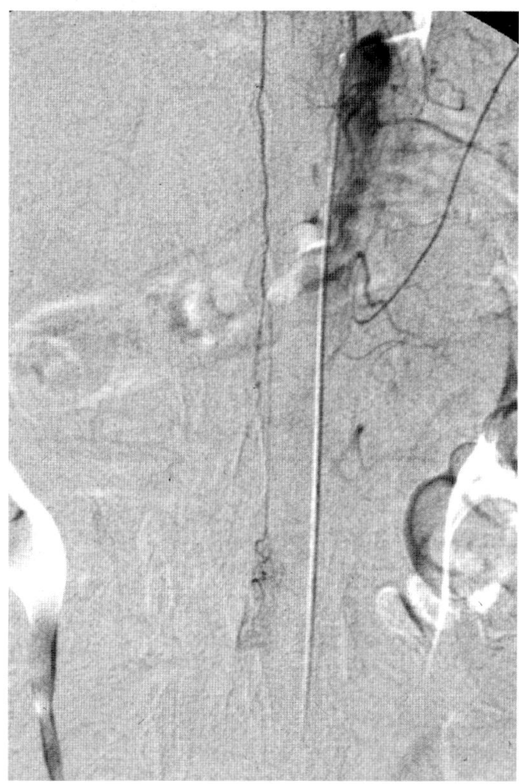

Fig. 6.39. Same patient. Spinal angiography showing intraspinal blush at L2-3 on the right. Intraoperative diagnosis of neurofibroma with venous congestion

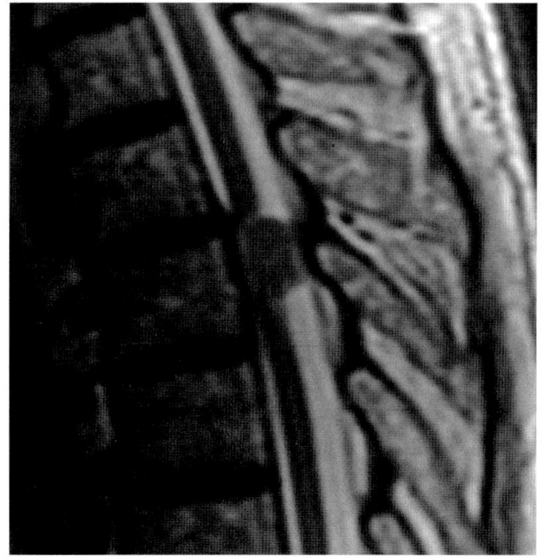

Fig. 6.40. Sagittal T2-weighted image showing a tumor isointense to the spinal cord with its base posteriorly and marked compression of the spinal cord at T4

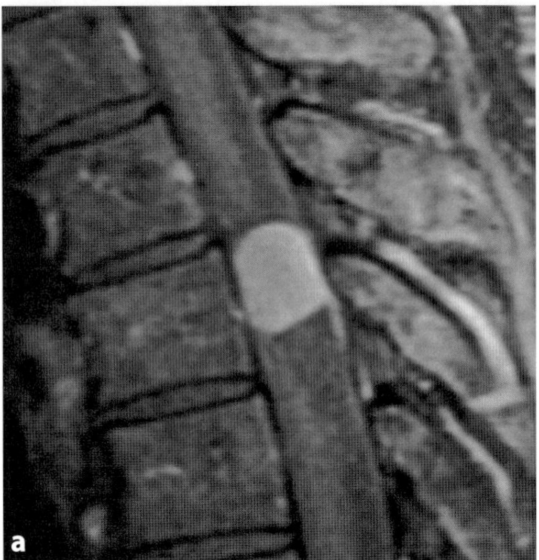

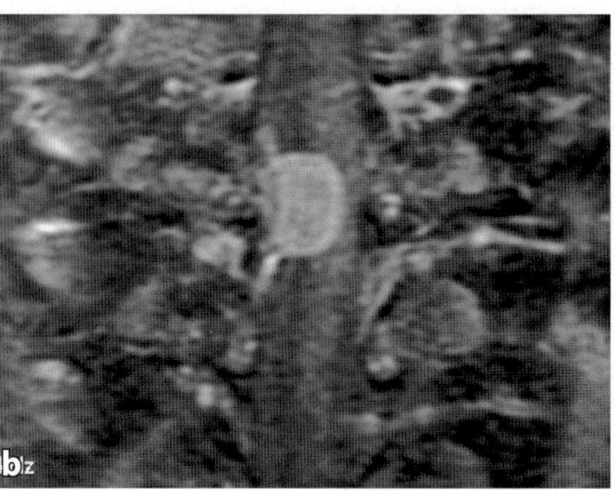

Fig. 6.41a, b. Same patient. Sagittal and coronal T1-weighted images with fat suppression after contrast administration. Depiction of a meningeal tail at the dural tumor base posteriorly (sagittal image) and at the right wall of the dural sheath (coronal image). Compression and displacement of the spinal cord

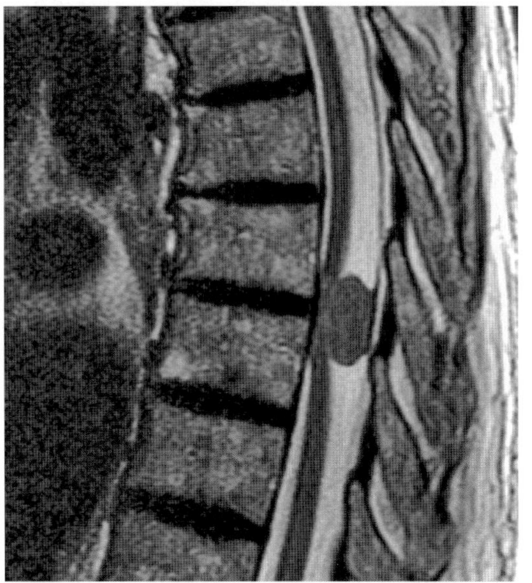

Fig. 6.42. Sagittal T2-weighted image showing oval tumor with pronounced compression of the spinal cord

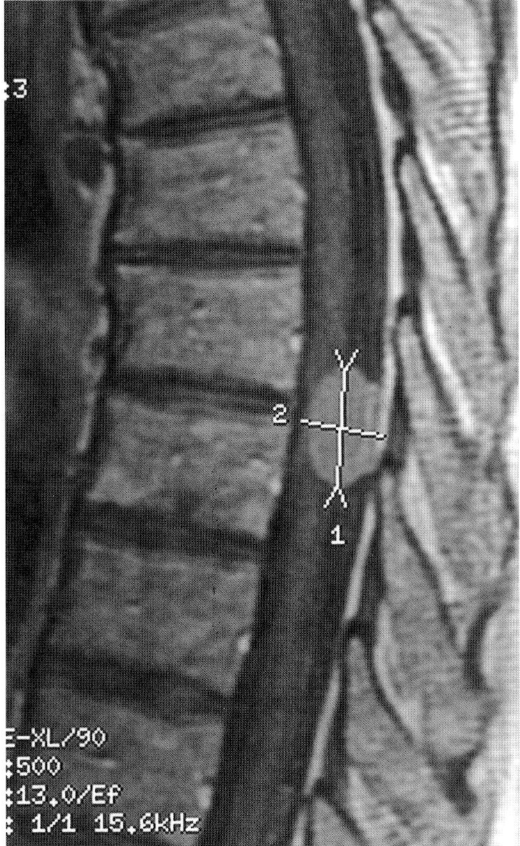

Fig. 6.43. Same patient. Sagittal T1-weighted image after contrast administration showing homogeneous enhancement of the tumor with its base at the posterior wall of the dural sheath

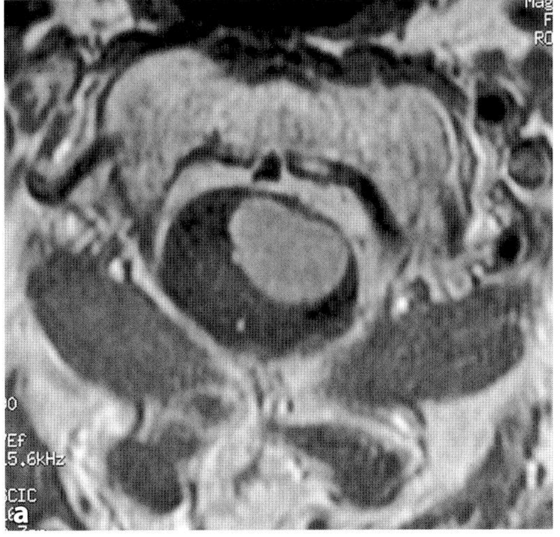

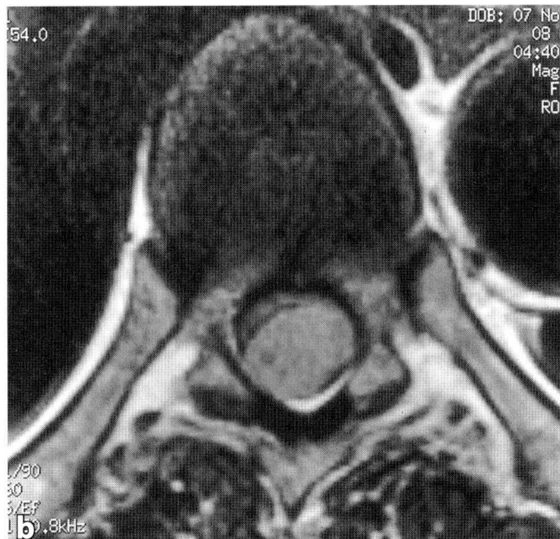

Fig. 6.44a,b. Demonstration of a second meningioma in the cervical spinal canal at the C2 level and transverse image documenting the thoracic meningioma at T8-9

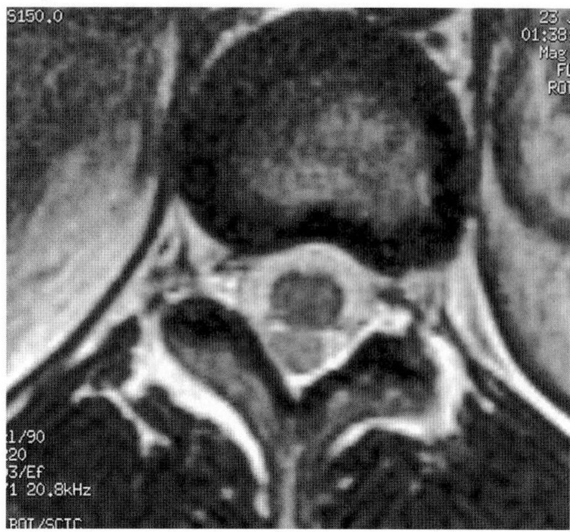

Fig. 6.45. Transverse T2-weighted spin echo image: demonstration of a small tumor behind the thoracic spinal cord

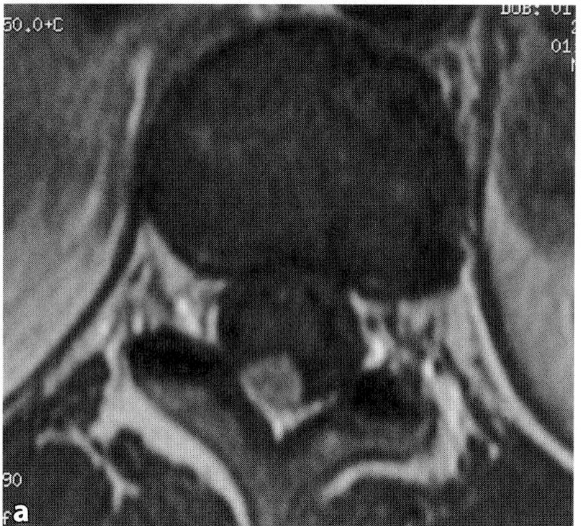

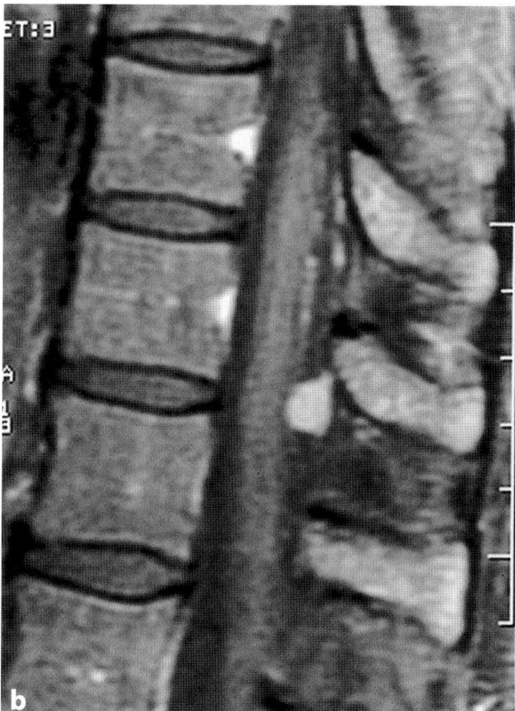

Fig. 6.46. **a** Transverse T1-weighted spin echo sequence after contrast administration and, **b**, sagittal T1-weighted spin echo sequence with fat suppression after contrast administration: homogeneous enhancement of the tumor, which has its base at the posterior wall of the dural sheath

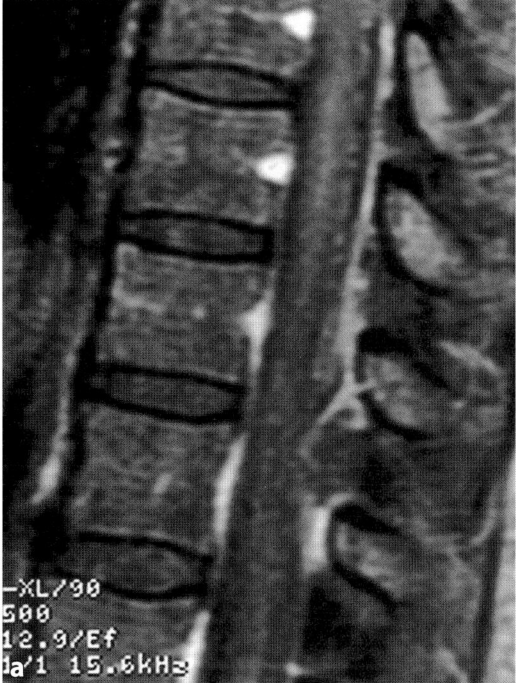

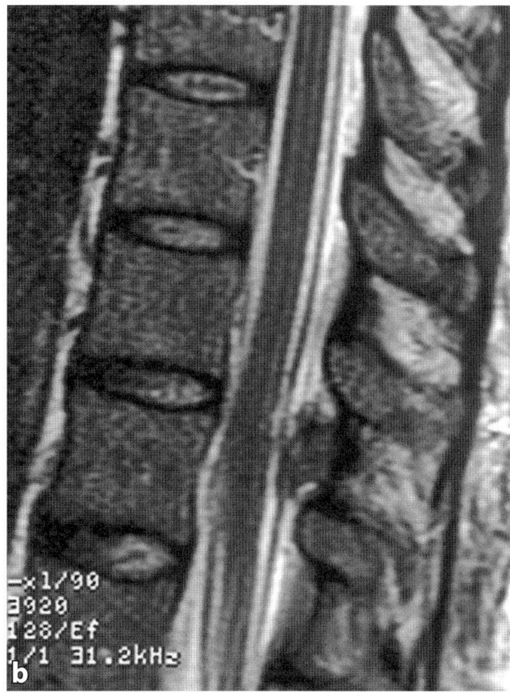

Fig. 6.47. Same patient, postoperative findings. **a** Sagittal T1-weighted image with fat suppression after contrast administration. No enhancing tumor but mild signal alteration at the posterior wall of the dural sheath. **b** Sagittal T2-weighted sequence

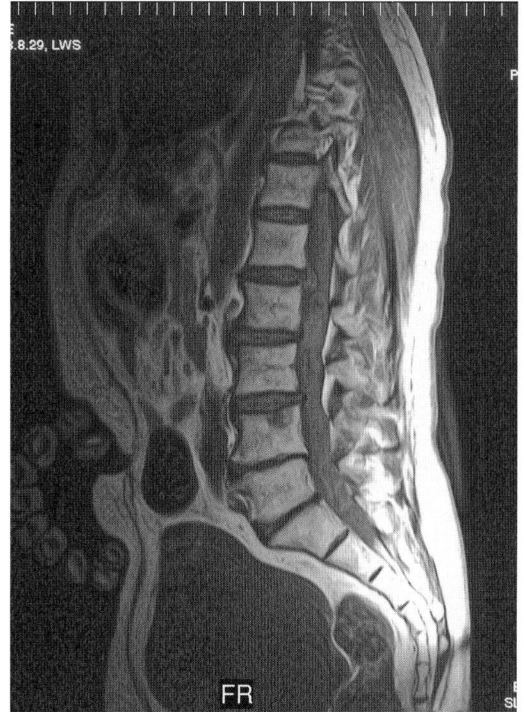

Fig. 6.48. Sagittal T1-weighted image of the lumbar spine in a 76-year-old patient with low back problems. Narrowing of L4-5 and herniations of L1-2 and L3-4. No definitive evidence of tumor

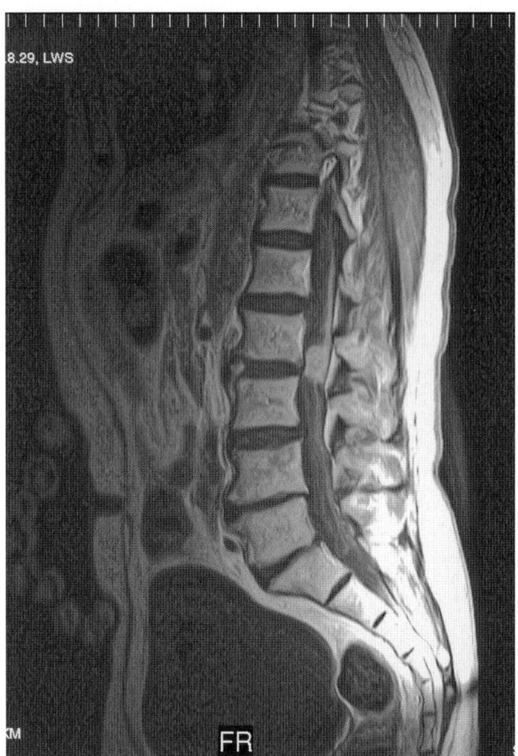

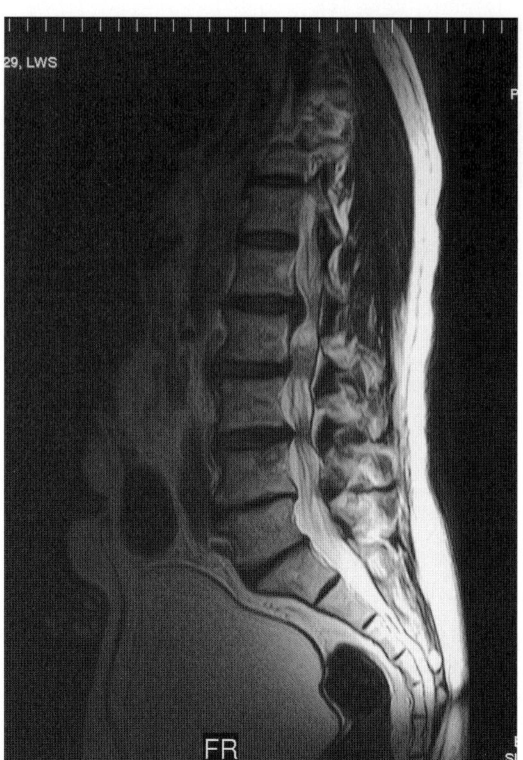

Fig. 6.49. Same patient as Fig. 6.48. Sagittal T1-weighted image after contrast administration showing an abnormally enhancing tumor at the L2-3 level. The tumor occupies most of the cross-sectional area of the spinal canal. The diagnosis was meningioma

Fig. 6.50. Sagittal T2-weighted image of the lumbar spine failing to clearly demonstrate the tumorous lesion at the L2-3 level. The disc herniations at L1-2 and L3-4 are seen more clearly

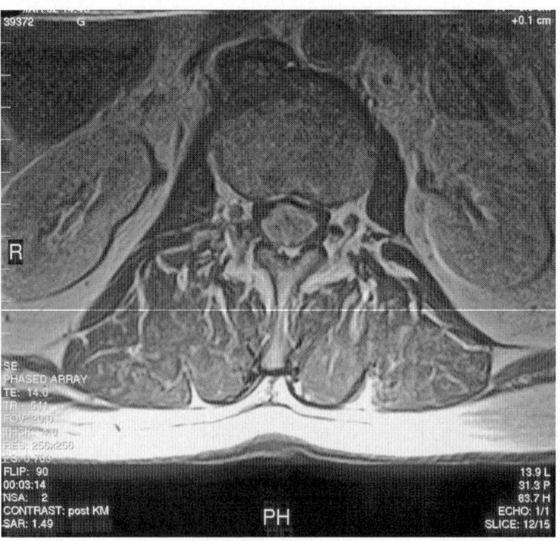

Fig. 6.51. Axial T1-weighted image through the L2-3 level after contrast administration. Large intraspinal and intradural tumor showing pronounced contrast enhancement in patient with known meningioma

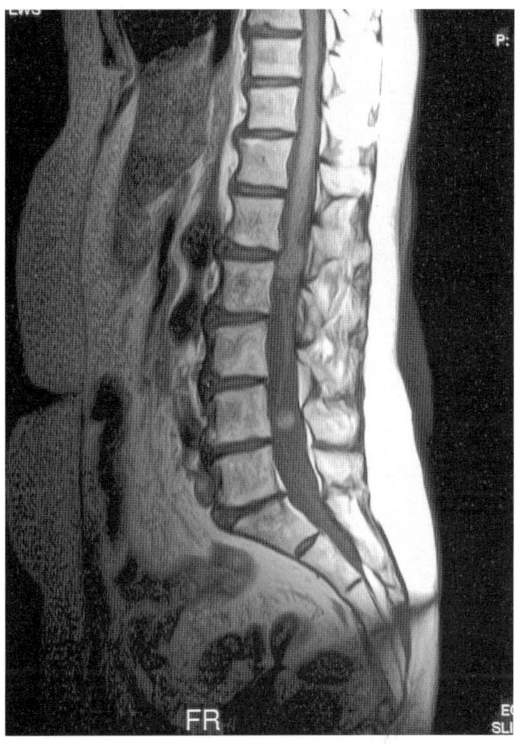

Fig. 6.52. Sagittal T1-weighted image of the lower thoracic and lumbar regions in a 62-year-old patient with low back symptoms. Intraspinal focal nodular lesions at the L1-2 and L4-5 levels. Wide spinal canal. Anterior disc herniations throughout the lumbar spine

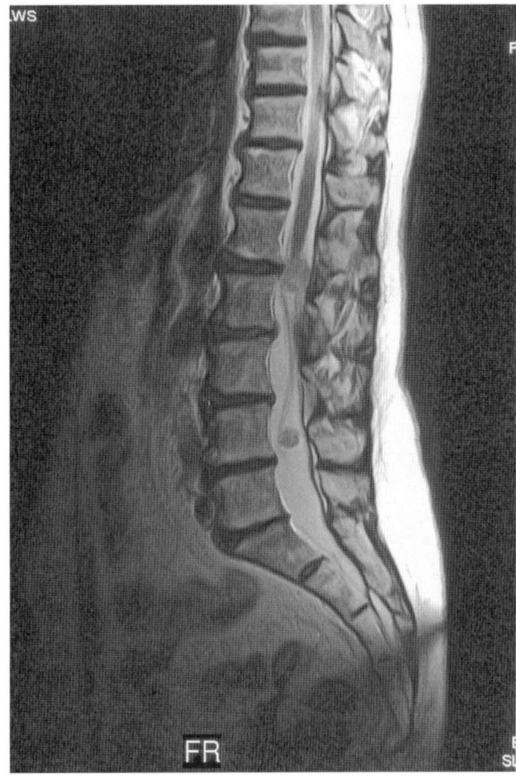

Fig. 6.53. Sagittal T2-weighted image of the lumbar spine showing the nodular lesions at L1-2 and L4-5

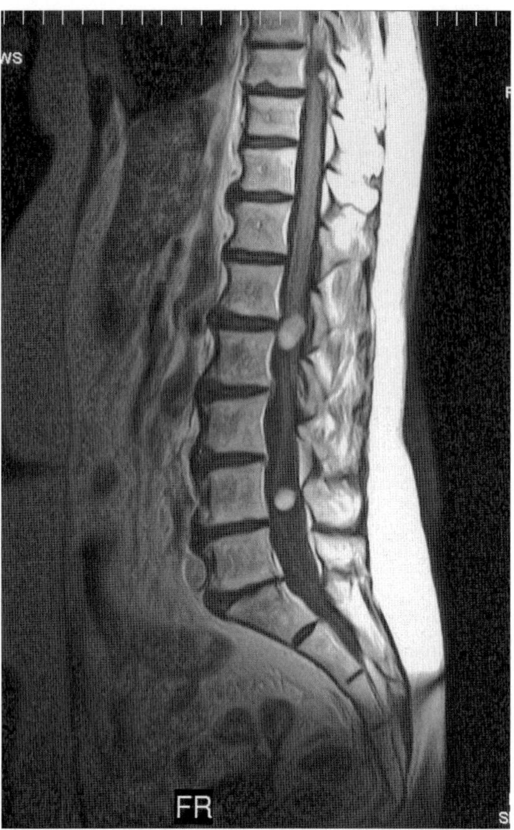

Fig. 6.54. Same patient. Sagittal T1-weighted image after contrast administration showing pronounced enhancement of the nodular lesions at L1-2 and L4-5, consistent with meningiomas

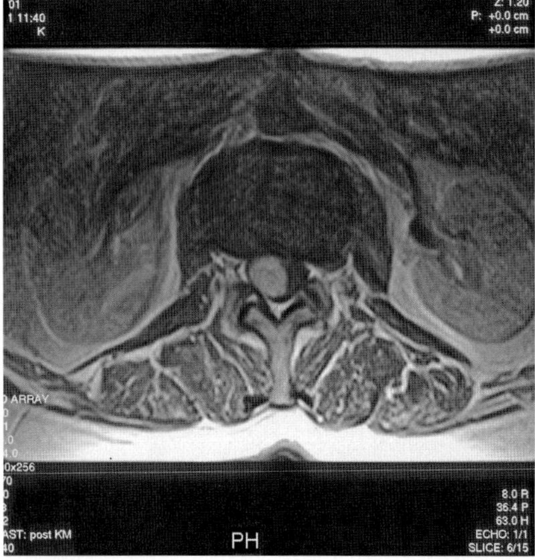

Fig. 6.55. Axial T1-weighted image showing the meningioma at the L1-2 level after contrast administration. Nodular intradural mass with pronounced enhancement

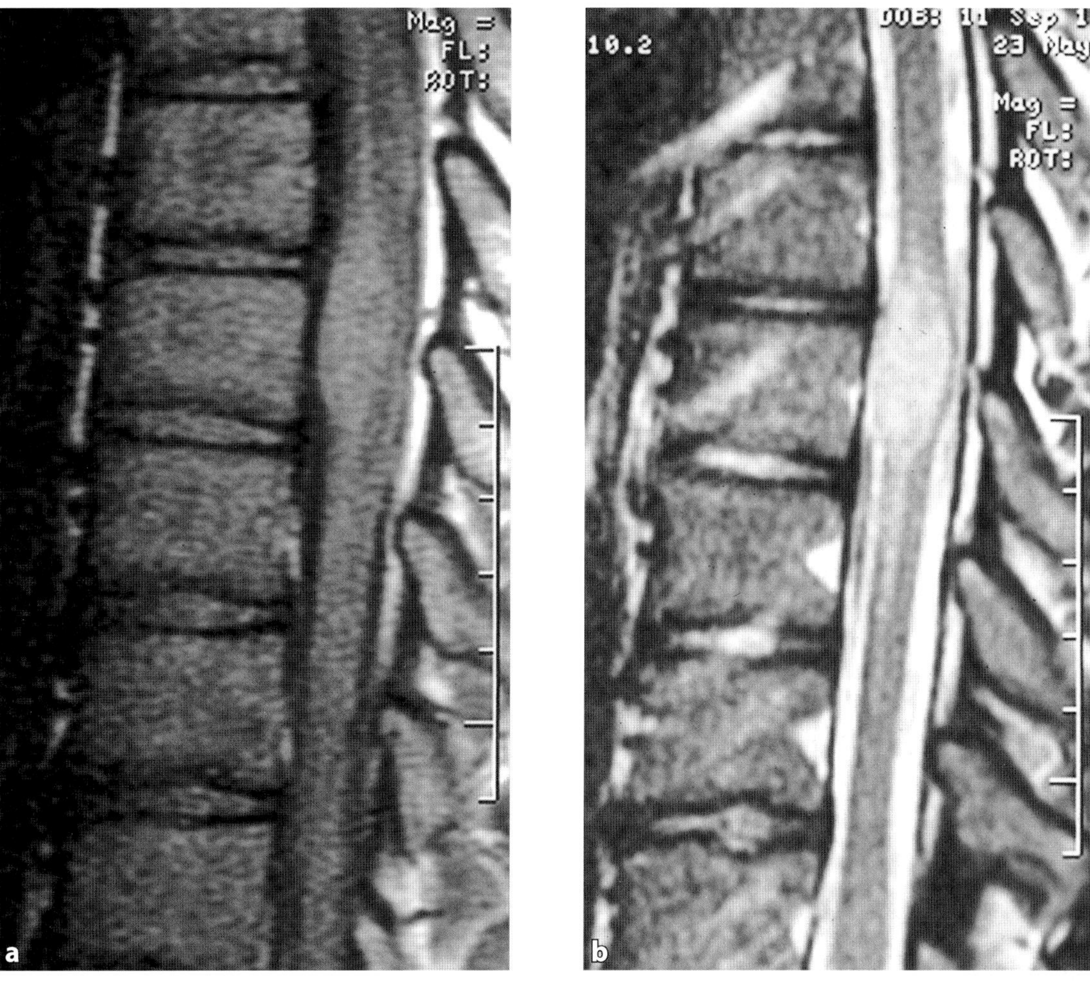

Fig. 6.56a, b. Intramedullary tumor. Sagittal proton-density- and T2-weighted images: spindle-shaped widening of the spinal cord by a tumor. Prominent central canal. Tumor and edema cannot be differentiated

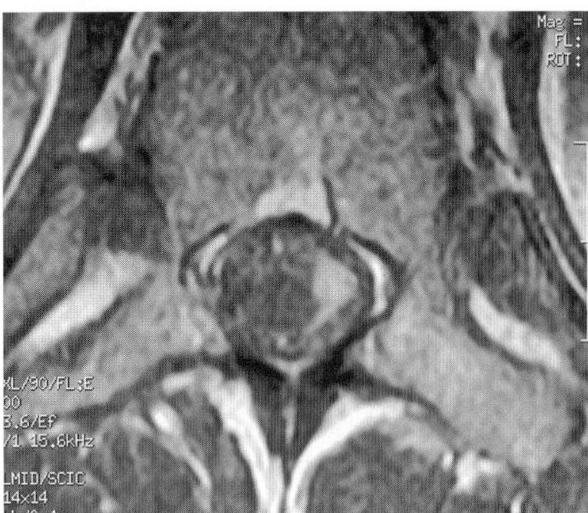

Fig. 6.57. Same patient. T1-weighted image after contrast administration showing eccentric tumor location in the left aspect of the spinal cord

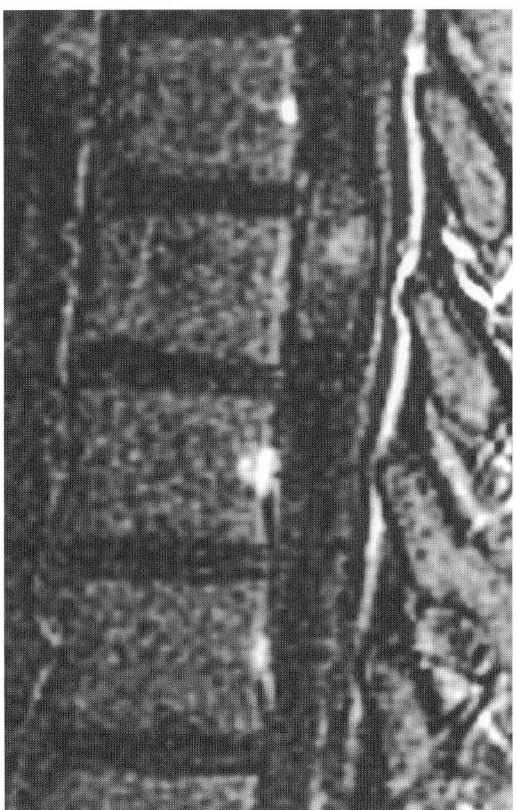

Fig. 6.58. T1-weighted contrast-enhanced subtraction image showing contrast-enhancing tumor focus in the center of the lesion

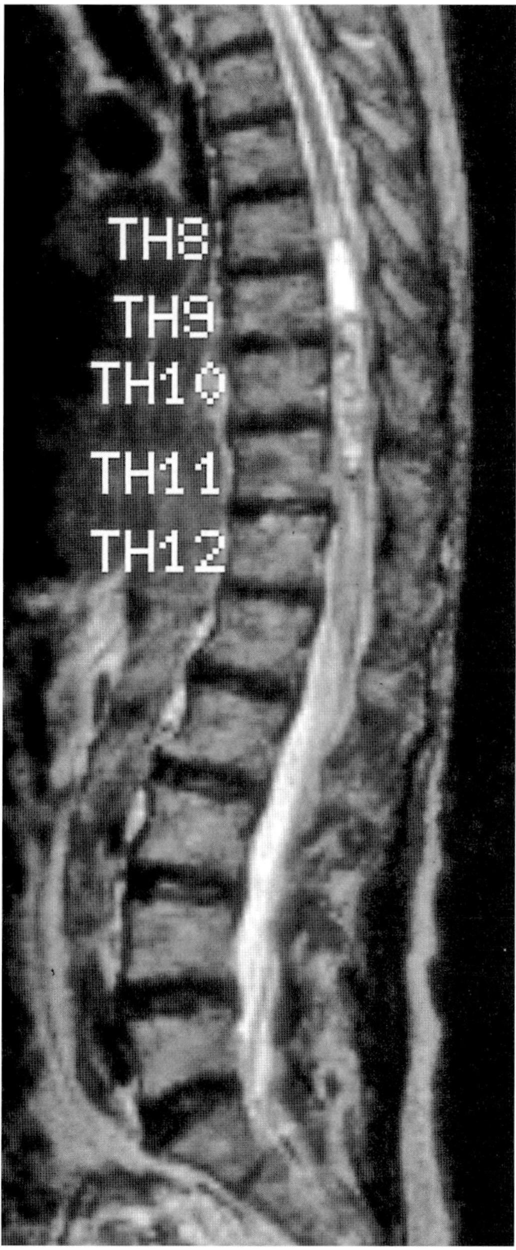

Fig. 6.59. T2-weighted scout image (body coil): good overview of the tumor and its cystic portions, predominantly at the upper end (T8 through T11)

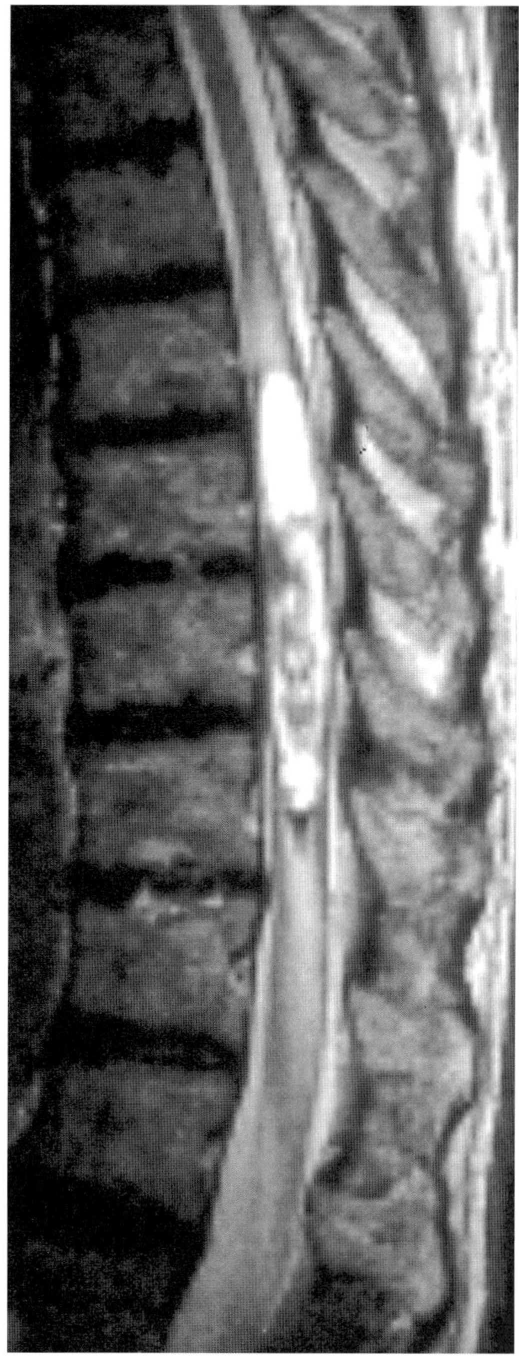

Fig. 6.60. Sagittal T2-weighted image showing heterogeneous tumor with a large, hood-shaped cyst superiorly and a rounded cystic area inferiorly. Longitudinal edema tapering off at both ends

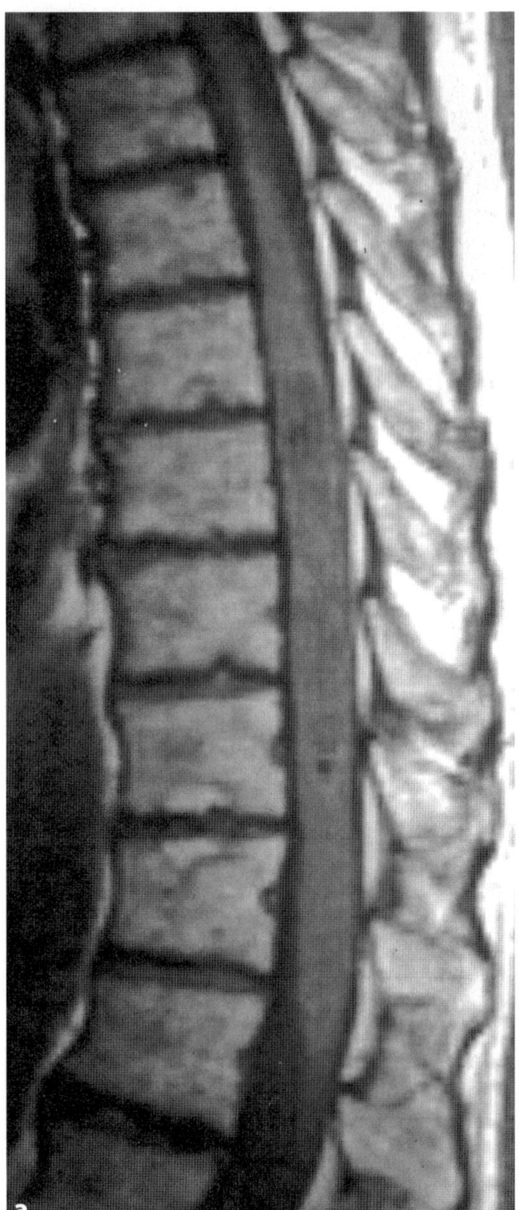

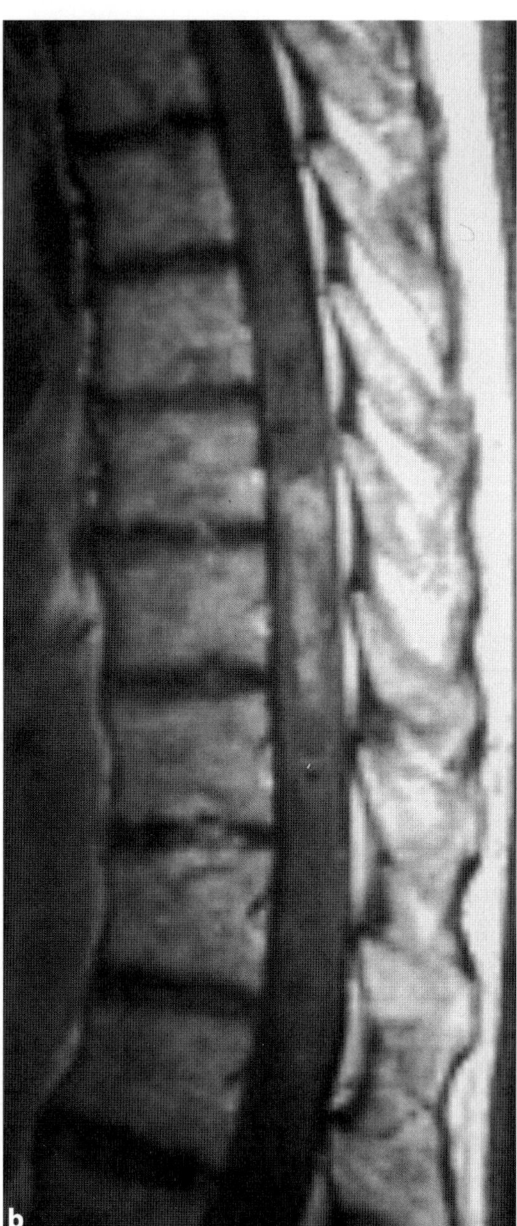

Fig. 6.61a, b. T1-weighted images before and after contrast administration: iso- to hypointense tumor on unenhanced image with poor demarcation of cystic components. Contrast-enhanced image allows differentiation of solid tumor portions. Appearance suggests blood sediment at the bottom of the small cyst below (low signal on T1 and T2)

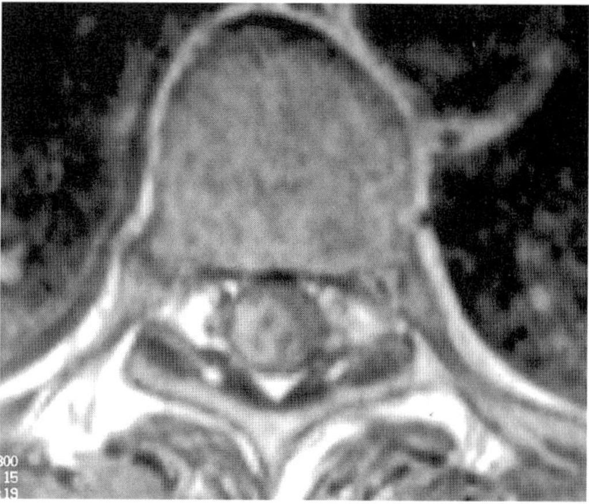

Fig. 6.62. Same patient as Fig. 6.61. Transverse T1-weighted image after contrast administration. Eccentric tumor in the thoracic spinal cord with partially necrotic cystic tumor portions

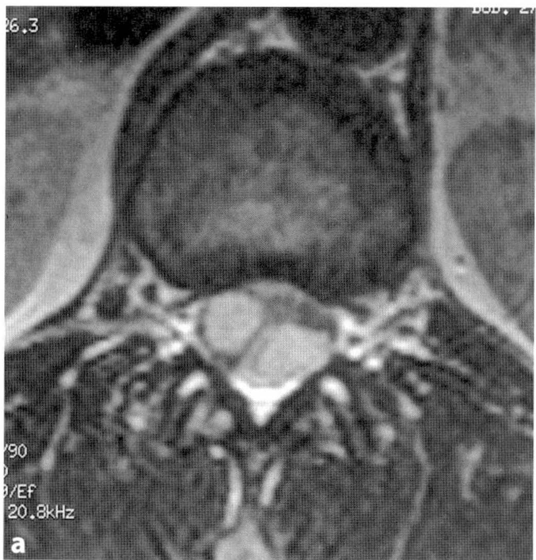

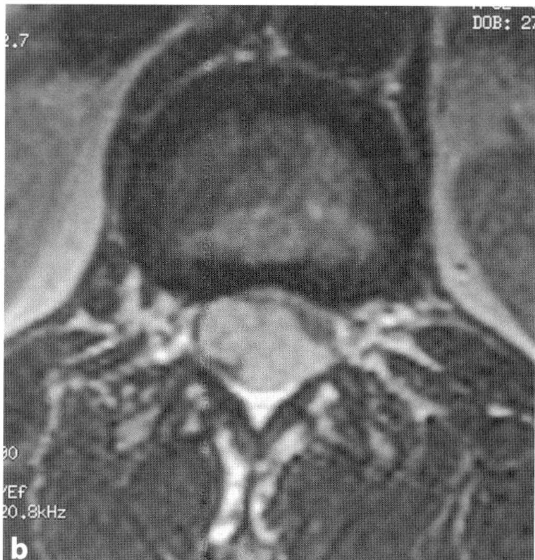

Fig. 6.63a, b. Transverse T2-weighted images: high-signal-intensity tumor occupying the entire cross-sectional area of the spinal cord

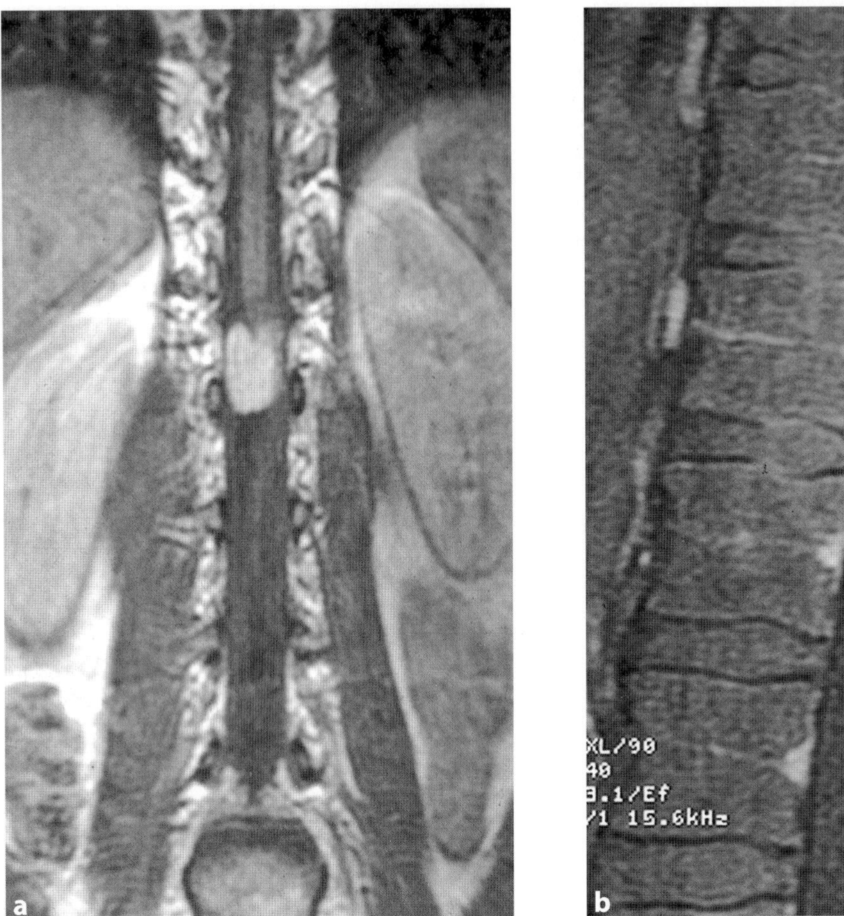

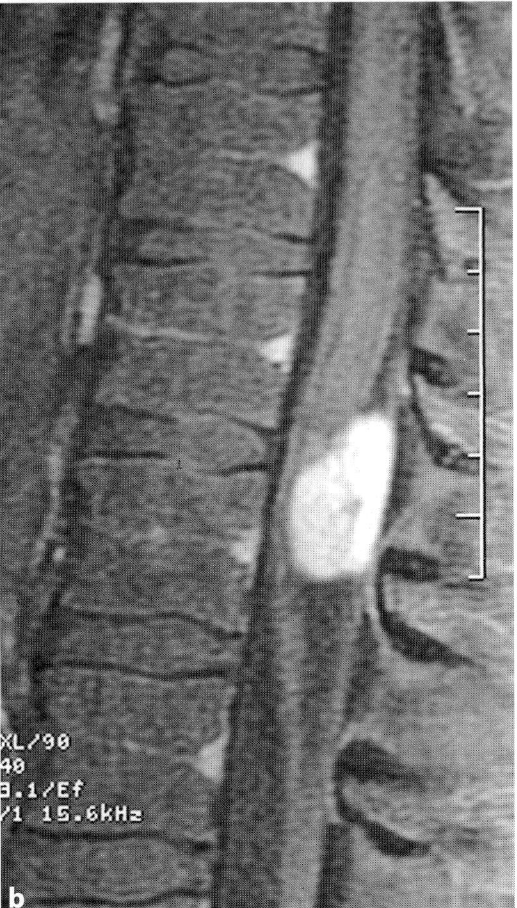

Fig. 6.64a, b. Coronal T1-weighted image and sagittal, fat-suppressed T1-weighted image showing pronounced, nearly homogeneous enhancement of the tumor

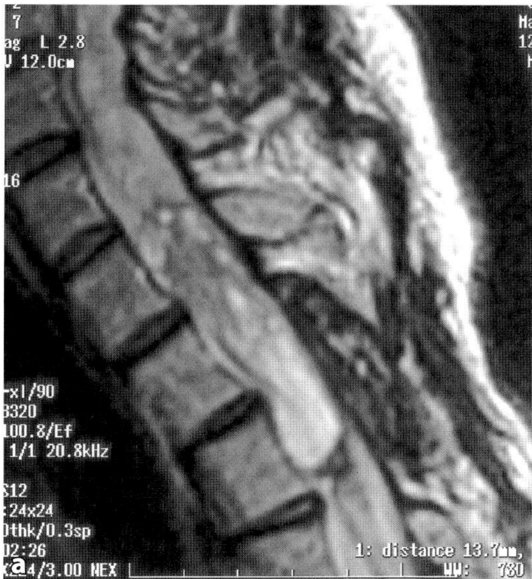

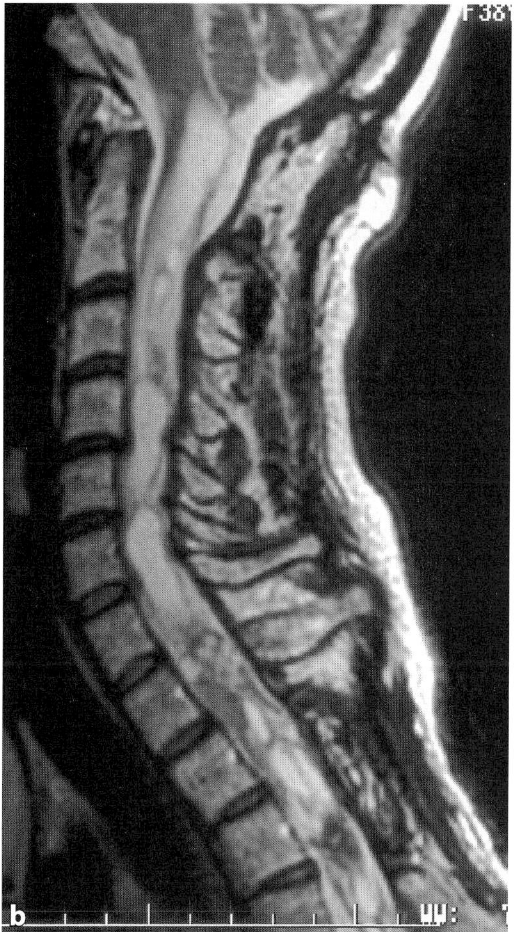

Fig. 6.65a, b. Sagittal T2-weighted image: recurrent ependymoma with hemorrhage containing hemosiderin and cystic areas. Large syrinx cavity above the tumor

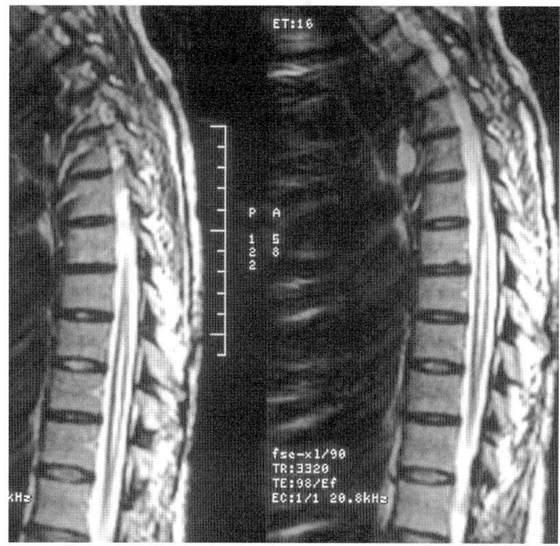

Fig. 6.66. Sagittal T2-weighted image of the thoracic spine showing syrinx extending downward from tumor

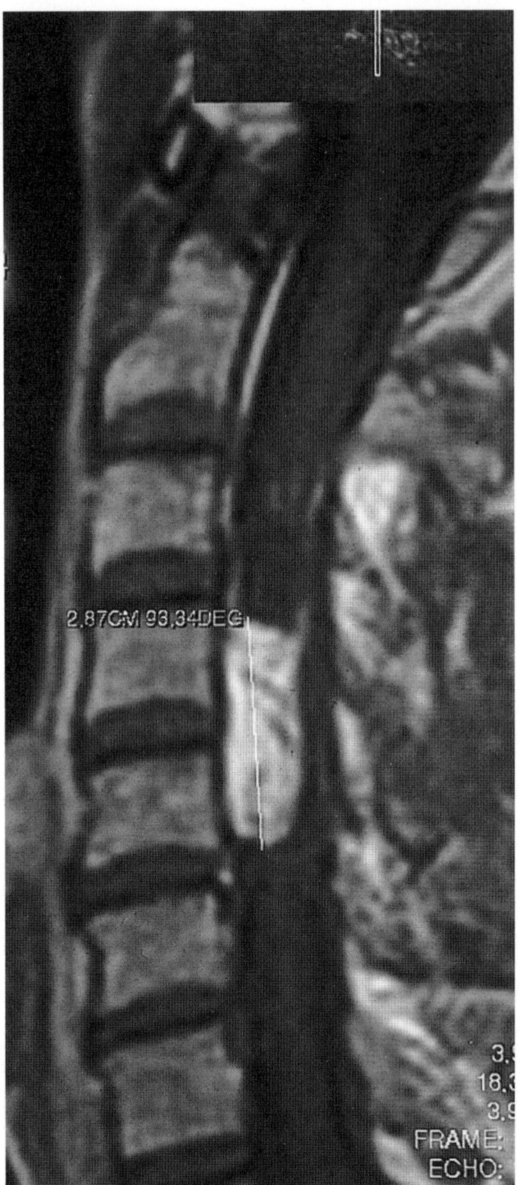

Fig. 6.67. Sagittal T1-weighted image after contrast administration showing intramedullary tumor with intradural extramedullary component. Strong contrast enhancement. Cystic portion at upper end of tumor

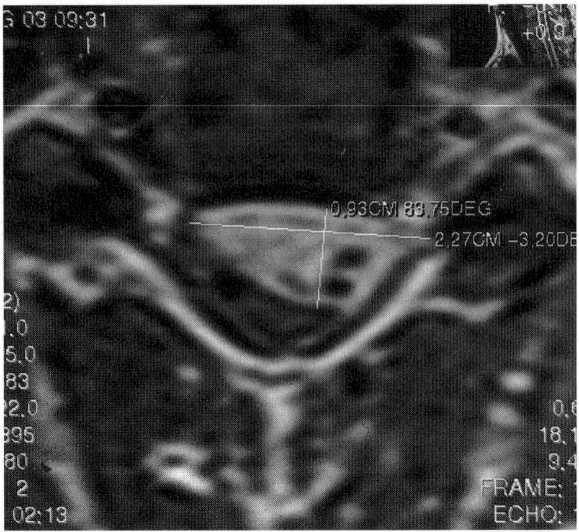

Fig. 6.68. Transverse T1-weighted image after contrast administration. Flow voids indicating arterial and venous supply

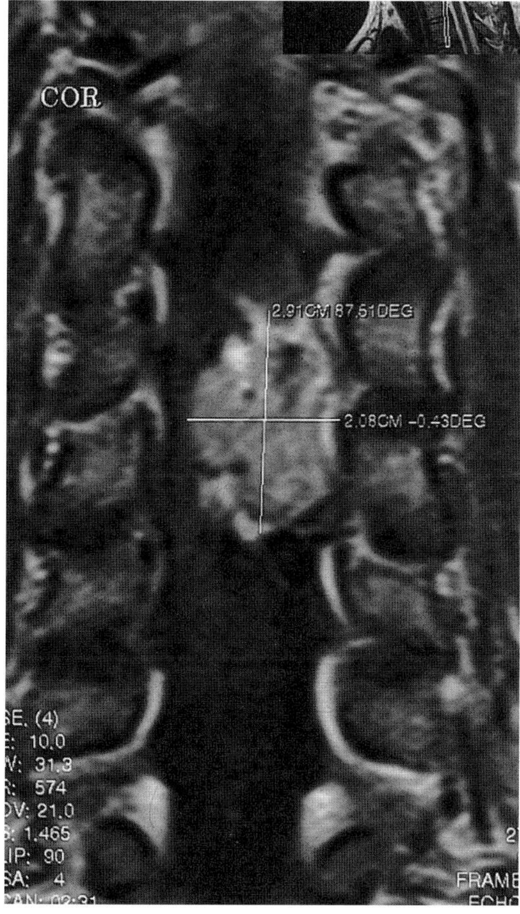

Fig. 6.69. Same patient. Coronal T1-weighted image after contrast administration

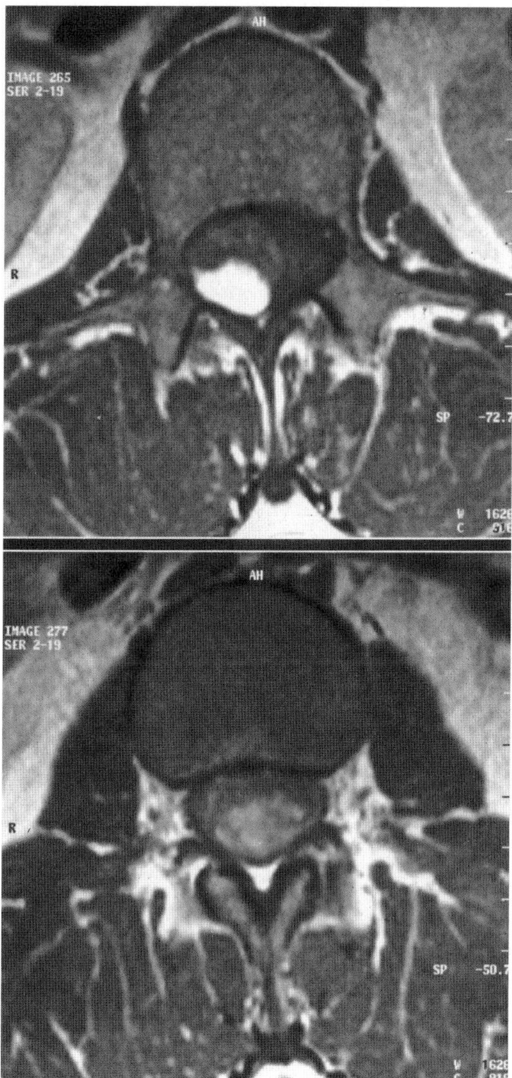

Fig. 6.70. Transverse T1-weighted image after IV contrast administration: tumor measuring 3 cm in length with fatty components in upper portion (intraoperative finding) and amorphous masses and hairs in lower portion. Tumor just beneath the conus medullaris in the filum terminale (typical sacral location of dermoid). Contrast administration does not contribute to tumor identification but may occasionally be helpful in evaluating concomitant (inflammatory) reactions

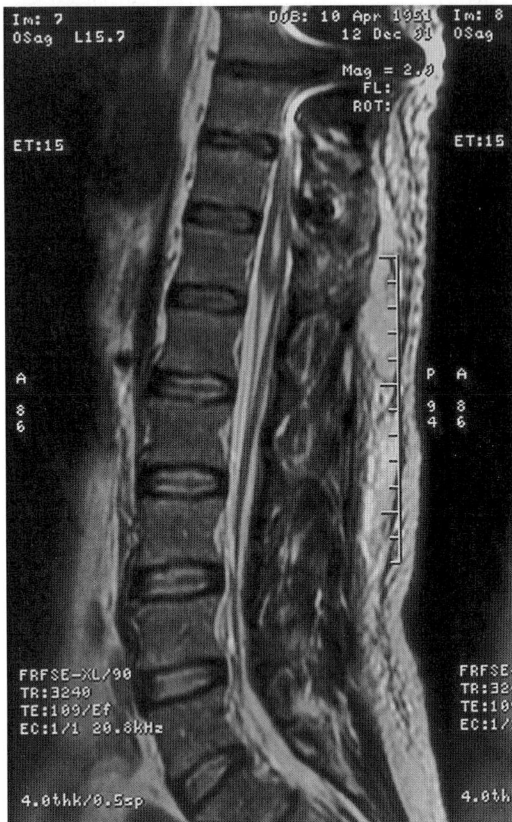

Fig. 6.71. Same patient. Sagittal T2-weighted image (follow-up 6 days postoperatively) showing the collapsed residual cyst in the conus medullaris from T11-12 to the inferior endplate of T12. Metal artifacts and image distortions at T9-10

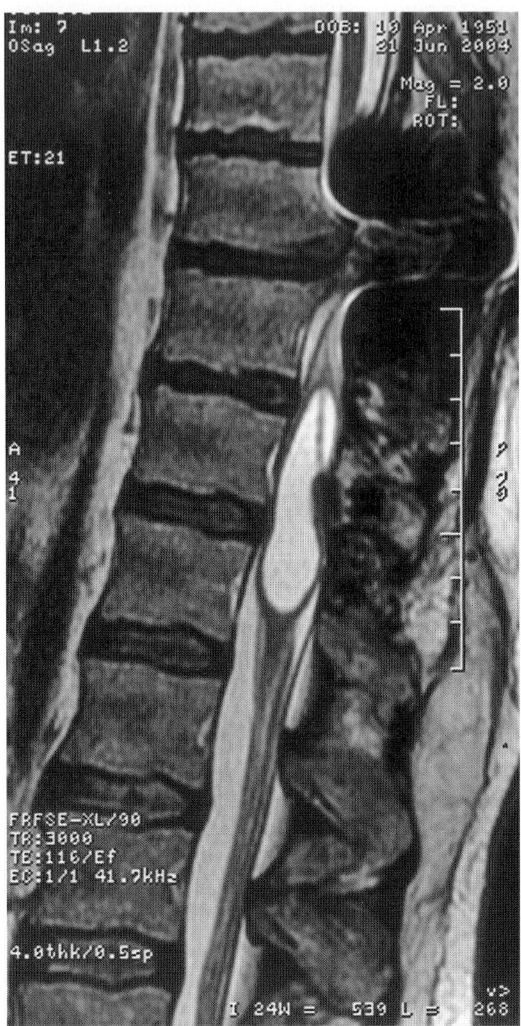

Fig. 6.72. T2-weighted image obtained 2 ½ years after surgery due to recurrent symptoms (back pain, paresthesia of the legs). Recurrence of the large cystic lesion, depicted with a slightly higher signal intensity than CSF

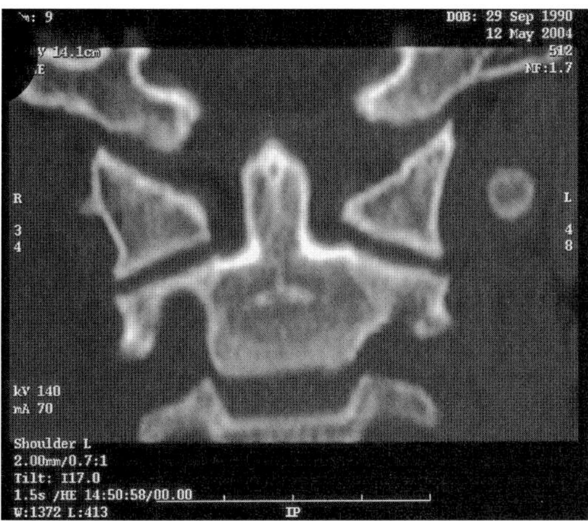

Fig. 6.73. Coronal reconstruction of computed tomography in a 13-year-old boy with symptoms in the craniocervical region. There is asymmetry of the C2 vertebra with possible erosion on the left

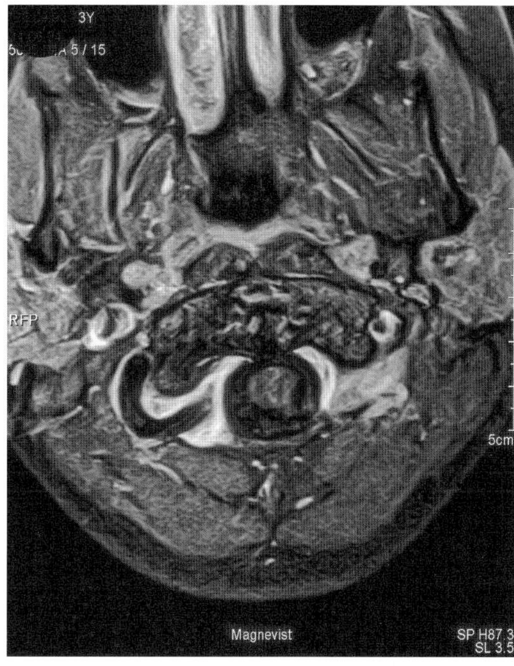

Fig. 6.74. Axial T2-weighted image of the craniocervical junction through the level of C2 showing pronounced ectasia of the right vertebral artery and a relatively small left vertebral artery

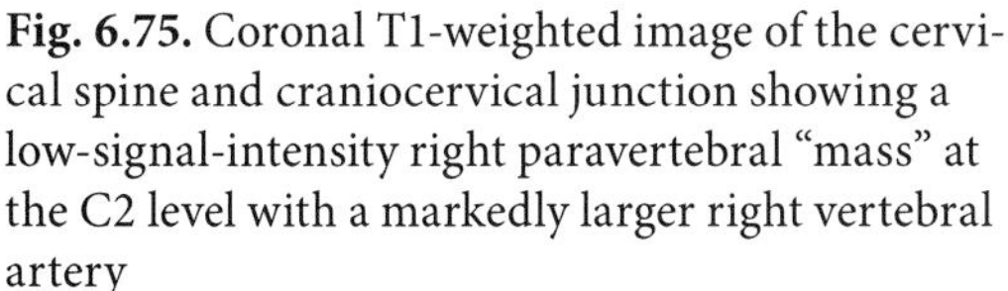
Fig. 6.75. Coronal T1-weighted image of the cervical spine and craniocervical junction showing a low-signal-intensity right paravertebral "mass" at the C2 level with a markedly larger right vertebral artery

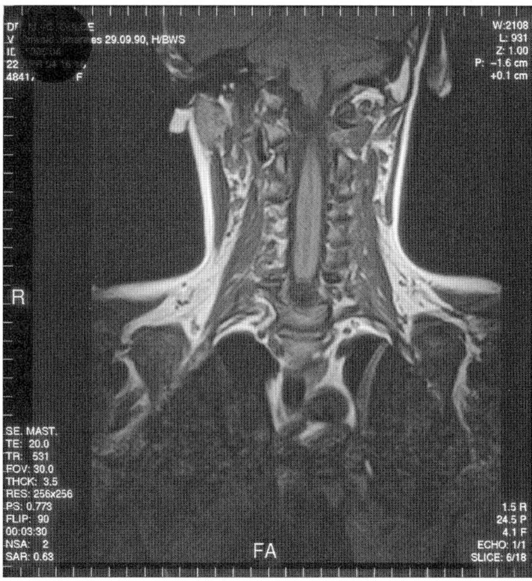

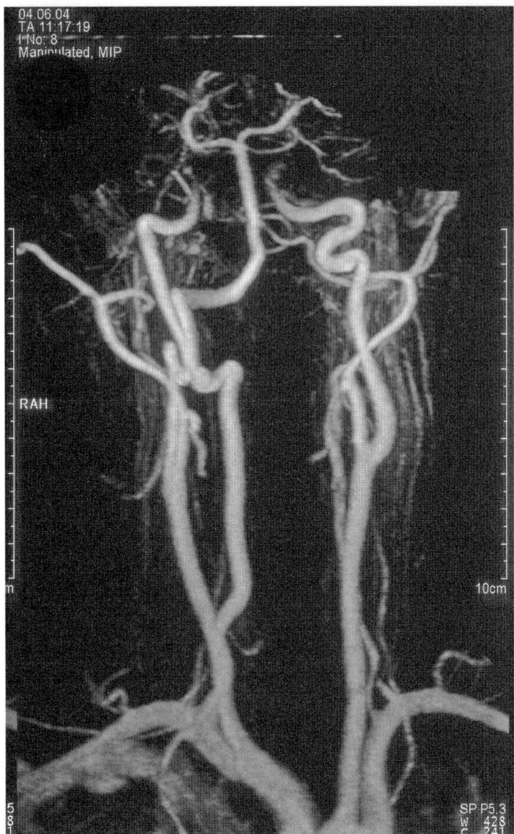

Fig. 6.76. Same patient. MR angiography of the supra-aortic branches confirming pronounced asymmetry of the vertebral arteries. The left artery is markedly hypoplastic, which explains the bony and soft tissue changes depicted by MRI

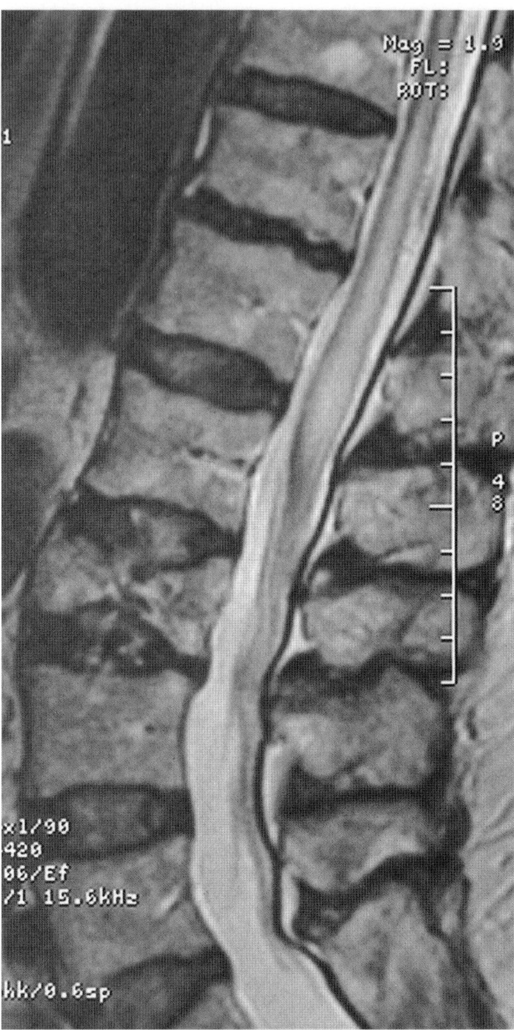

Fig. 6.77. Sagittal T2-weighted image. Spindle-shaped widening of the spinal cord beginning at T10 and increasing toward the conus at T12-L1. Spinal cord edema due to increased pressure in the draining venous arm. Incidental finding: vertebral compression/spontaneous deformation of L2

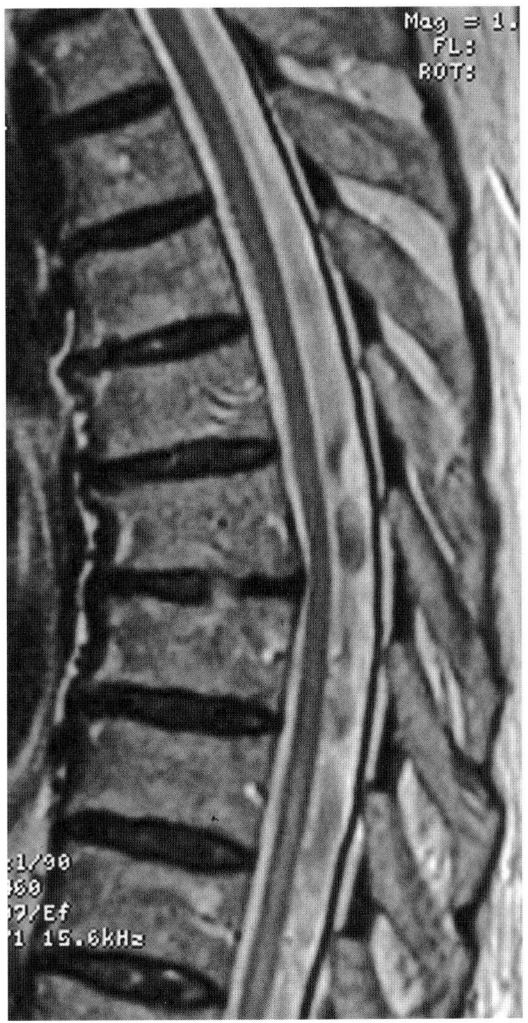

Fig. 6.78. T2-weighted image of the thoracic region: ectasia and increased pulsation of intradural draining veins

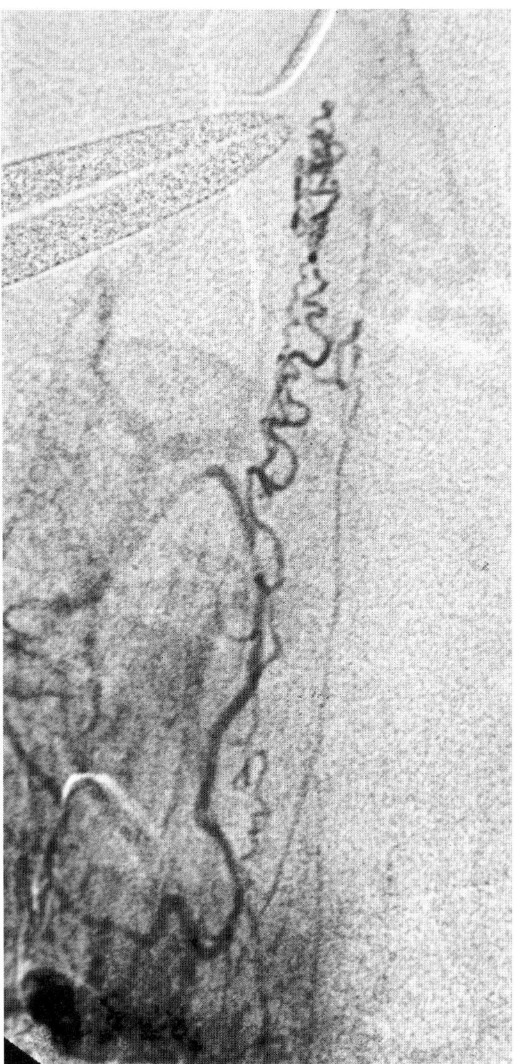

Fig. 6.79. Spinal angiography showing the feeding artery of the dural fistula at T5, which is opacified through the artery of Adamkiewicz

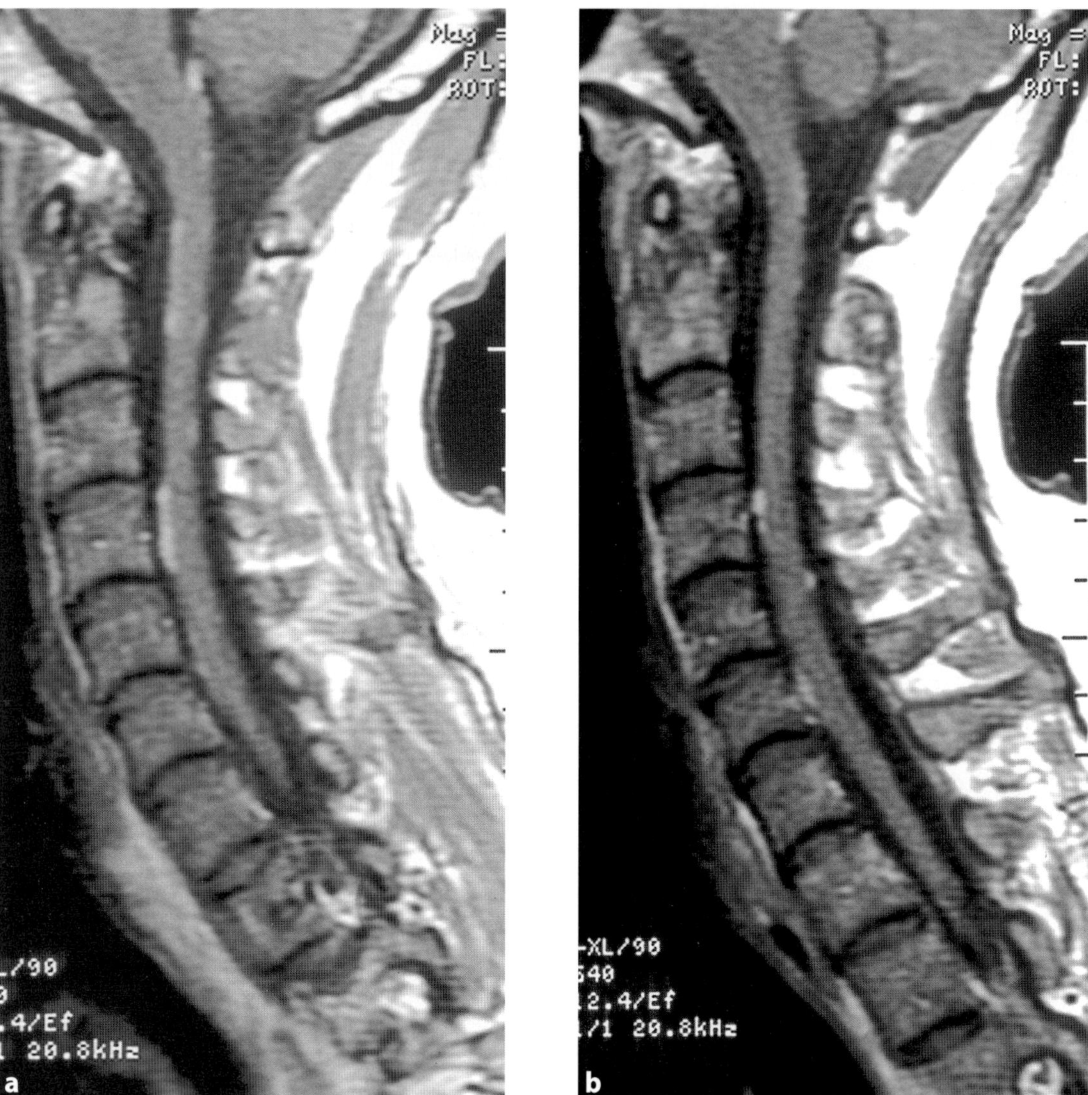

Fig. 6.80a, b. Spinal sarcoidosis. Sagittal T1-weighted images after contrast administration. Multiple foci of contrast enhancement in the cervical meninges

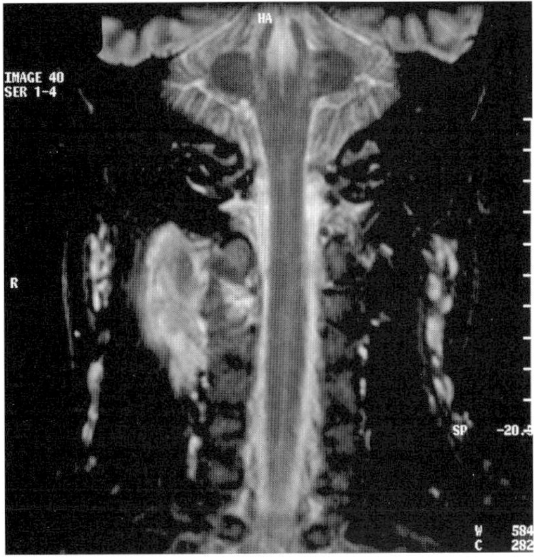

Fig. 6.81. Coronal T2-weighted image of the cervical region with fat saturation (STIR) in a patient with osteoid osteoma of the right transverse process of C4. Large edematous fluid collection in the affected transverse process and surrounding soft tissue structures

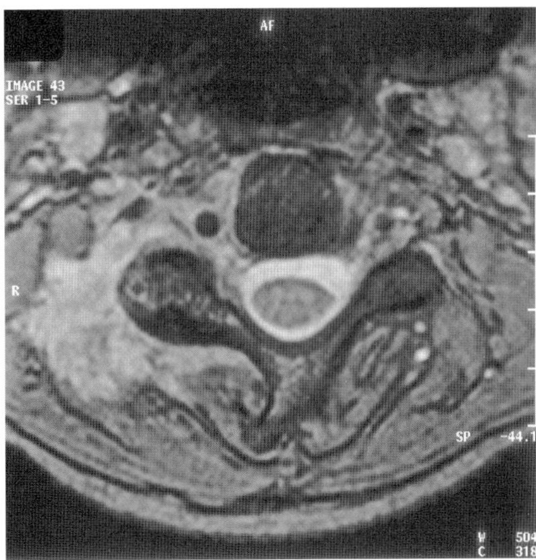

Fig. 6.82. Axial T2-weighted image through the C4 level showing a low-signal-intensity nidus in the C4 transverse process surrounded by high-signal-intensity edema. In addition, there is thinning of adjacent cortical bone

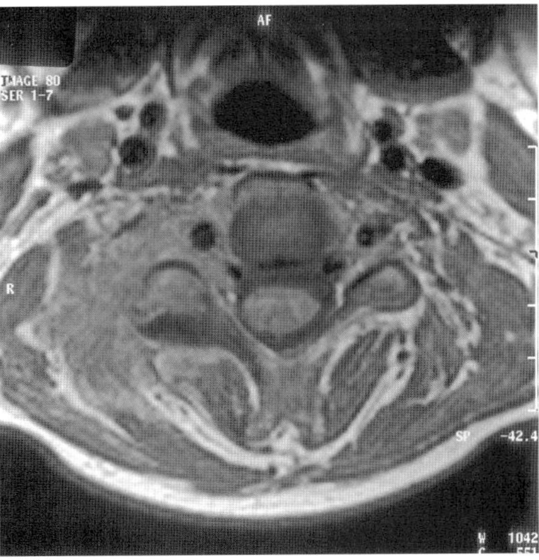

Fig. 6.83. Axial T1-weighted image through the C4 level. The nidus is not well-defined, while the surrounding edema is indicated by the reduced signal intensity relative to surrounding soft tissue. The cortical bone of the right transverse process is blurred and partially disrupted

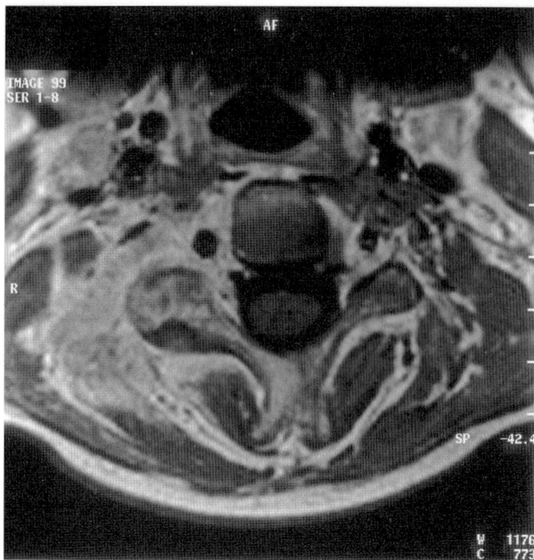

Fig. 6.84. Same patient. Axial T1-weighted image of the cervical spine through the C4 level. Pronounced enhancement of the osteoid osteoma in and around the right transverse process. The nidus is still not clearly visible. The enhancing structures extend into the right C4 foramen and to the right vertebral artery

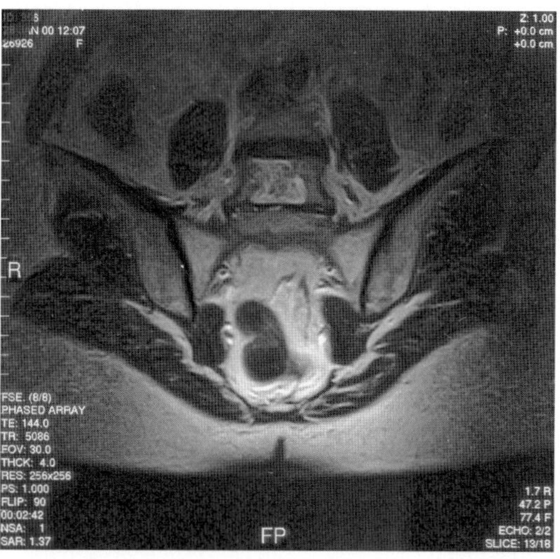

Fig. 6.85. Coronal T2-weighted image of the lumbar and sacral regions in a 65-year-old patient with osteoblastoma. Sharply demarcated area of high signal intensity with slight central inhomogeneities in the right aspect of L5 without enlargement of the vertebral body

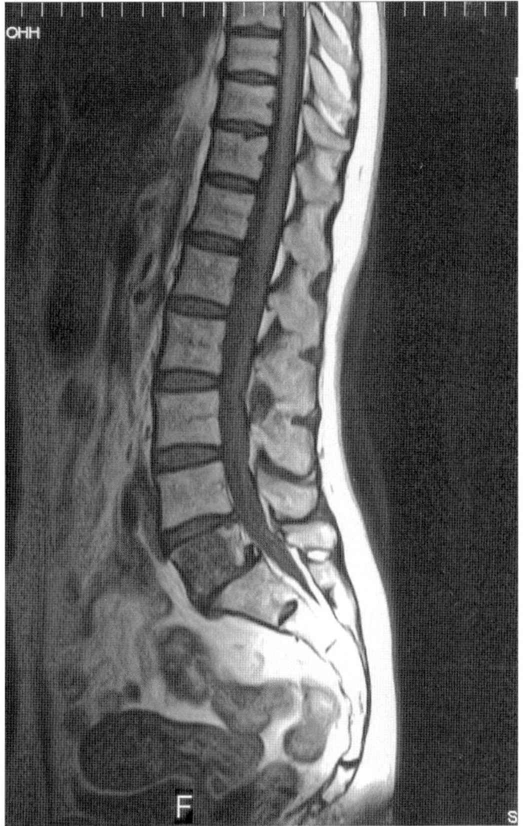

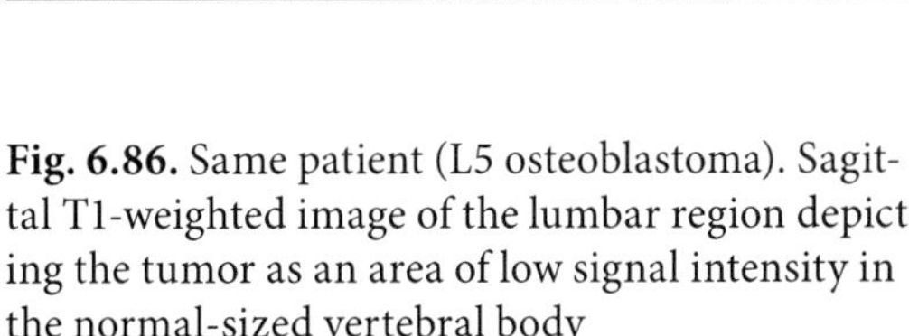
Fig. 6.86. Same patient (L5 osteoblastoma). Sagittal T1-weighted image of the lumbar region depicting the tumor as an area of low signal intensity in the normal-sized vertebral body

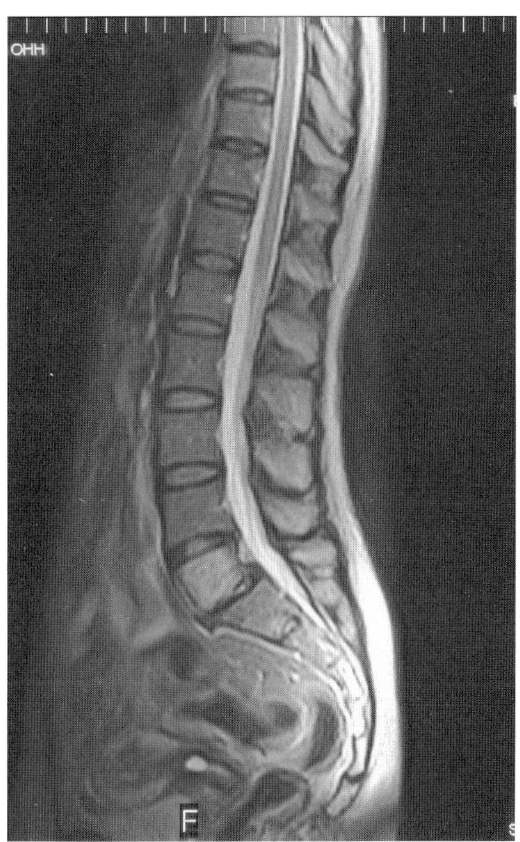

Fig. 6.87. L5 osteoblastoma. Sagittal T2-weighted image showing high signal intensity of the normal-sized L5 vertebral body

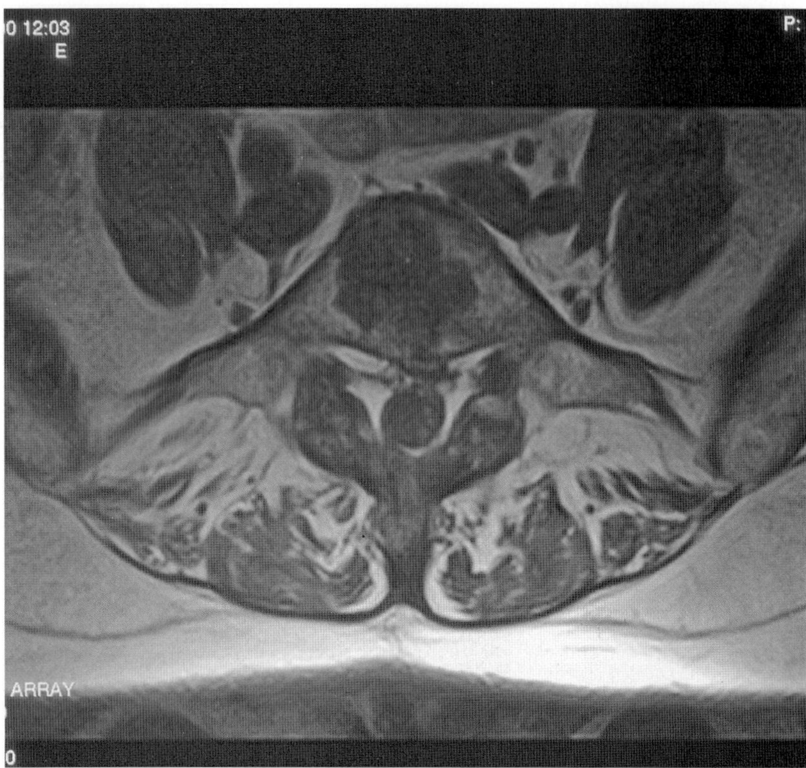

Fig. 6.88. Same patient. Axial T1-weighted image of the L5 osteoblastoma showing a slightly irregular, low-signal-intensity tumor in the L5 vertebral body without cortical destruction

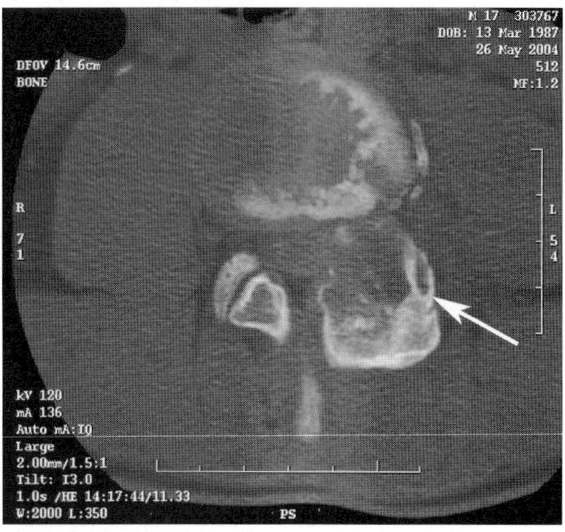

Fig. 6.89. Axial CT scan through the L3-4 level of the patient with osteoblastoma showing tumorous expansion of the left pedicle and posterolateral portions of the vertebral body

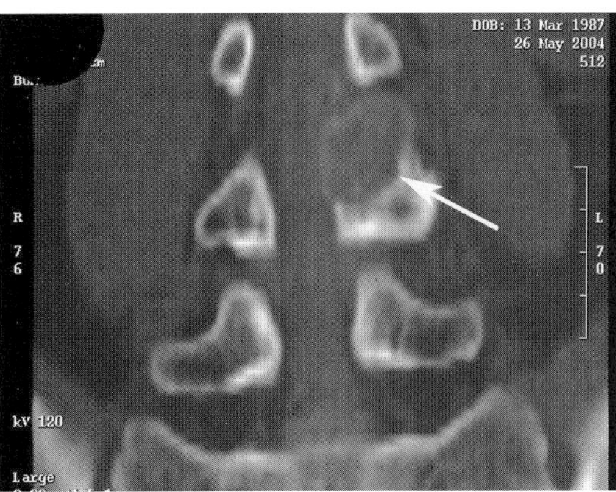

Fig. 6.90. Same patient. Coronal CT reconstruction showing the osteoblastoma with soft tissue density at the L4 pedicle

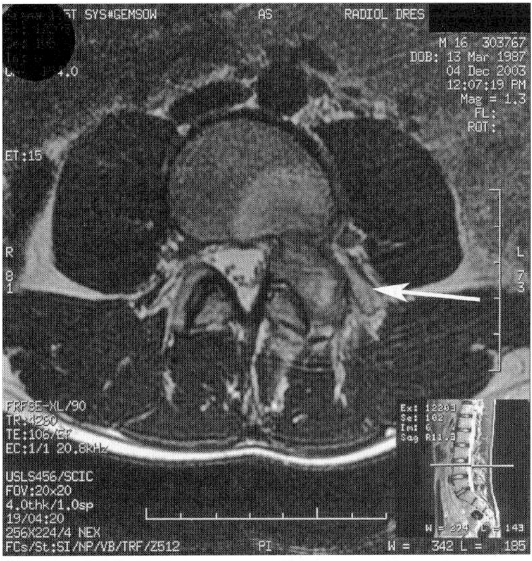

Fig. 6.91. Axial T2-weighted image of the osteoblastoma. The image through the L3-4 level shows involvement of the left posterolateral portions of the vertebral body and left arch. The tumor has slightly higher signal intensity than normal bone marrow

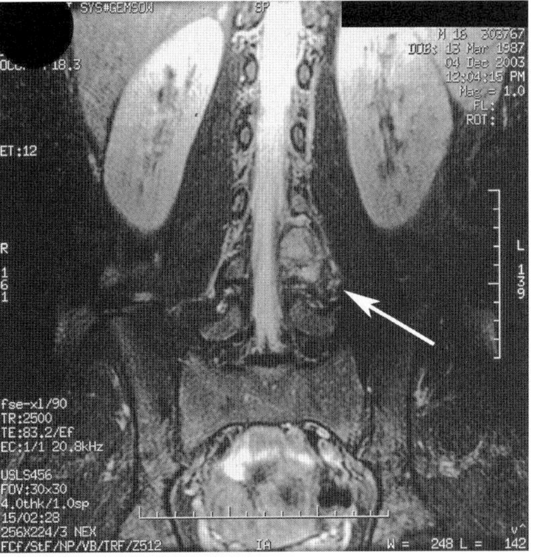

Fig. 6.92. Coronal T2-weighted image with fat saturation depicting the osteoblastoma above the left L4 pedicle

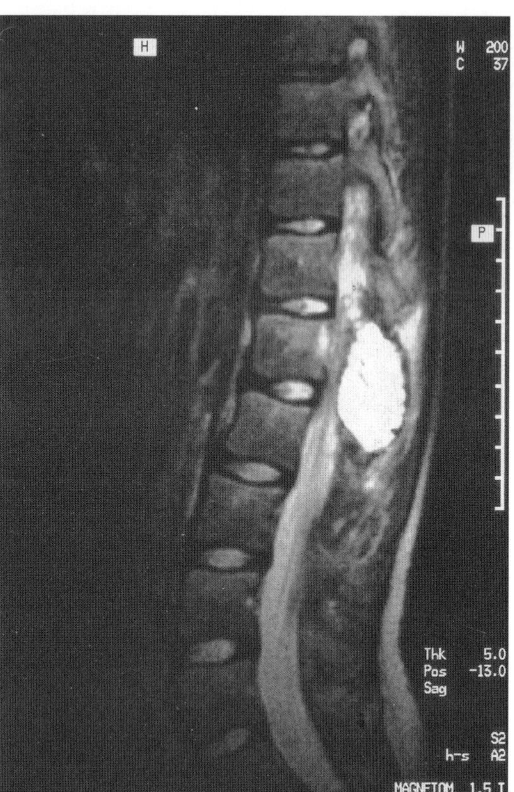

Fig. 6.93. Aneurysmal bone cyst at T12. Sagittal T2-weighted image with fat saturation at the level of the thoracolumbar junction showing a bright cystic lesion of the posterior elements of the T12 vertebra with partial involvement of the pedicle

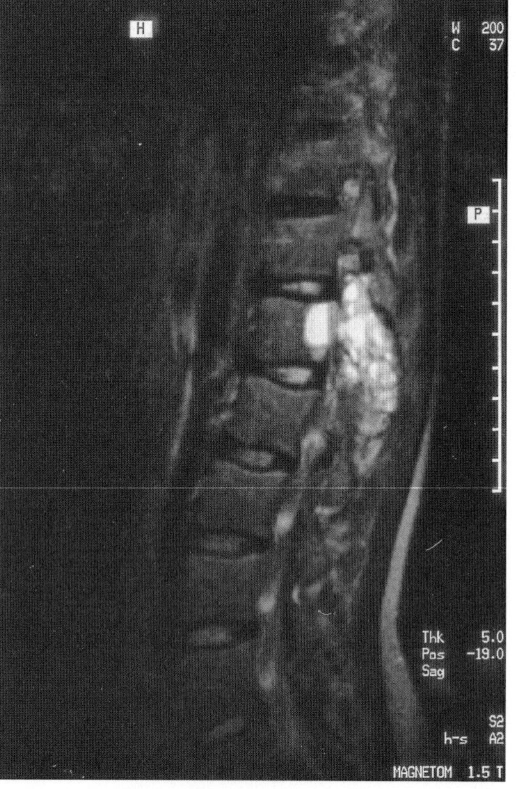

Fig. 6.94. Right parasagittal T2-weighted image with fat saturation of the T12 aneurysmal bone cyst already shown in the preceding figure. Lobulated cystic lesion involving the posterior elements of T12. The intravertebral component is seen more clearly

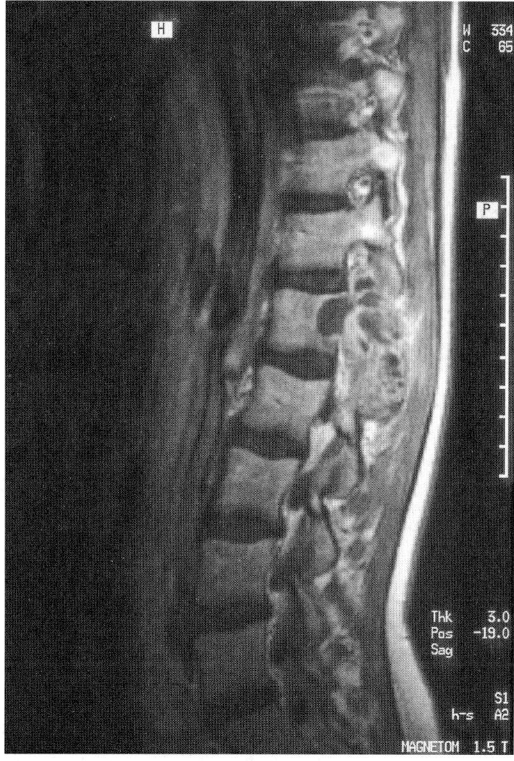

Fig. 6.95. Same patient. Sagittal T1-weighted image of the T12 aneurysmal bone cyst after contrast administration demonstrating the lobulated cystic lesion with involvement of the T12 vertebral body, right pedicle, inferior articular process, and spinous process.

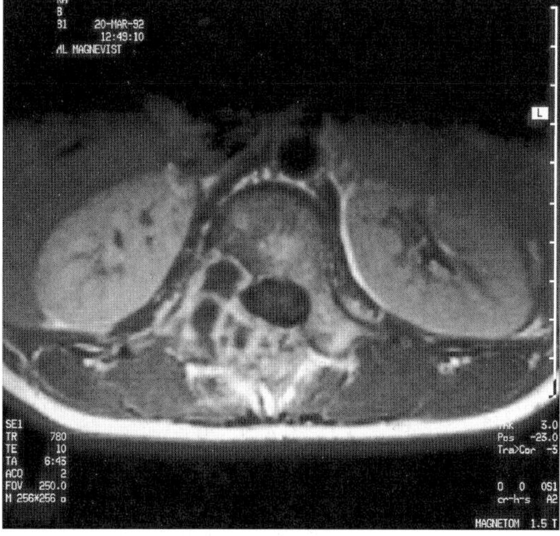

Fig. 6.96. Axial T1-weighted image of the T12 aneurysmal bone cyst after contrast administration. The cyst is depicted as a lobulated lesion with pronounced peripheral enhancement and a poorly perfused center. There is slight posterior indentation and narrowing of the spinal canal

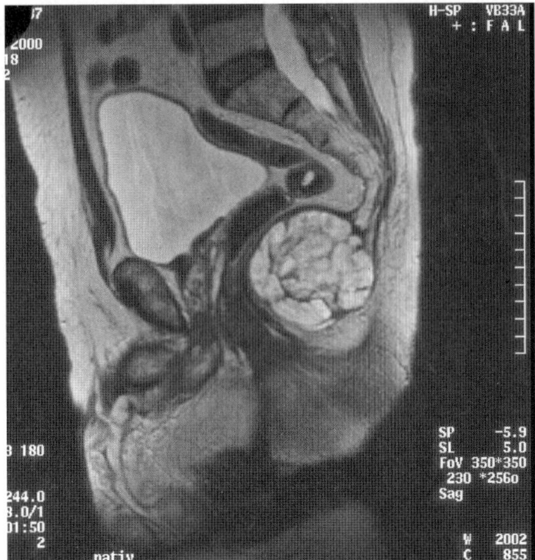

Fig. 6.97. Sagittal T2-weighted image of the lower lumbar region and sacrum showing a large tumor with a diameter of about 5 cm in the area of the coccygeal bone. The tumor has high signal intensity with lower-intensity septae and is clearly delineated from surrounding fatty tissue

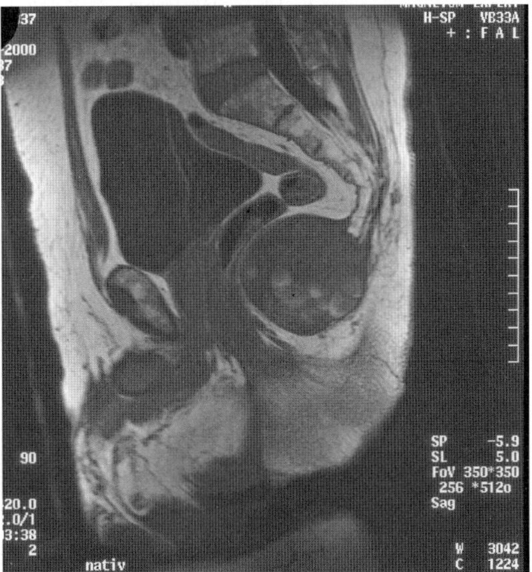

Fig. 6.98. Sagittal T1-weighted image. Coccygeal chordoma with low signal intensity and some hyperintensities in the posterobasal portions suggesting fresh hemorrhage

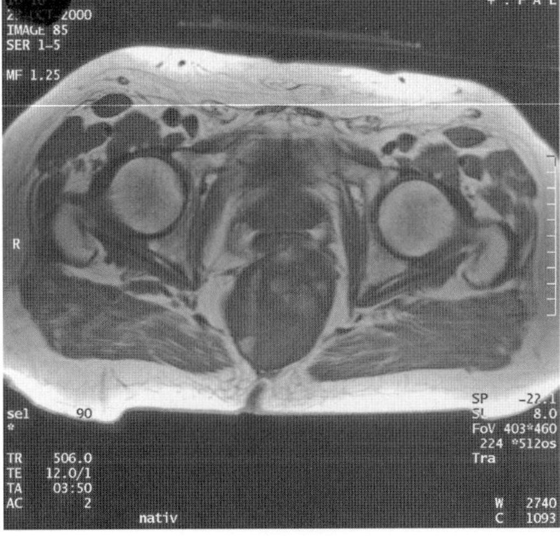

Fig. 6.99. Axial T1-weighted image of the chordoma at the coccygeal level. Well-defined tumor with mostly low signal intensity

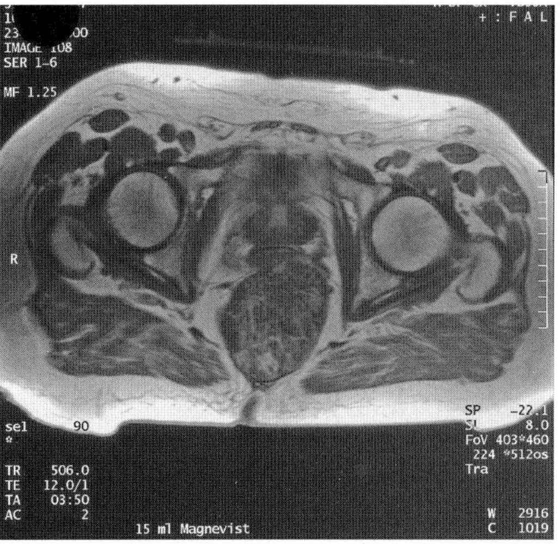

Fig. 6.100. Same patient as in preceding figures. Contrast-enhanced axial T1-weighted image at the level of the coccygeal chordoma. There is only slight, inhomogeneous enhancement

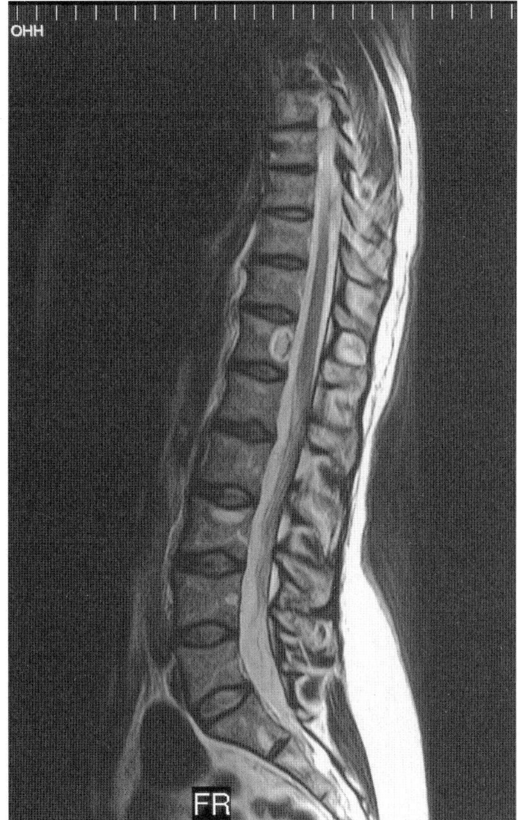

Fig. 6.101. Sagittal T2-weighted image of the lower thoracic spine and lumbar region in a 53-year-old patient with eosinophilic granuloma of the T12 vertebra. Well-defined oval lesion of high signal intensity in the posterior portion of the T12 vertebral body without endplate destruction. The high-signal-intensity tumor is surrounded by a rim of even higher signal intensity

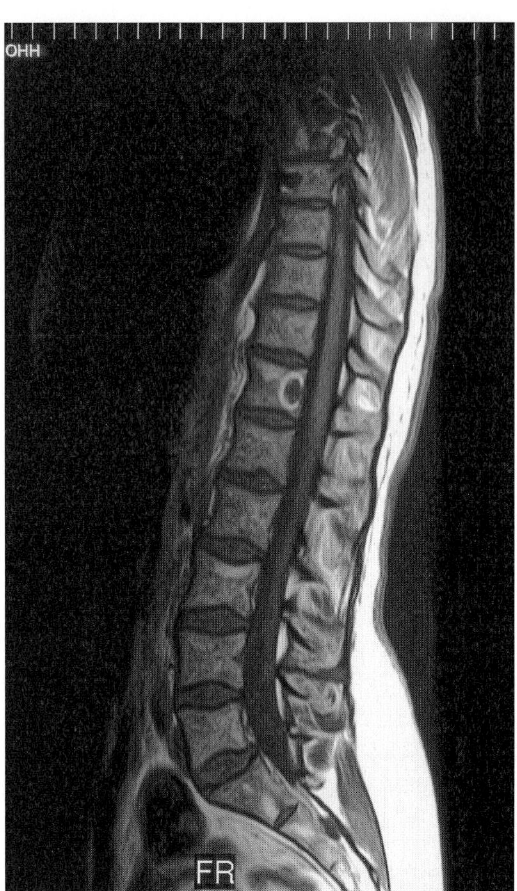

Fig. 6.102. Same patient. Sagittal T1-weighted image of the T12 eosinophilic granuloma. Low signal intensity in the center, while the rim is markedly hyperintense, consistent with peripheral hemorrhage

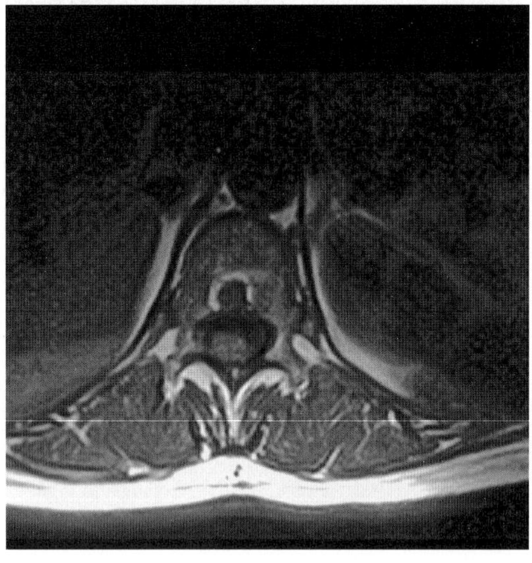

Fig. 6.103. Axial T1-weighted image through the T12 level. The low-signal-intensity center of the eosinophilic granuloma is surrounded by a hemorrhagic rim

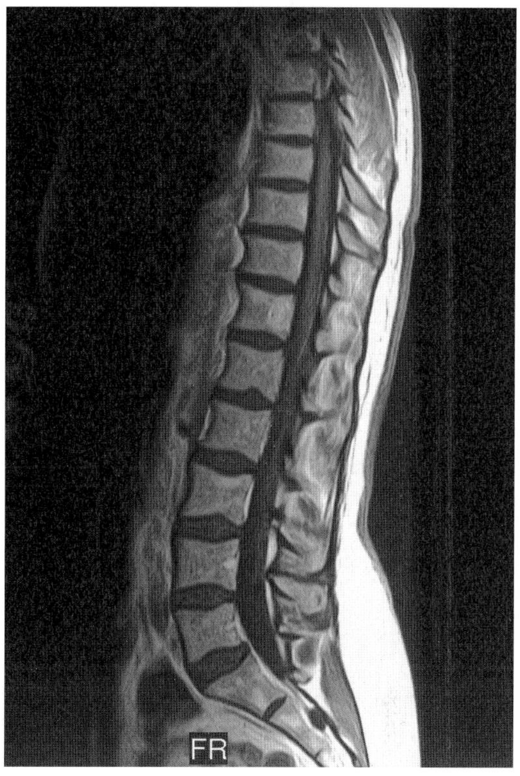

Fig. 6.104. Same patient. Sagittal T1-weighted image of the eosinophilic granuloma in the posterior portion of the T12 vertebral body after contrast administration. Central enhancement of the lesion results in isointensity with the rim, which already had a high signal on unenhanced images

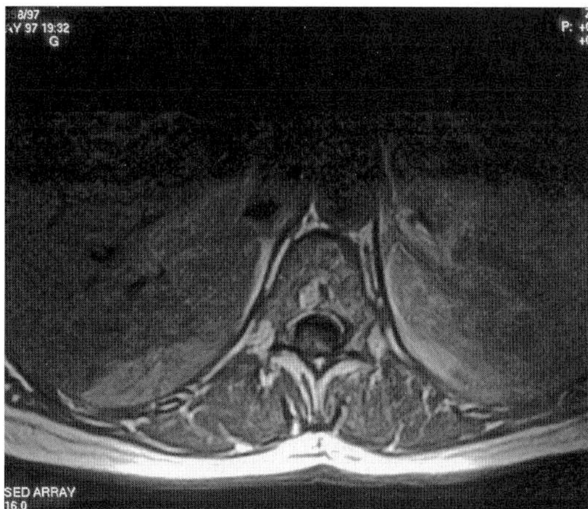

Fig. 6.105. Axial T1-weighted image through T12 after contrast administration showing pronounced enhancement of the eosinophilic granuloma directly beneath the posterior edge of the vertebra

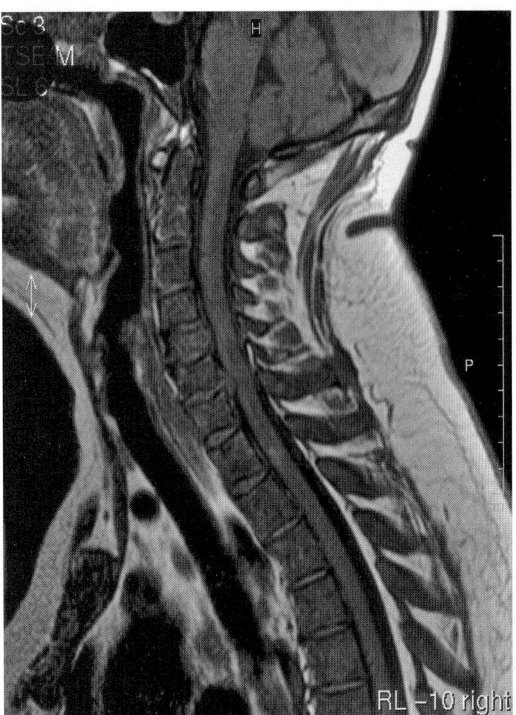

Fig. 6.106. Sagittal T1-weighted image of the cervical region in a 73-year-old man with known plasmocytoma. Low signal intensity of all vertebral bodies and bony elements, indicating replacement of the normal fatty marrow. C6-7 disc herniation with displacement of the spinal cord. Loss of height of C5

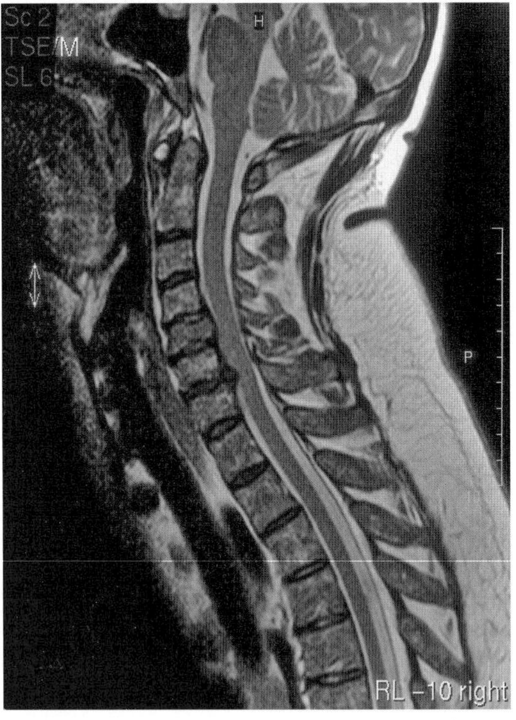

Fig. 6.107. Sagittal T2-weighted image of the patient with diffuse plasmocytoma. There is loss of height of C5, most prominent in the posterior portion, with inhomogeneously reduced bone marrow signal intensity. C6-7 disc herniation indenting the spinal cord

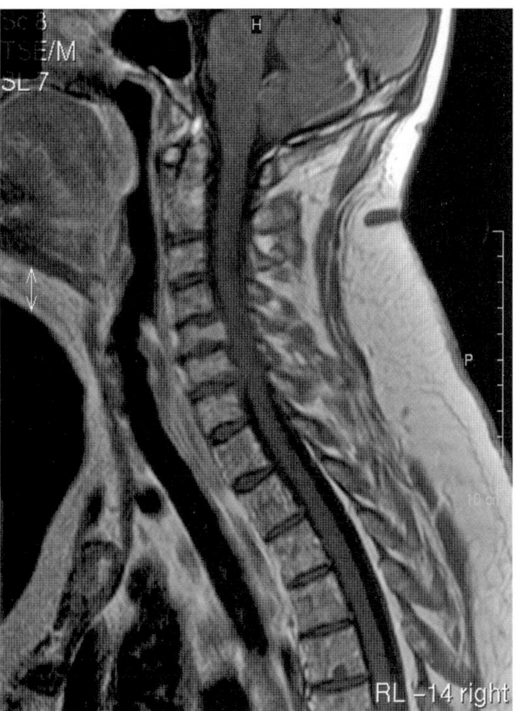

Fig. 6.108. Sagittal T1-weighted image of the plasmocytoma patient after contrast administration. Diffuse plasmocytoma is confirmed by enhancement of all bony structures depicted. Partial destruction of C5 and loss of height

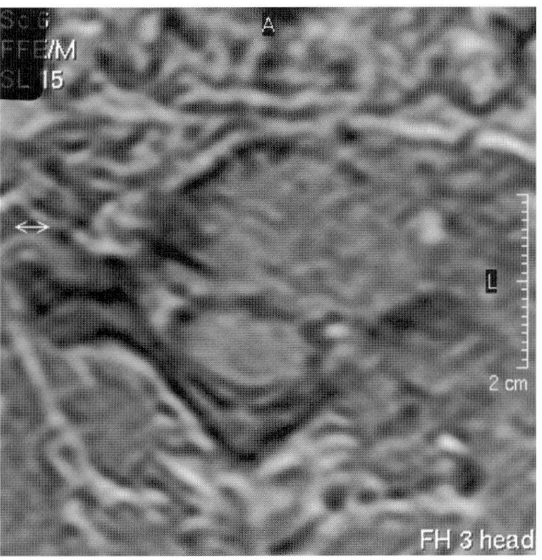

Fig. 6.109. Axial T1-weighted image through C5 showing slightly hyperintense expansion and destruction of the left portion of C5

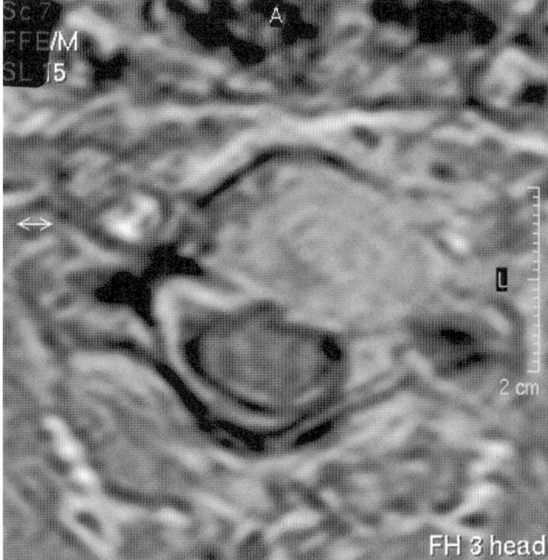

Fig. 6.110. Axial T1-weighted image through C5 after contrast administration showing bony destruction of the posterior edge and left portion of the C5 vertebral body. There is partial occlusion of the left C5 neural foramen and posterior displacement of the spinal cord

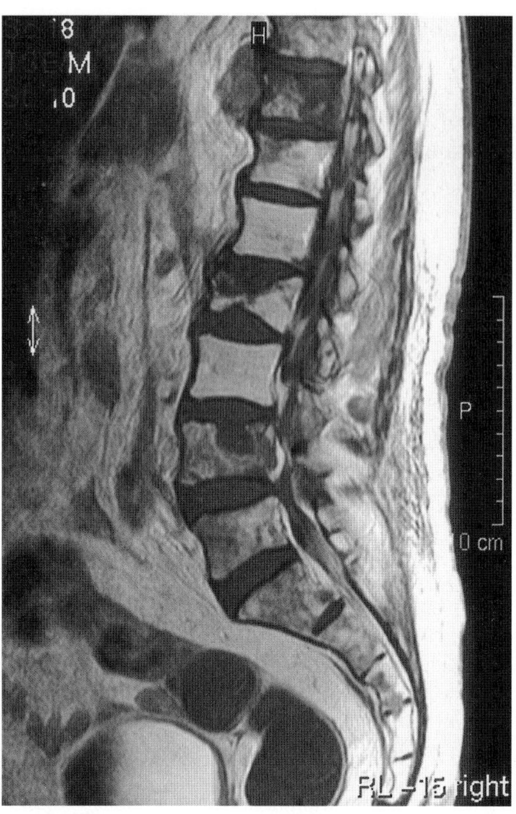

Fig. 6.111. Sagittal T1-weighted image of the lumbosacral region in a patient with plasmocytoma. The image shows butterfly deformity of the L2 vertebral body and diffuse signal alterations of T12, L4-5, S1, and S2. L4 endplate impression. The inhomogeneous and slightly reduced signal of these vertebral bodies indicates partial displacement of the normal fatty marrow

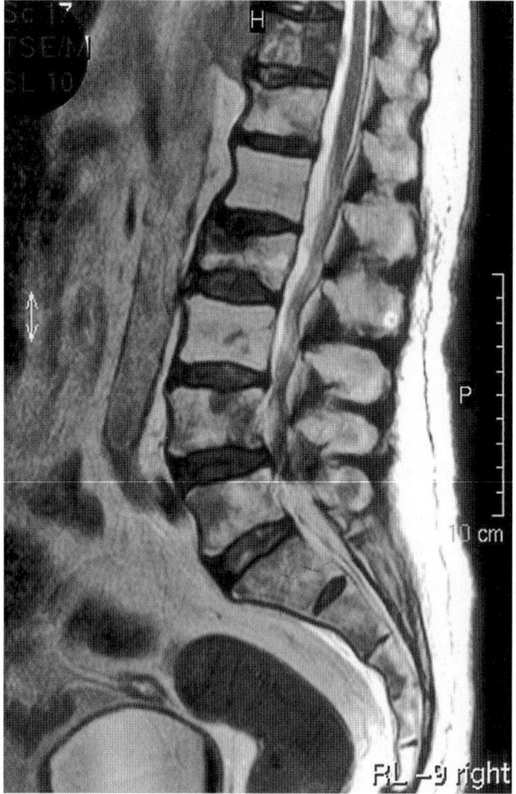

Fig. 6.112. Sagittal T2-weighted image of the same patient. Plasmocytoma with tumorous infiltration of T11, L2, L4, L5, S1, and S2 as indicated by the reduced signal intensity of the vertebral marrow

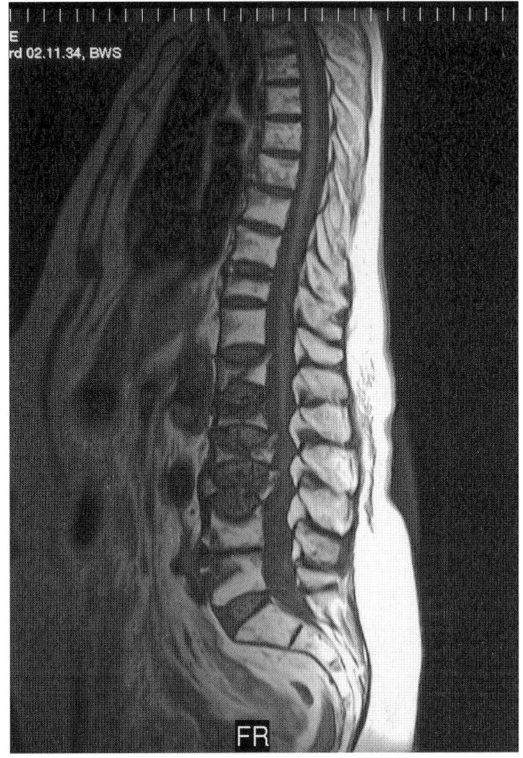

Fig. 6.113. Sagittal T1-weighted image of the thoracolumbar region showing a plasmocytoma with partially very inhomogeneous vertebral body signal in the middle and lower thoracic spine. In addition, the image shows impression fracture of T10, butterfly deformity of T12, complex fractures and compression fractures of L1 through L3, impression of the superior endplate of L4, and abnormal signal alterations of the anterior edge of L5

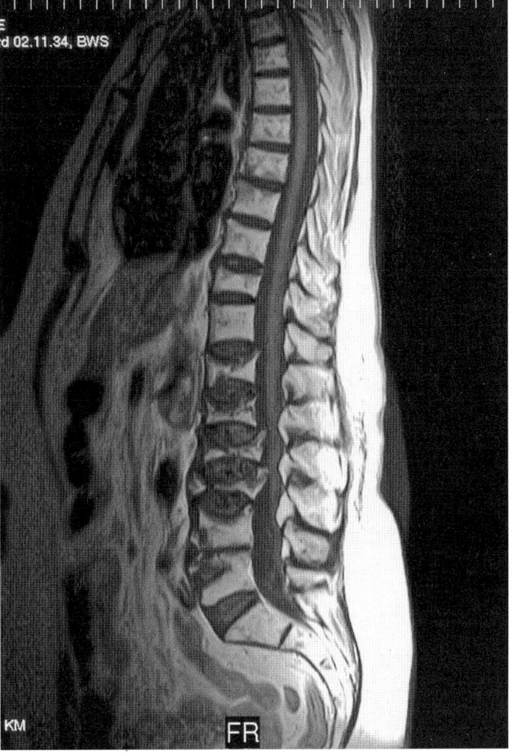

Fig. 6.114. Sagittal T1-weighted image of the plasmocytoma after contrast administration. There is enhancement of the abnormal areas in T10, T12, L1 through L3, and L5. Displacement of the posterior walls of L2 and L3 toward the spinal canal and the resulting spinal stenosis are more conspicuous on this image

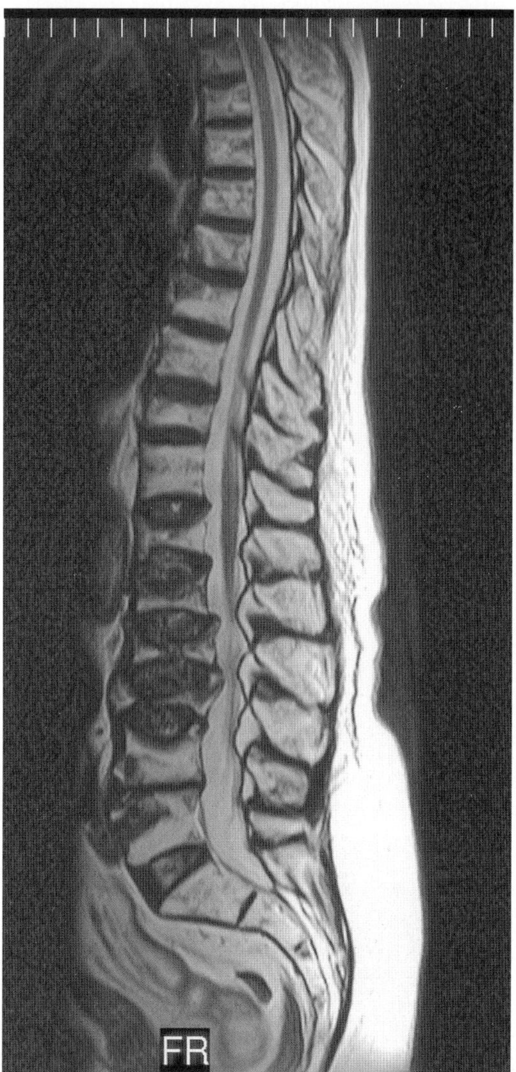

Fig. 6.115. Same patient. Sagittal T2-weighted image of the plasmocytoma of the thoracolumbar spine showing low signal intensity of the involved vertebral bodies of T10, T12, L1 through L3, and superior endplate of L4 and anterior edge of L5. In addition, part of the affected vertebrae are compressed and fractured

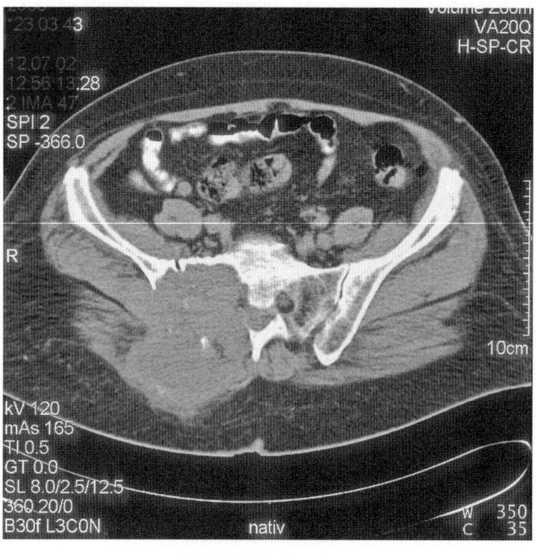

Fig. 6.116. Axial pelvic CT scan of a 60-year-old patient presenting with severe pain in the upper sacral region. Large tumor in the area of the sacroiliac joint on the right with partial destruction of the posterior portions of the medial ilium and sacrum. Malignant fibrous histiocytoma measuring approximately 8×7×6 cm

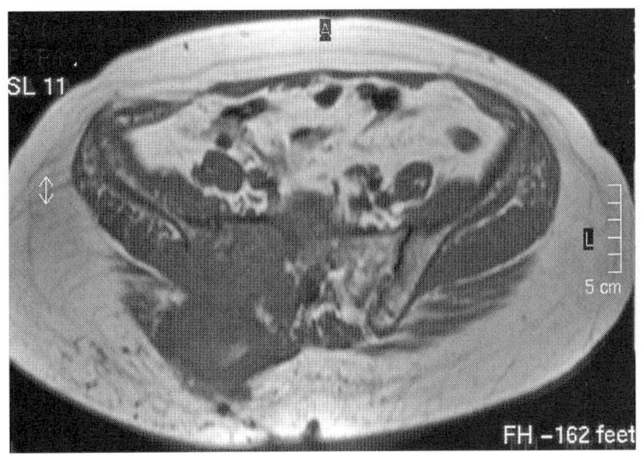

Fig. 6.117. Same patient. Axial T1-weighted image of the malignant fibrous histiocytoma at the level of the sacroiliac joint. The image shows a poorly defined, low-signal-intensity tumor on the right with partial destruction of the sacrum and ilium

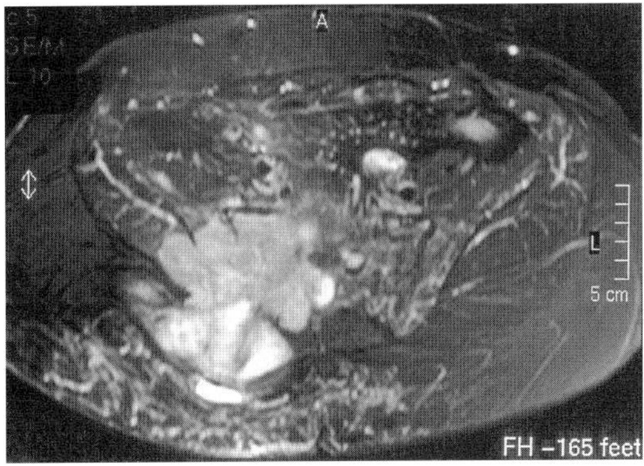

Fig. 6.118. Axial T2-weighted image with fat saturation (STIR). The malignant fibrous histiocytoma is shown as a high-signal-intensity mass in the area of the sacral and iliac bones on the right. The tumor appears lobulated but is relatively well-defined

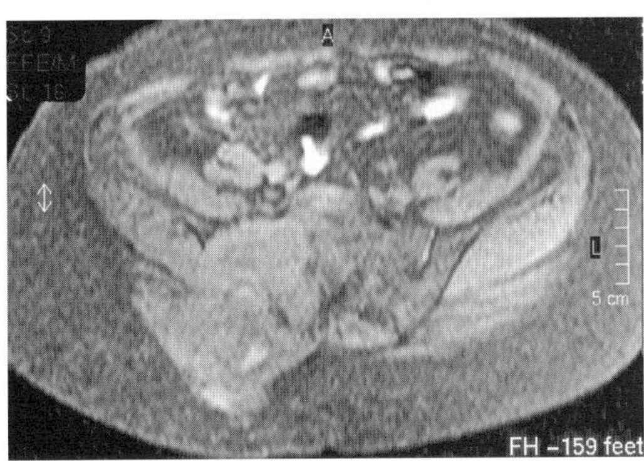

Fig. 6.119. Axial T1-weighted image with fat saturation of the malignant fibrous histiocytoma at the sacroiliac joint on the right

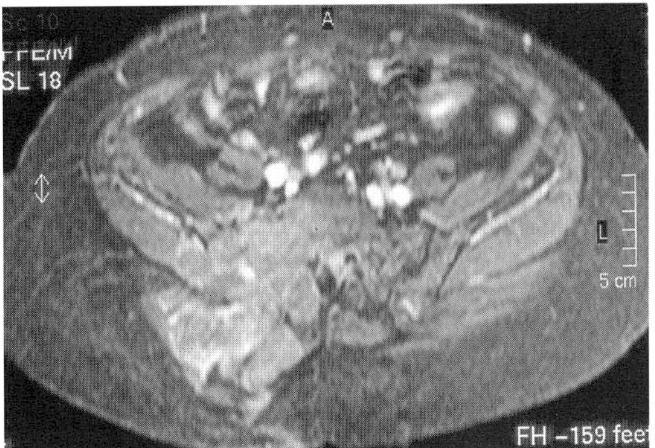

Fig. 6.120. Axial T1-weighted image of the malignant fibrous histiocytoma at the level of the sacroiliac joint after contrast administration. The tumor shows altogether moderate enhancement with slightly more pronounced peripheral enhancement. There is better delineation of intraspinal structures on the contrast-enhanced image. The extent of bony destruction is seen less clearly than on CT

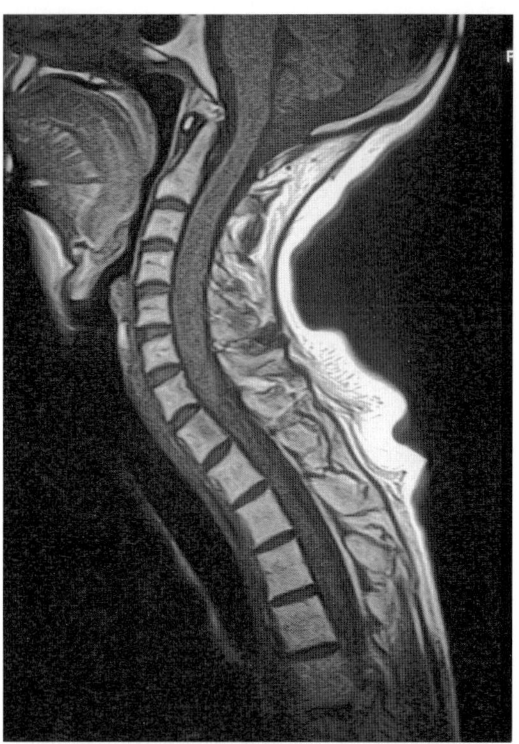

Fig. 6.121. Sagittal T1-weighted image of the cervical region in a 41-year-old patient with breast cancer and spinal cord metastasis extending from C2 through C6-7. Widening of the cervical cord and slight increase in signal intensity

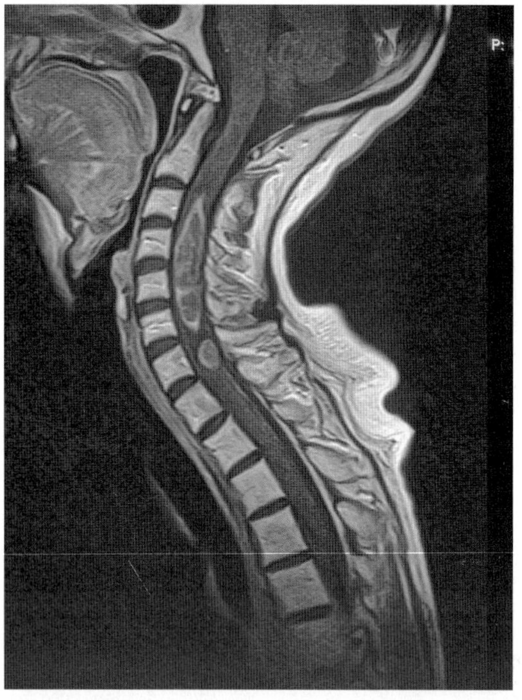

Fig. 6.122. Sagittal T1-weighted image of the same patient after contrast administration. Marked peripheral enhancement of the intramedullary metastases from C2-3 through C6-7 and at C7. The metastases have a slight mass effect

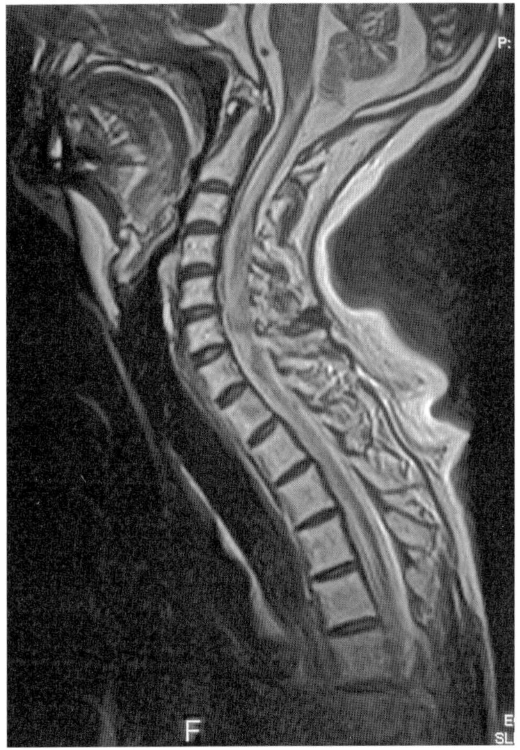

Fig. 6.123. Same patient. Sagittal T2-weighted image of the cervical region with intramedullary metastases from C2-3 through C7. The band of increased signal in the spinal cord extending from the base of skull down to the T4-5 level reflects large perifocal edema associated with intramedullary metastases

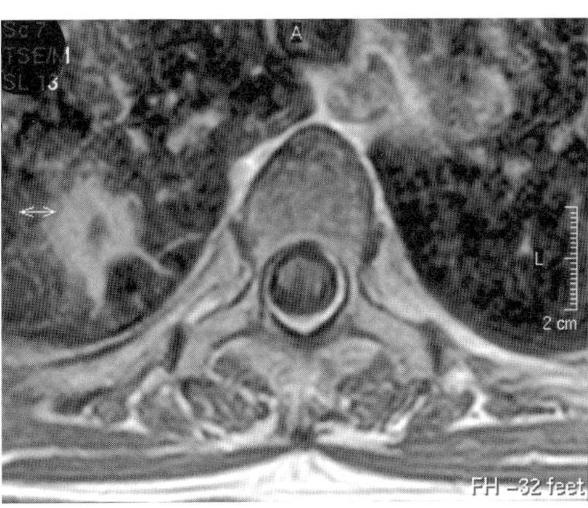

Fig. 6.124. Axial T1-weighted image of a 70-year-old patient with bronchial cancer seen to the right of the spine as a streaky high-signal-intensity mass with reticular extensions

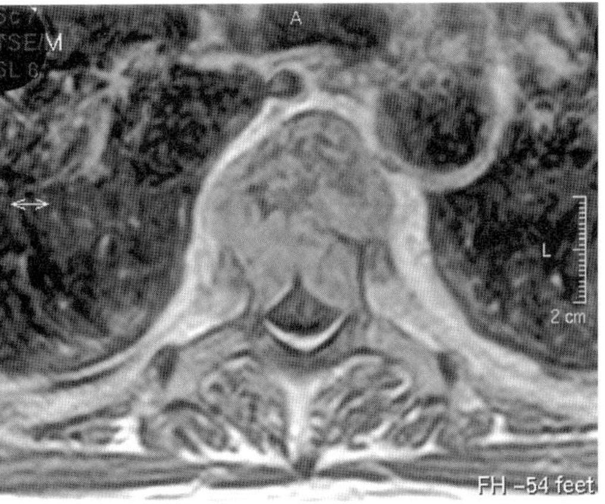

Fig. 6.125. Contrast-enhanced axial T1-weighted image through the T6 level showing a bone metastasis expanding the T6 vertebral body anteriorly and laterally and extending into the spinal canal from the right and left (so-called draped curtain sign)

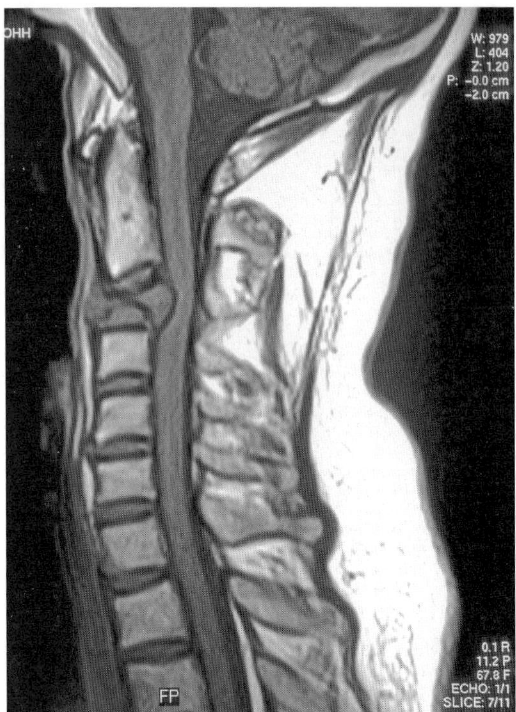

Fig. 6.126. Sagittal T1-weighted image of the cervical spine in a 60-year-old patient with bronchial cancer. The image shows a tumor-induced compression fracture of C3 with low signal intensity of the residual vertebral body portions as well as convex deformity of the posterior surface which protrudes into the spinal canal with marked displacement and indentation of the spinal cord

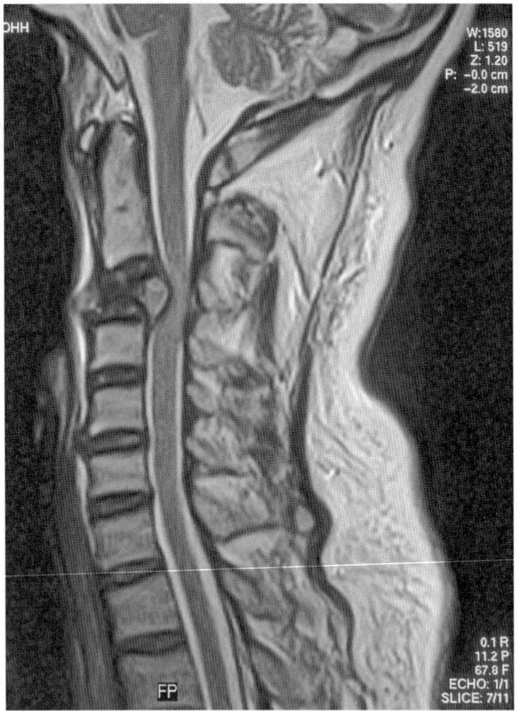

Fig. 6.127. Sagittal T2-weighted image of the cervical spine in the patient with lung cancer and C3 fracture/destruction. There is pronounced deformity of the cervical spinal cord but no definitive signal alteration of the vertebral body

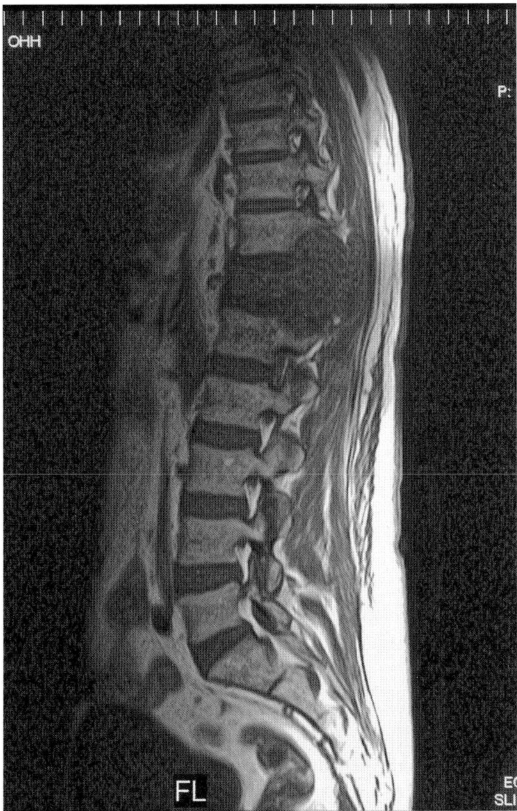

Fig. 6.128. Sagittal T1-weighted image of a 60-year-old patient with lung cancer. Bone metastasis of T12 with low signal intensity of the vertebral body and posterior extension of the tumor

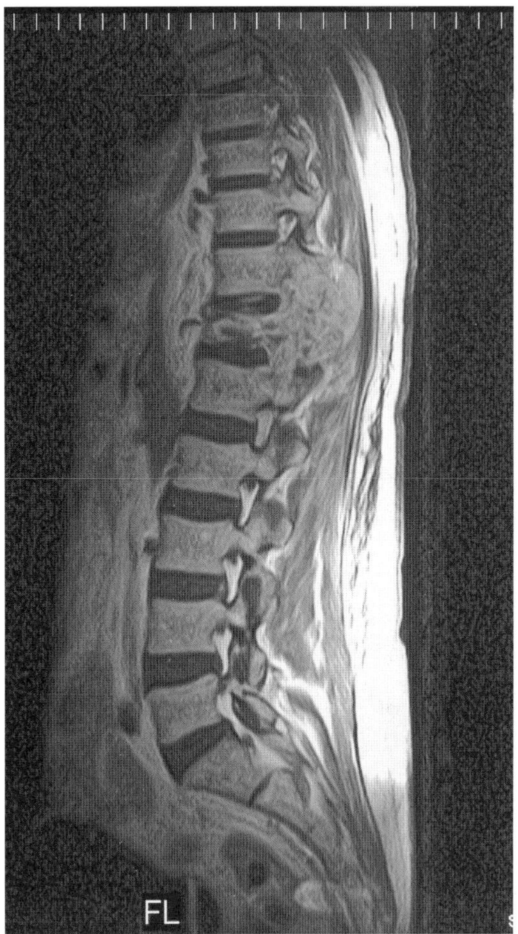

Fig. 6.129. Sagittal T1-weighted image of the lower thoracic and lumbar regions with T12 metastasis from bronchial cancer. There is pronounced contrast enhancement of the collapsed and partially destroyed T12 vertebral body and of the extraosseous components of the metastasis posterior to T12 and T11

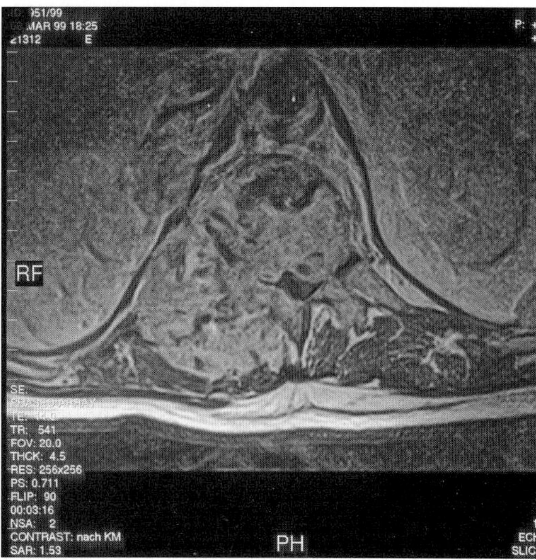

Fig. 6.130. Same patient. Axial T1-weighted image of the T12 bone metastasis from bronchial cancer. Tumorous destruction of the vertebral body and extravertebral tumor extension to the right and posteriorly. There is marked narrowing of the spinal canal with a faint draped curtain sign

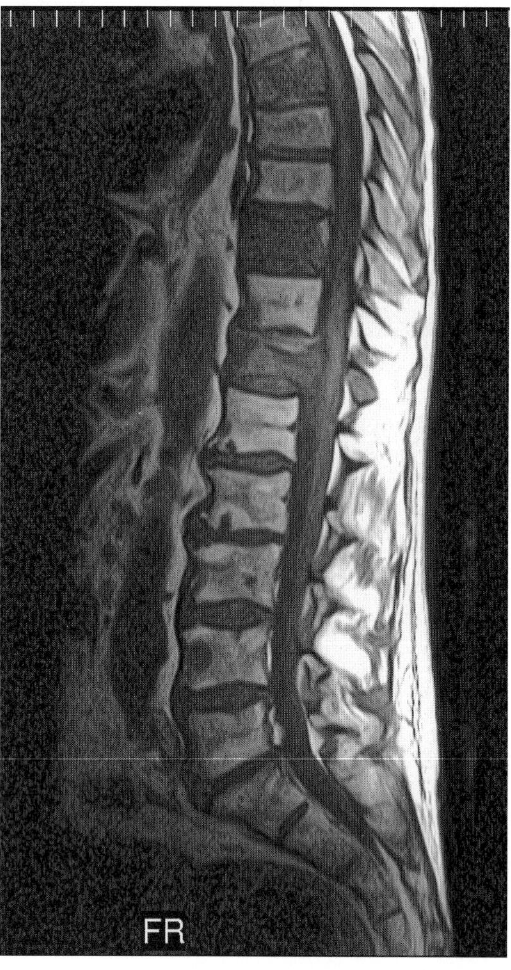

Fig. 6.131. Sagittal T1-weighted image of the lower thoracic spine and lumbar region in an 81-year-old patient with bone metastases from bronchial cancer. Low signal intensity of T7, T10, and T12 and of the anterior portion of L4 with less pronounced signal reduction also of T8 and T9. Posterior displacement of the posterior edge of T12 and low signal of the T12 pedicle

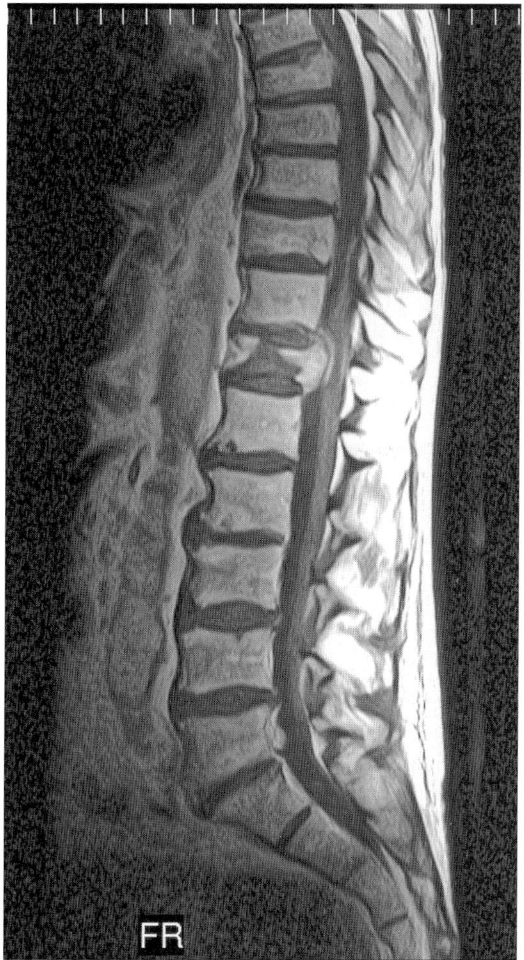

Fig. 6.132. Sagittal T1-weighted image of the lower thoracic spine and lumbar region in the patient with multiple metastases from lung cancer after contrast administration. There is marked enhancement of all metastases except for the central portions of T12. Spinal stenosis at T12 through posterior displacement of the tumorous posterior edge

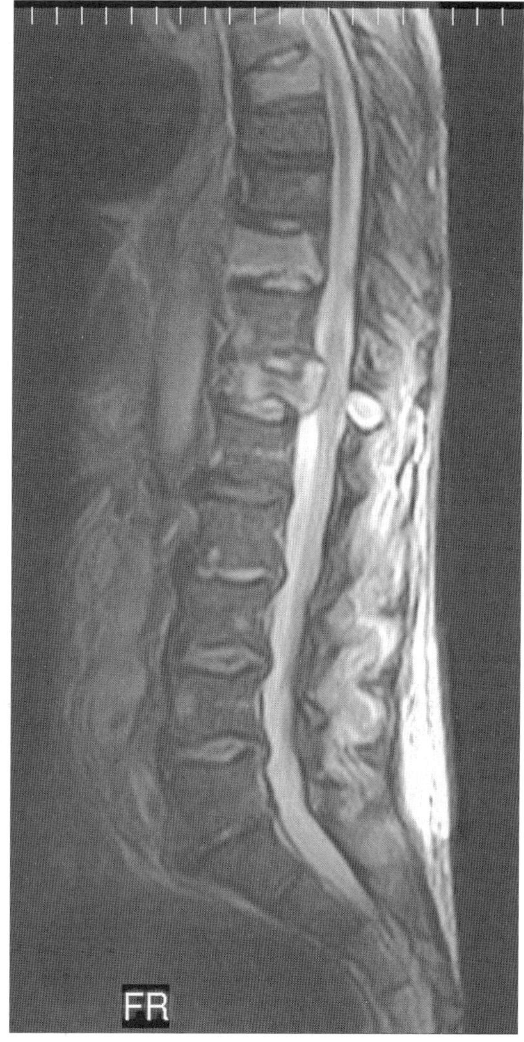

Fig. 6.133. Sagittal T2-weighted image with fat saturation. High signal intensity of the metastatic T7, T10, and T12 vertebral bodies (including the T12 pedicle) and spinal stenosis at T12. Mild signal enhancement of the focal metastasis in the anterior portion of the L4 vertebral body

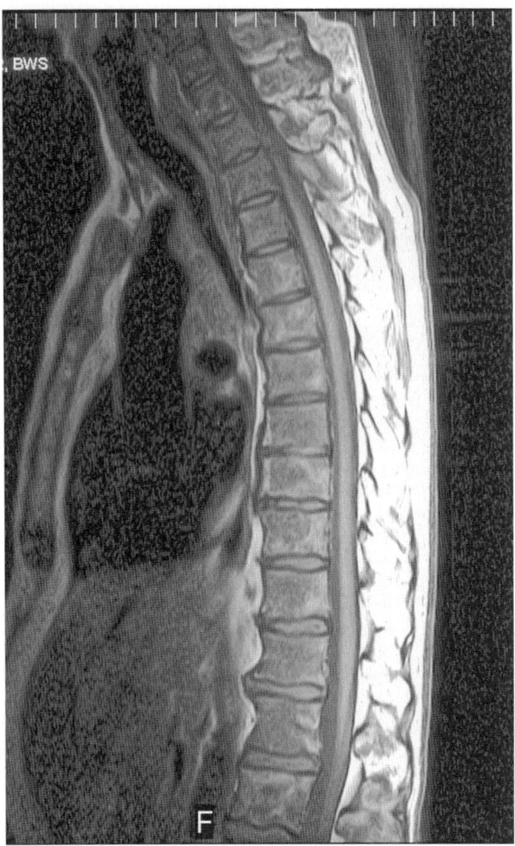

Fig. 6.134. Sagittal T1-weighted image of the thoracic region in a patient with bronchial cancer with diffuse metastatic spread to all vertebrae shown. There is inhomogeneous low signal intensity of the marrow in all vertebral bodies without signs of destruction

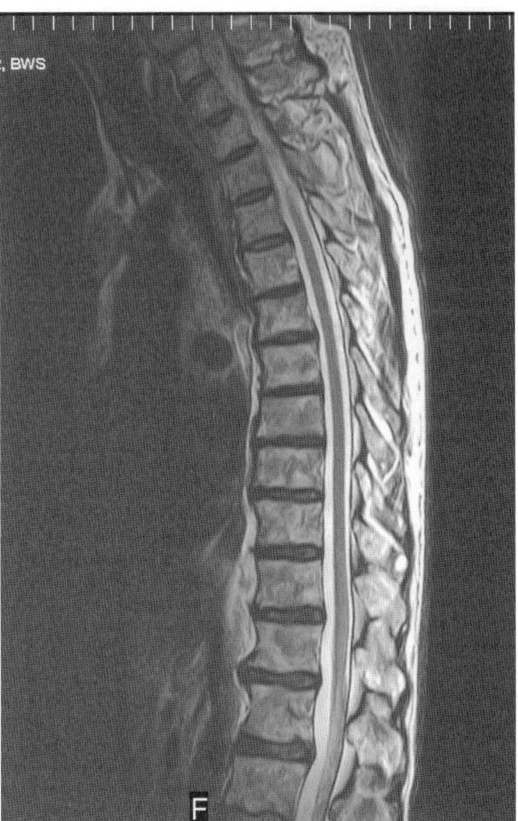

Fig. 6.135. Sagittal T2-weighted image of the thoracic region of the same patient. There is diffuse metastatic spread from bronchial cancer to all vertebral bodies. Again, the bone marrow is very inhomogeneous but there is no vertebral destruction

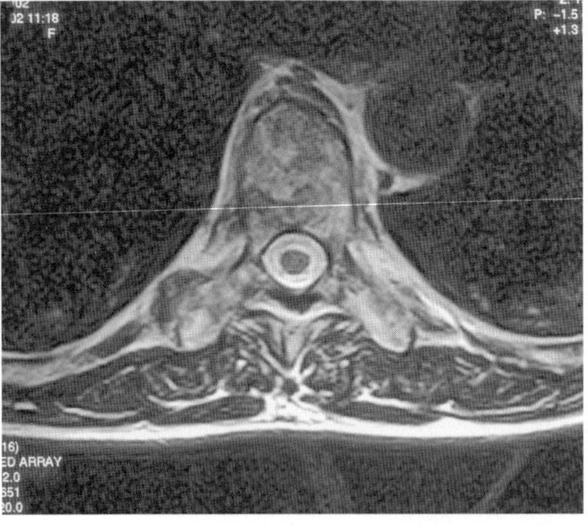

Fig. 6.136. Same patient. Axial T2-weighted image through the T7 level showing slight expansion of the right transverse process with very inhomogeneous, mostly hypointense, bone marrow but no signs of invasion of the spinal canal

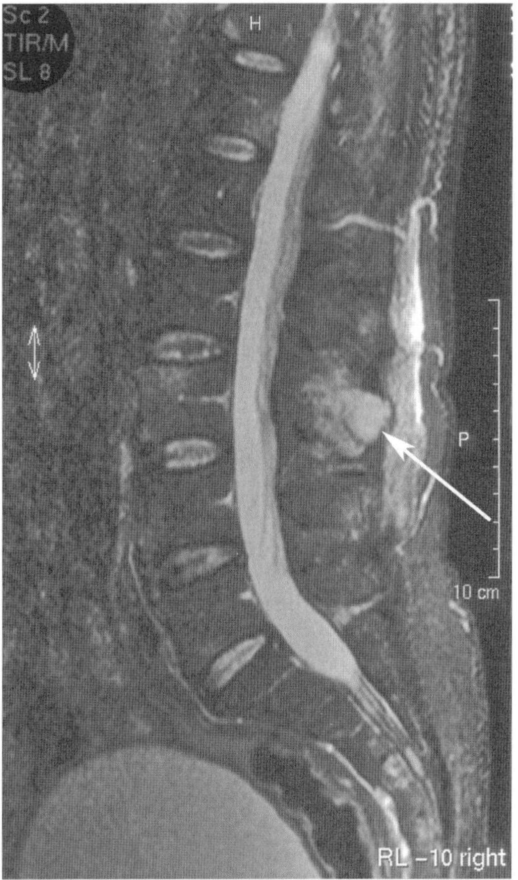

Fig. 6.137. Sagittal T2-weighted image with fat saturation of the lumbar region in a 48-year-old patient with a single spinous process metastasis from bronchial cancer. The image shows an ill-defined, high-signal-intensity lesion in the area of the L3 spinous process with mild edema of surrounding soft tissue structures

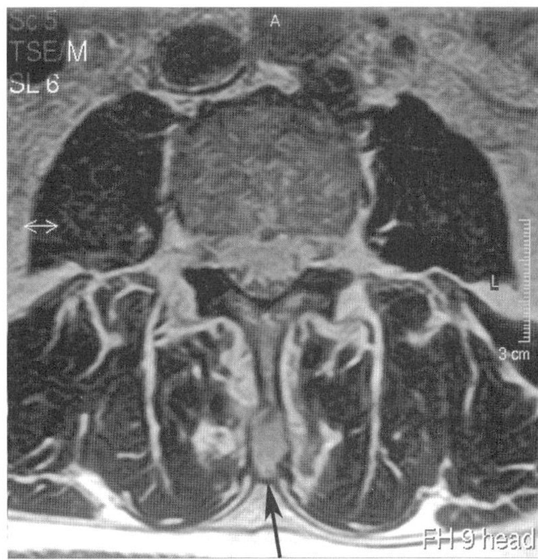

Fig. 6.138. Axial T2-weighted image of the L3 spinous process metastasis. Increased signal intensity of the posterior portions of the spinous process expanded by the metastasis

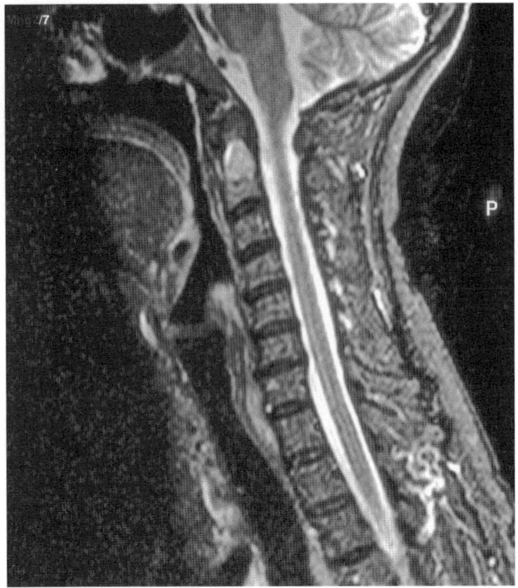

Fig. 6.139. Sagittal T2-weighted image with fat saturation showing metastasis from bronchial cancer in the dens axis. The metastasis is seen as a relatively well-defined focal lesion of increased signal intensity in the area of the dens

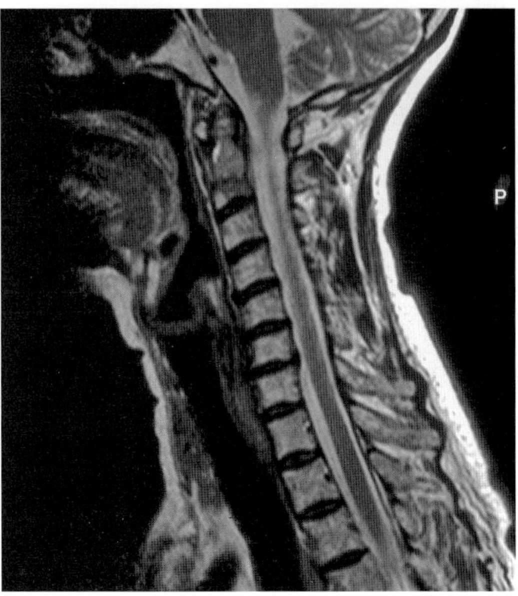

Fig. 6.140. Sagittal T2-weighted image of the dens metastasis, which is much less conspicuous on this image obtained without fat saturation

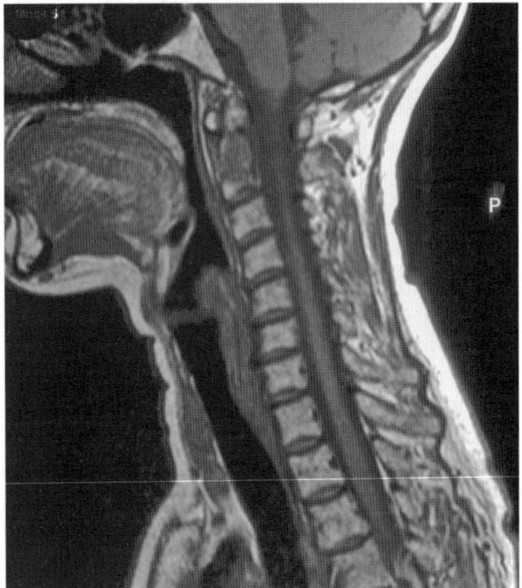

Fig. 6.141. Sagittal T1-weighted image (unenhanced) of the dens metastasis. The metastasis is seen as a low-signal-intensity bone lesion in the area of the dens. There is no fracture

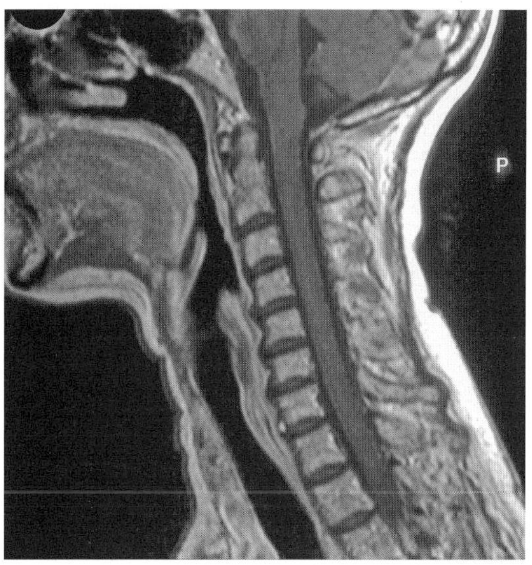

Fig. 6.142. Same patient. Sagittal T1-weighted image of the dens metastasis after contrast administration. Approximation of the bone marrow signal to that of the metastasis effaces contrast and the metastasis is no longer discernible

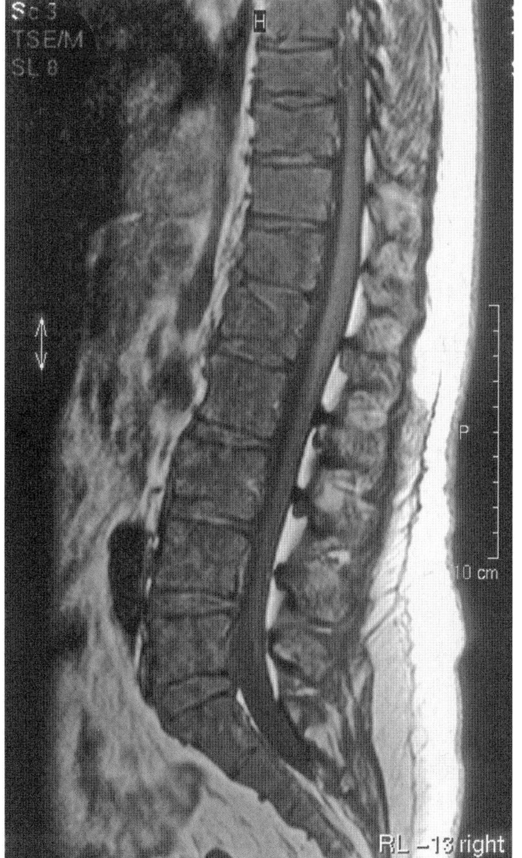

Fig. 6.143. Sagittal T1-weighted image of the thoracolumbar junction and lumbar region in a 44-year-old patient with unspecific back complaints. Low signal intensity of all vertebrae including the arches and spinous processes, consistent with replacement of the normal fat marrow

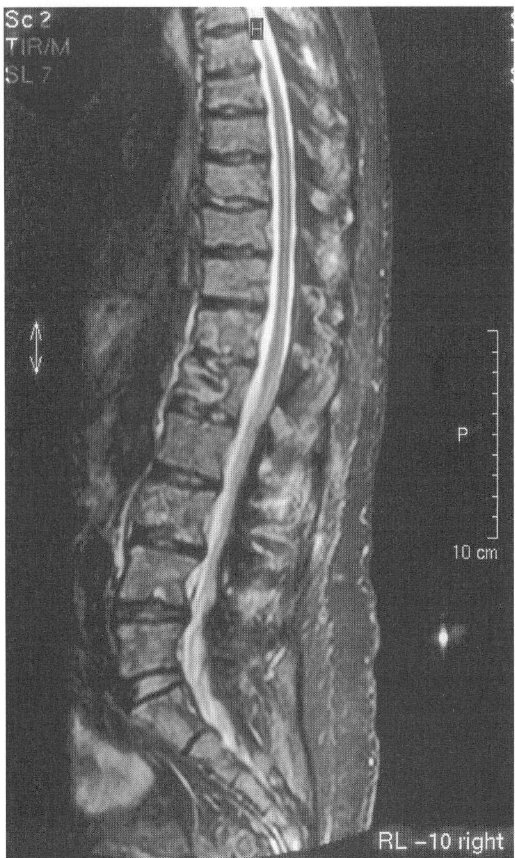

Fig. 6.144. Same patient. Sagittal T2-weighted image with fat saturation showing inhomogeneous, slightly increased signal intensity of all vertebrae depicted including the sacrum with inhomogeneous appearance of the endplates of T12, L1, and L3, consistent with early vertebral compression

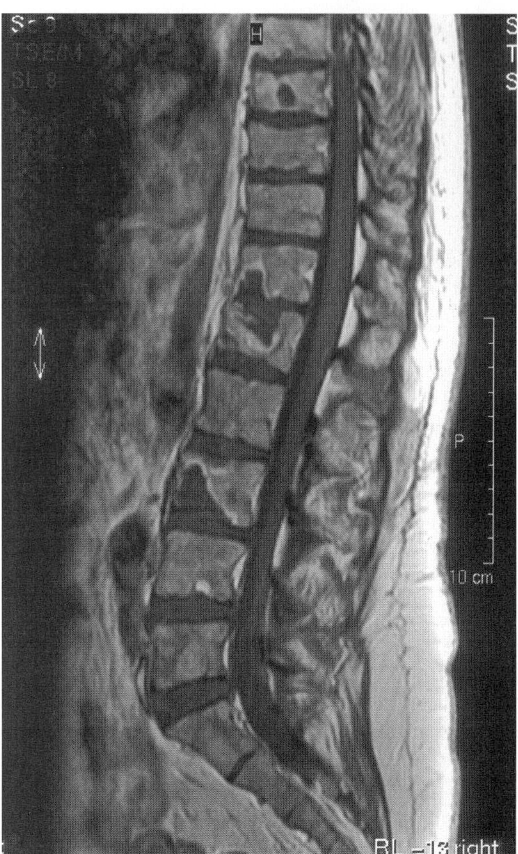

Fig. 6.145. Sagittal T1-weighted image after contrast administration. Diffuse invasion of the bone marrow by bronchial cancer with early erosion and destruction of the endplates of T12, L1, L3, and T9

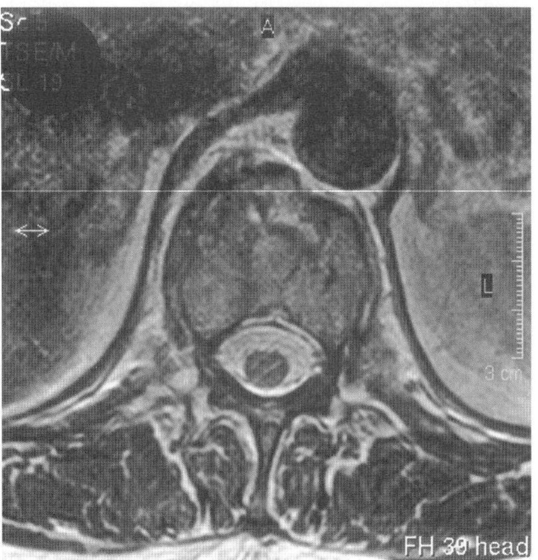

Fig. 6.146. Same patient. Axial T2-weighted image through the L1 level showing early signs of destruction of the L1 vertebral body near the superior endplate with incomplete fracture of the posterior edge

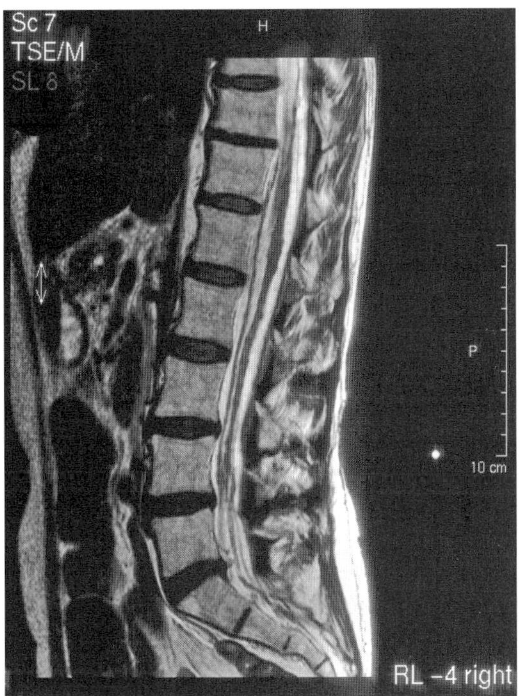

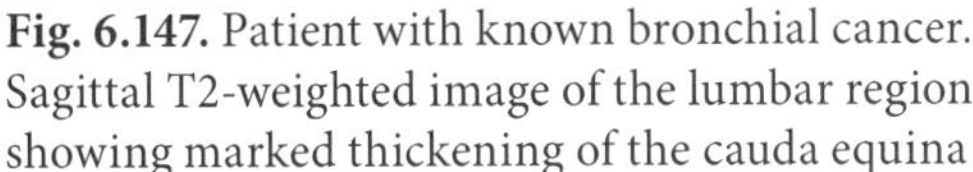

Fig. 6.147. Patient with known bronchial cancer. Sagittal T2-weighted image of the lumbar region showing marked thickening of the cauda equina

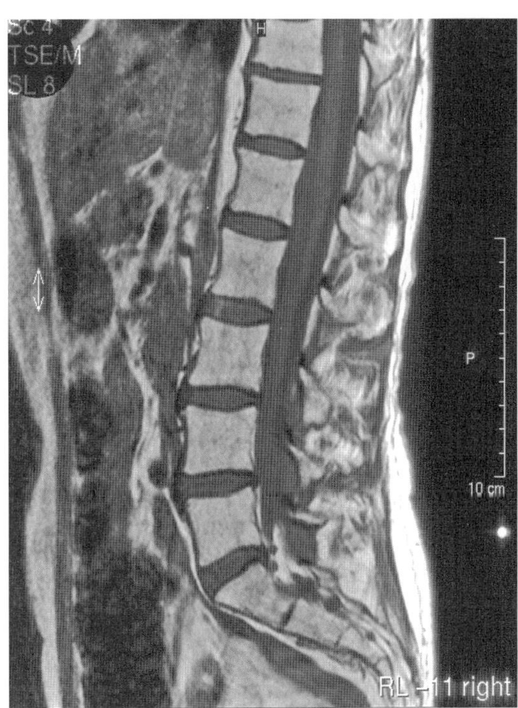

Fig. 6.148. Sagittal T1-weighted image of the patient with bronchial cancer and meningiosis carcinomatosa. Thickening of the cauda equina is just barely seen

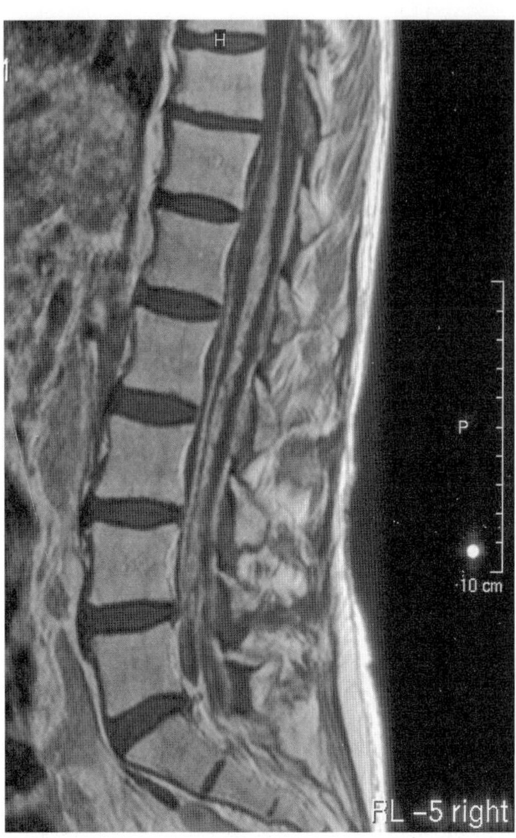

Fig. 6.149. Same patient (meningiosis carcinomatosa). Sagittal T1-weighted image after contrast administration. Marked enhancement in the area of the dura and cauda equina fibers from T12 through L5

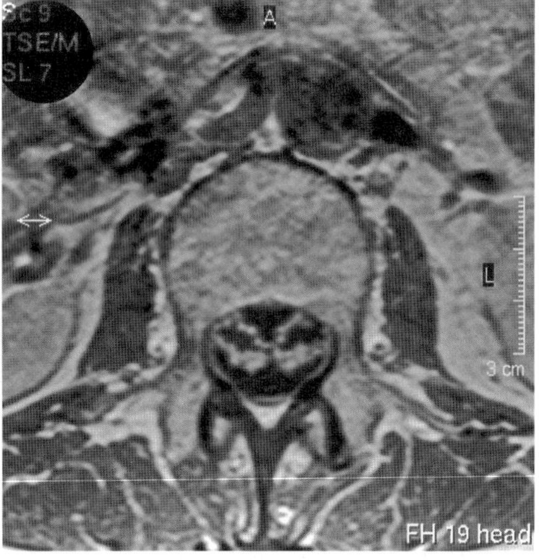

Fig. 6.150. Axial T1-weighted image through the L4 level after contrast administration showing marked ring enhancement around the cauda equina fibers in the patient with meningiosis carcinomatosa from metastatic bronchial cancer

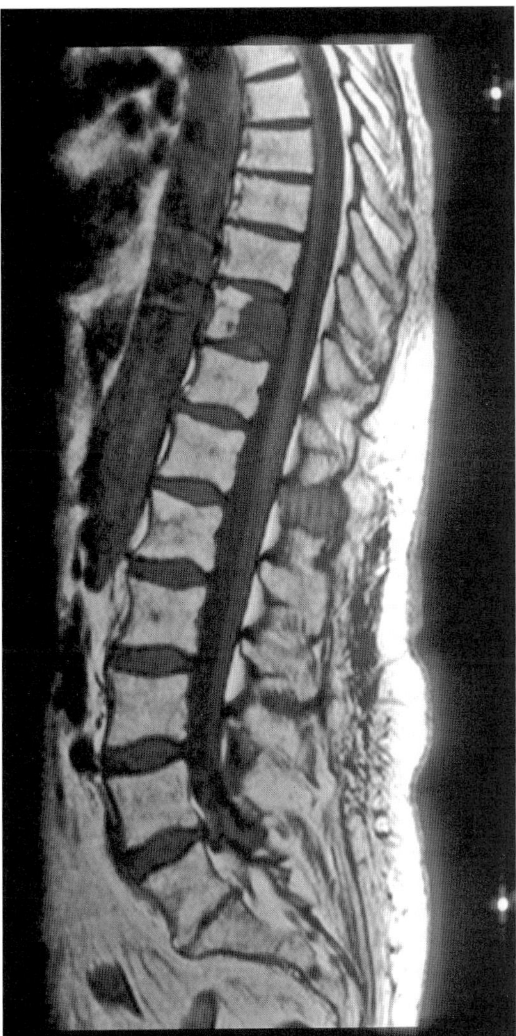

Fig. 6.151. Sagittal T1-weighted image of the lumbar region in a patient with metastasis of the L1 spinous process and T11 vertebral body. The metastatic bone areas have a lower signal intensity than the normal vertebrae

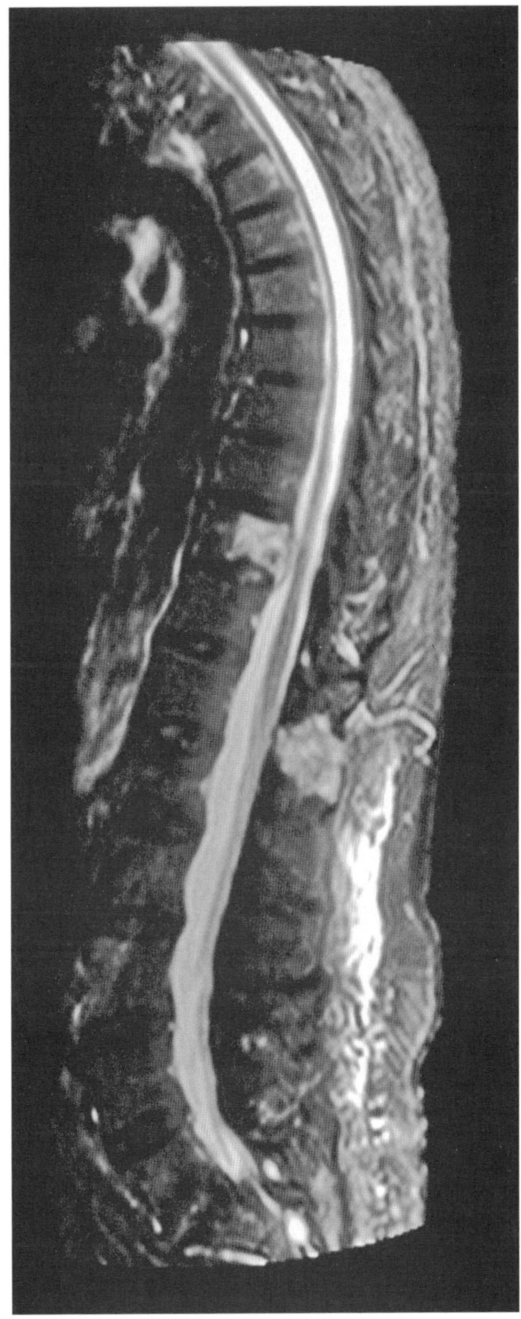

Fig. 6.152. Sagittal T2-weighted image with fat saturation showing high signal intensity of the metastatic portions of T11 and L1

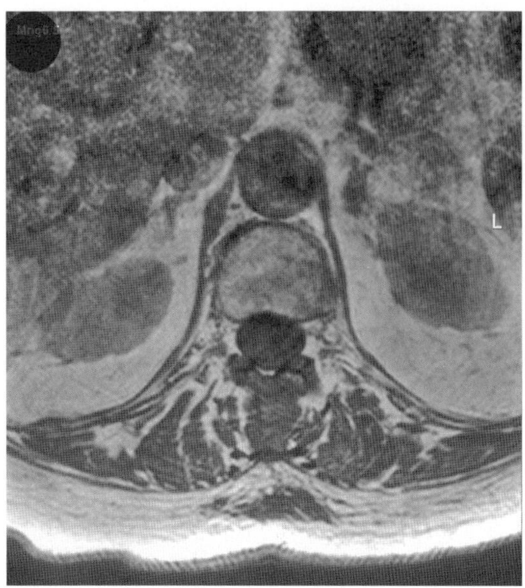

Fig. 6.153. Axial T1-weighted image through the L2 level. Low-signal-intensity metastasis with irregular margins

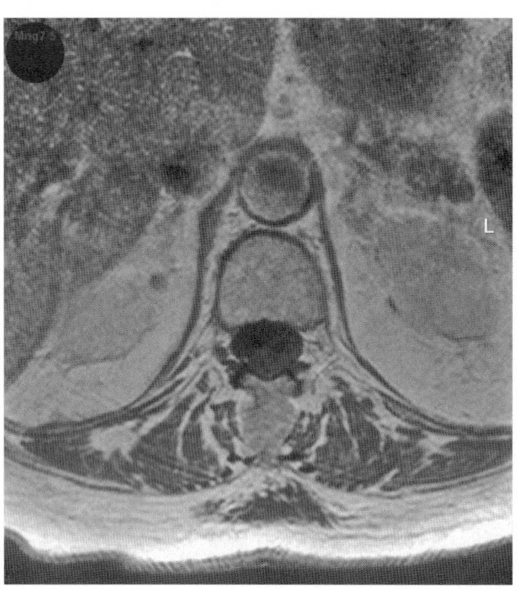

Fig. 6.154. Axial T1-weighted image after contrast administration showing marked enhancement of the metastatic spinous process of L2. Contrast enhancement effaces the difference in intensity between the metastasis and marrow

7 The Postoperative Spine

7.1 Scars

Contrast-enhanced MRI is the most suitable imaging tool for differentiating postoperative scars from other changes such as recurrent disc herniation (Figs. 7.1–7.6).

7.2 Recurrent Disc Herniation

See Figs. 7.7–7.13.

7.3 Bone Defects/Fenestration

CT is more reliable than MRI in evaluating bony defects in the postoperative spine (Figs. 7.14–7.16).

7.4 Seroma/Hematoma

Fluid collection in the area of the surgical access is consistently seen in postoperative patients even for longer periods. Reliable characterization is not possible. This is true especially for the differentiation of older hematoma/seroma and bacterial infection unless other typical changes are present (e.g. characteristic MR changes of spondylitis) (Figs. 7.17-7.24).

7.5 Bone Grafting

MRI is very useful for assessing the proper position of a bone chip, for example, in patients who underwent surgical fusion with chip grafting as well as for demonstrating bony consolidation in the further course (Figs. 7.25–7.35).

7.6 Vertebroplasty

See Figs. 7.36–7.38.

7.7 Osteosynthesis

MRI is limited in the postoperative evaluation of patients with a titanium implant because metal artifacts impair the evaluation of the osteosynthesis. CT is more suitable for checking the proper position of a titanium implant (Figs. 7.39 and 7.40).

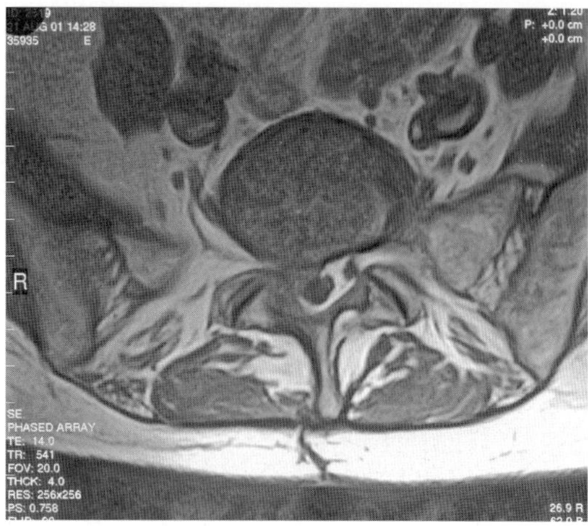

Fig. 7.1. Postoperative scar at L5-S1 on the right. Axial T1-weighted image showing soft-tissue-signal structure in the right lateral recess and medial portion of the right L5 foramen. There is only slight displacement of the dural sac posteriorly toward the right. A laminectomy defect is not seen at this level. Normal appearance of the left S1 nerve root. The right S1 root is obscured by the soft tissue mass

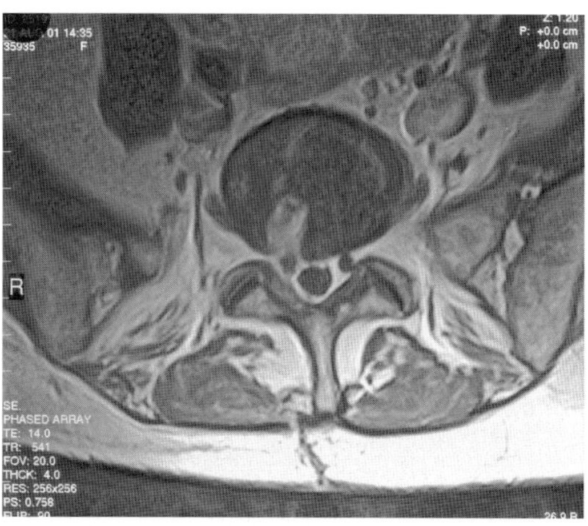

Fig. 7.2. Axial T1-weighted image through the L5-S1 level in the same patient after contrast administration. The proximal segment of the right S1 nerve root is now seen and the mass in the right lateral recess shows pronounced contrast enhancement. Appearance consistent with a large, well-perfused scar

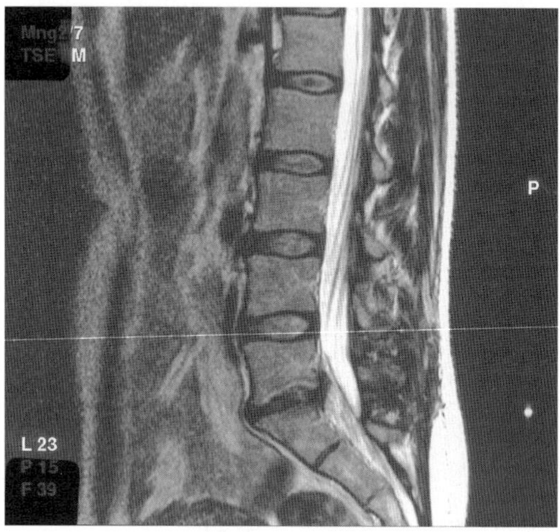

Fig. 7.3. Postoperative scar in the posterior soft tissue and intraspinally after L5-S1 disc surgery. Sagittal T2-weighted image showing a low-signal-intensity epidural mass posterior to the L5-S1 interspace and the inferior portion of the L5 vertebral body. Inhomogeneous appearance of the posterior soft tissue structures with very minute metal artifacts postoperatively. Normal vertebral size and shape. Reduced height of the L5-S1 disc

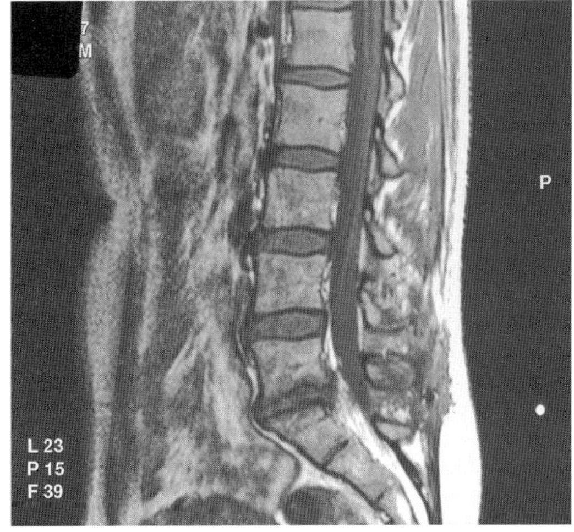

Fig. 7.4. Same patient. Sagittal T1-weighted image of the lumbar region showing a mass of the same signal intensity as the disc posterior to the L5-S1 disc. Inhomogeneous appearance of the posterior soft tissue structures at this level with minute susceptibility artifacts, consistent with presence of metal particles after surgery

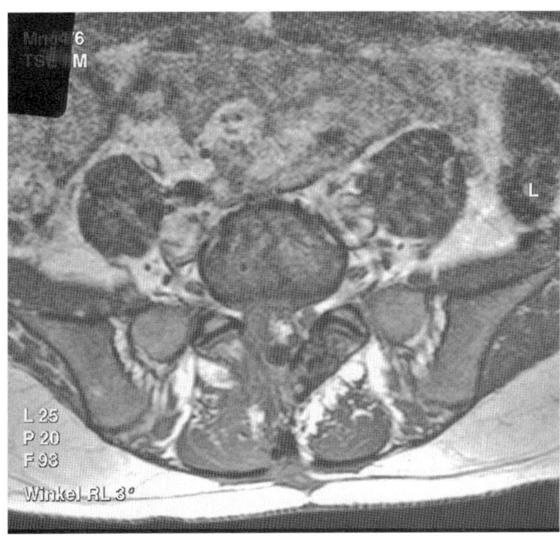

Fig. 7.5. Axial T1-weighted image through the L5-S1 level showing low-signal-intensity scar tissue in the spinal canal on the right near the laminotomy defect identified on this unenhanced image by the low signal intensity relative to the higher fat marrow signal of the remaining anterior portion of the vertebral arch. Susceptibility artifacts in the posterior soft tissue

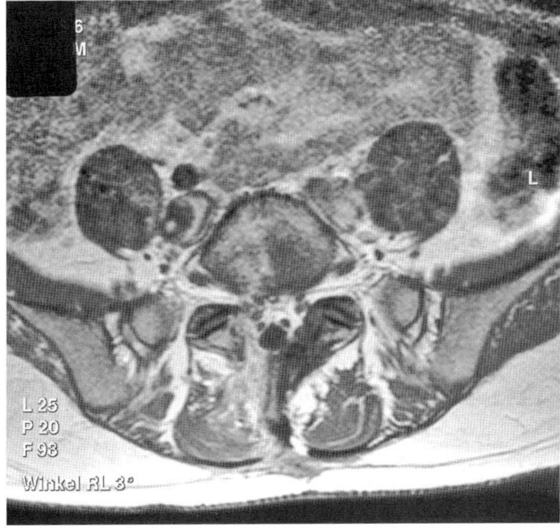

Fig. 7.6. Axial T1-weighted image through L5-S1 after contrast administration. There is marked enhancement of the scar tissue and the nerve roots on the right are now discernible as punctate structures. They are similar in appearance to their counterparts on the left. There is also enhancement of the scar structures at the level of the osteotomy defect posterior to the disc space on the right and in the posterior soft tissue. Status after L5-S1 disc operation

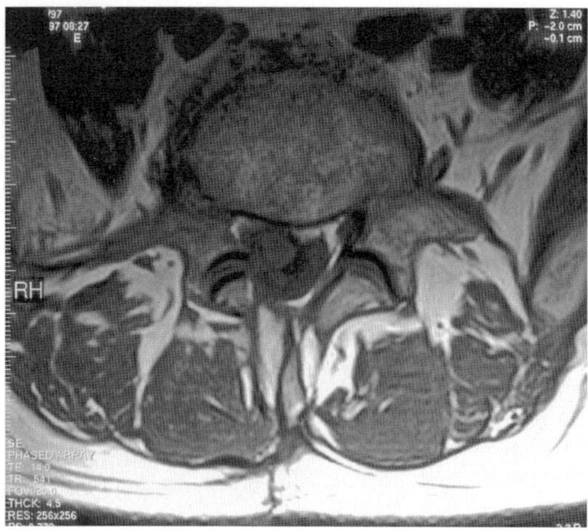

Fig. 7.7. Axial T1-weighted image showing recurrent herniation at L5-S1. There is a rounded mass of low signal intensity in the right lateral recess, which appears to indent and displace the dural sac. Right posterolateral osteotomy defect after surgery

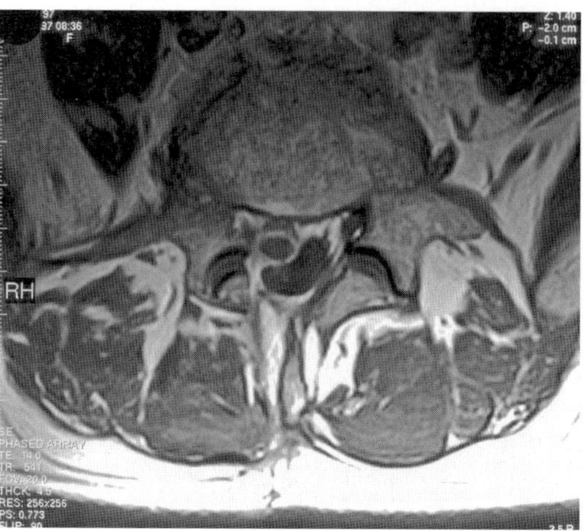

Fig. 7.8. Axial T1-weighted image through the L5-S1 level after contrast administration. The free disc fragment anteriorly to the right of the dural sac is seen more clearly due to pronounced contrast enhancement of scar tissue around the fragment and in the area of the osteotomy defect. There is marked deformity of the dural sac and displacement to the left

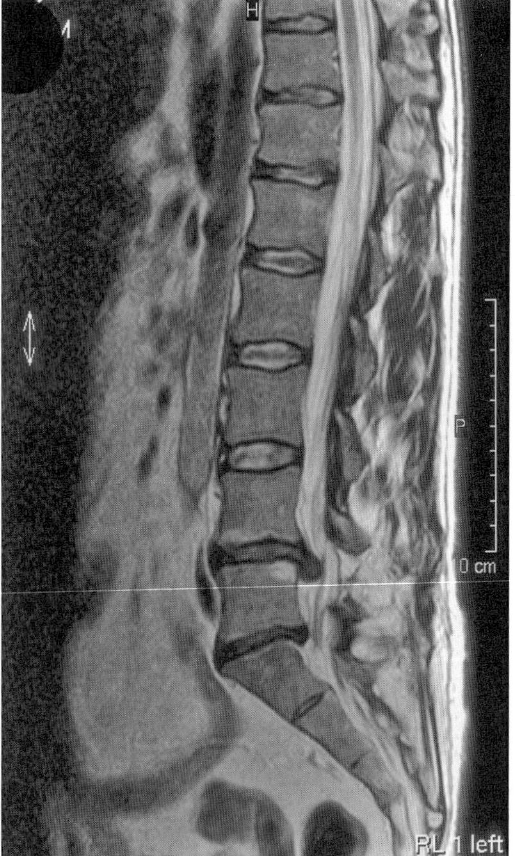

Fig. 7.9. Recurrent herniation at L4-5. Sagittal T2-weighted image of the lumbar region showing downward extension of the herniated disc and postoperative signal alterations and contour irregularities in the soft tissue posterior to L4-5. Additional herniation of the L5-S1 disc with signs of dehydration and degeneration of the L4-5 and L5-S1 discs

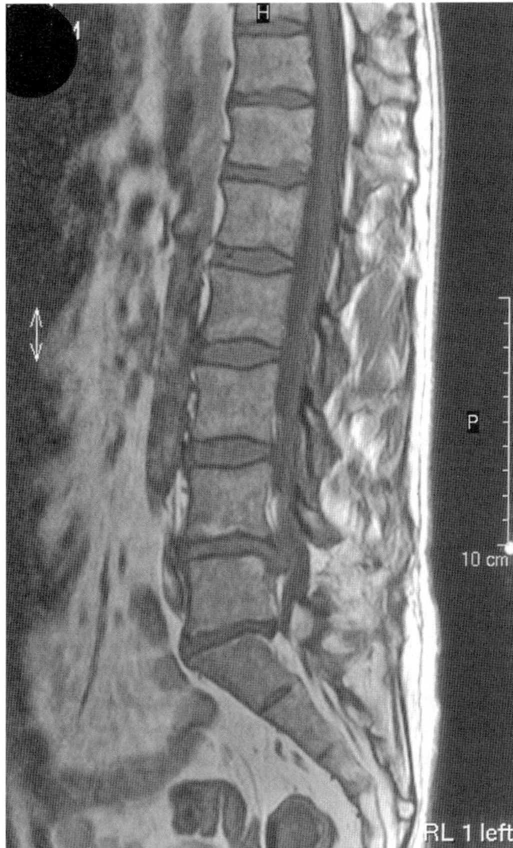

Fig. 7.10. Same patient. Sagittal T1-weighted image of the recurrent L4-5 disc herniation. Tongue-shaped mass behind and below the L4-5 disc space

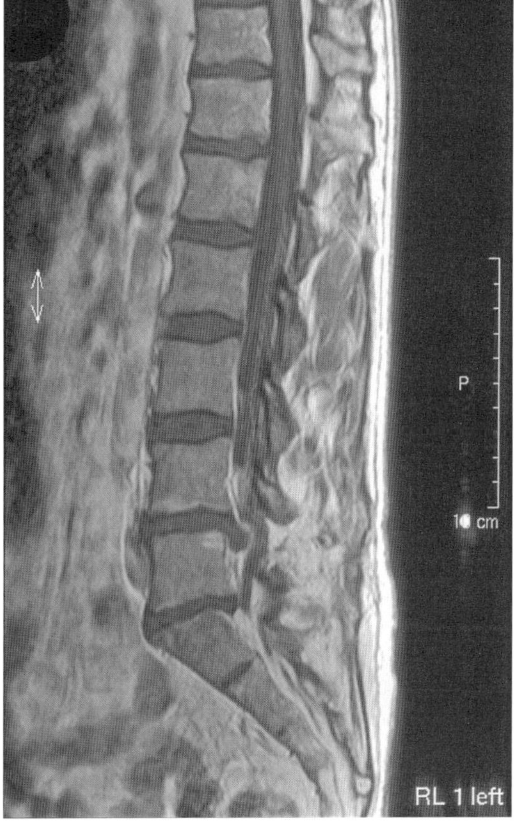

Fig. 7.11. Sagittal T1-weighted image after contrast administration. No enhancement of the tongue-shaped mass with mild enhancement of the posterior soft tissue structures, which also appear slightly inhomogeneous

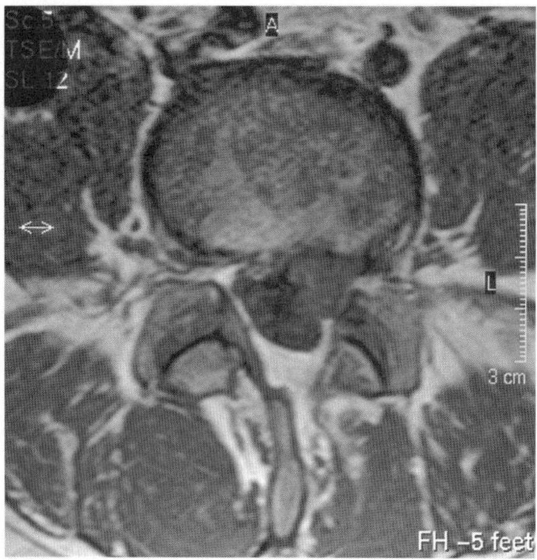

Fig. 7.12. Same patient. Axial T1-weighted image through L4-5. Low-signal-intensity mass in the left lateral recess and left L4-5 foramen with deformity and displacement of the dural sac posteriorly to the right

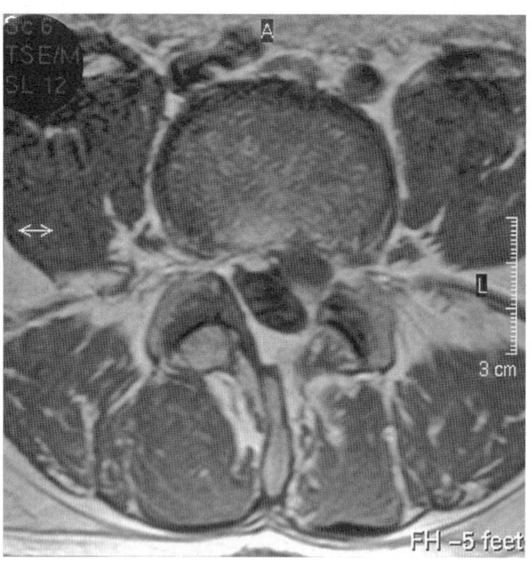

Fig. 7.13. Axial T1-weighted image after contrast administration showing peripheral enhancement of the herniated disc described in the preceding figures with a nonenhancing central portion in the left lateral recess. Consistent with recurrent left posterolateral herniation. Left posterior osteotomy defect from surgery performed some years earlier

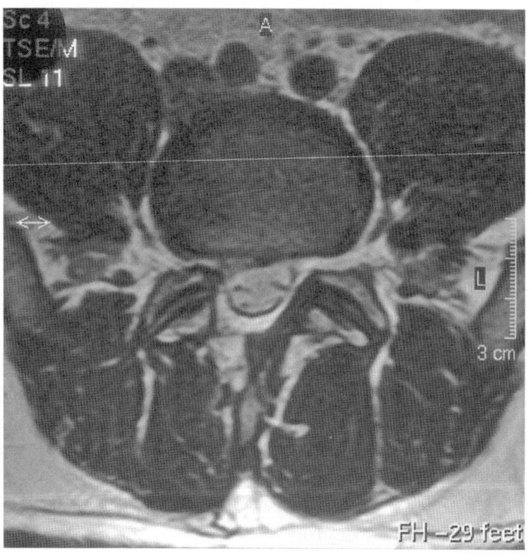

Fig. 7.14. Status after disc surgery with osteotomy defect of the right vertebral arch. Axial T2-weighted image through the L5-S1 level showing the osteotomy defect posteriorly on the right. The ligamentum flavum on the right is not depicted, while the posterior portions of the arch and the ligamentum flavum on the left appear normal. Degenerative hypertrophy of the facet joints. Discreet soft-tissue-intensity mass anteriorly to the right of the dural sac with slight deformity of the dural sac

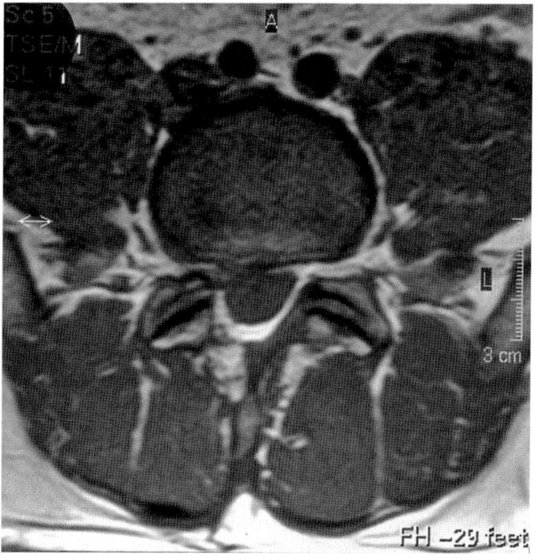

Fig. 7.15. Same patient. Axial T1-weighted image through L5-S1 showing the osteotomy defect posteriorly on the right with only negligible distortion of the dural sac. Small mass of disc intensity anteriorly to the right of the dural sac

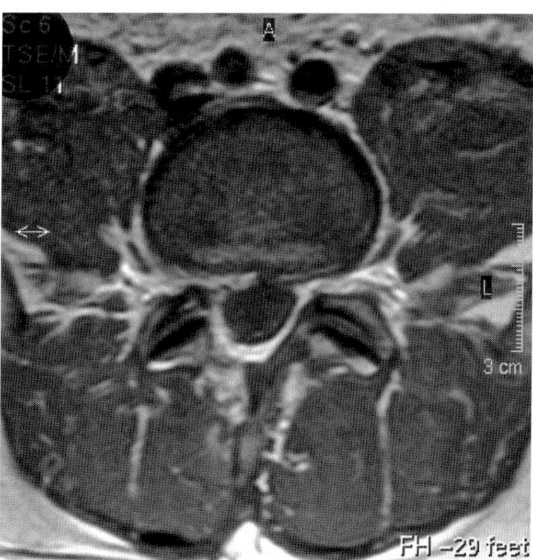

Fig. 7.16. Axial T1-weighted image after contrast administration showing minimally enhancing scar tissue anteriorly to the right of the dural sac and discreet enhancing structures between the facet joint and spinous process posterior to the osteotomy defect of the right arch. Status after disc surgery

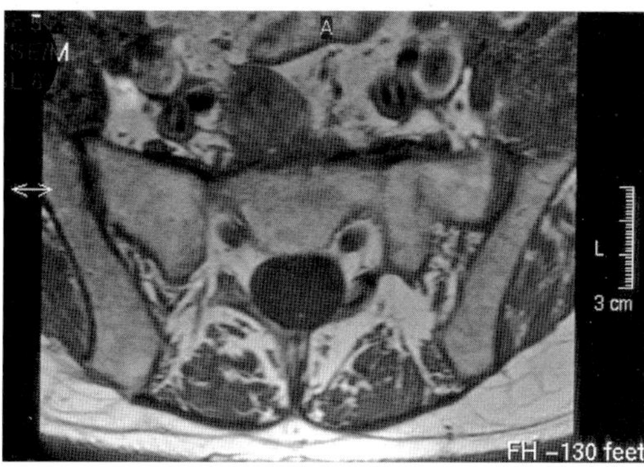

Fig. 7.17. Postoperative hematoma anterior to S1. Axial T1-weighted image through the S1 level showing a mass anterior to the sacrum. The mass is of muscle intensity and measures about 2x2.5 cm. Large susceptibility artifact in the area of the spinal canal after surgery

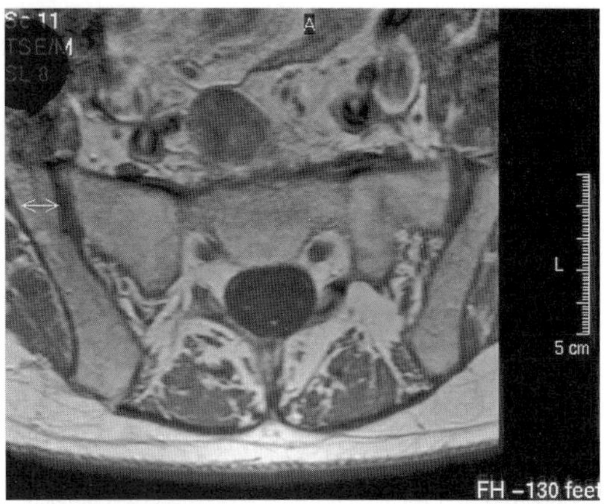

Fig. 7.18. Same patient. Axial T1-weighted image through S1 after contrast administration. The absence of contrast enhancement suggests an older hematoma

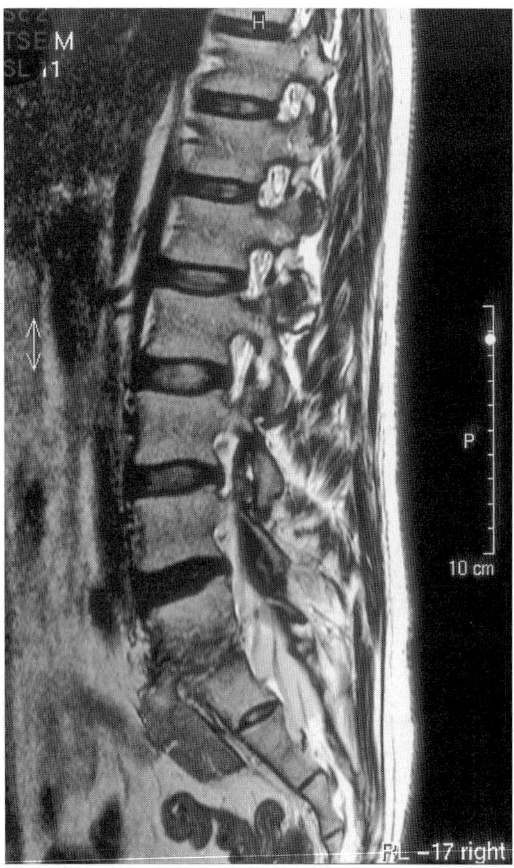

Fig. 7.19. Sagittal T2-weighted image of the lumbosacral junction in the patient with hematoma anterior to S1. Larger, tongue-shaped mass arising from the L5-S1 disc operated on using an anterior approach. Low-signal-intensity lesion anterior to S1 consistent with old hemorrhage/old hematoma

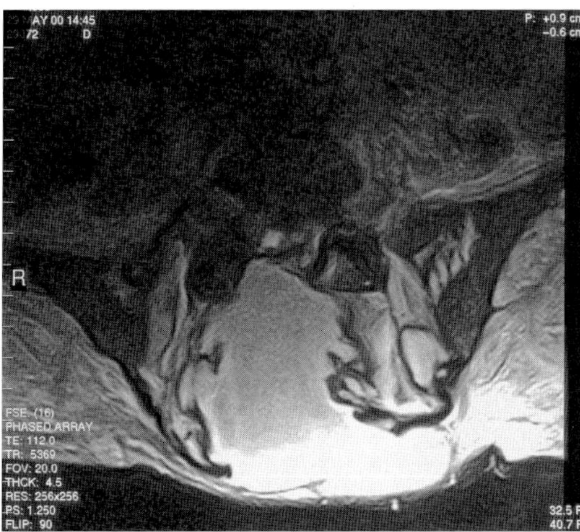

Fig. 7.20. Postoperative seroma in posterior soft tissue. Axial T2-weighted image through L5-S1 showing a lobulated and sharply marginated mass of homogeneously high signal intensity posterior to the L5-S1 interspace. Absence of the posterior portions of the L5 arch after posterior fenestration at L5-S1

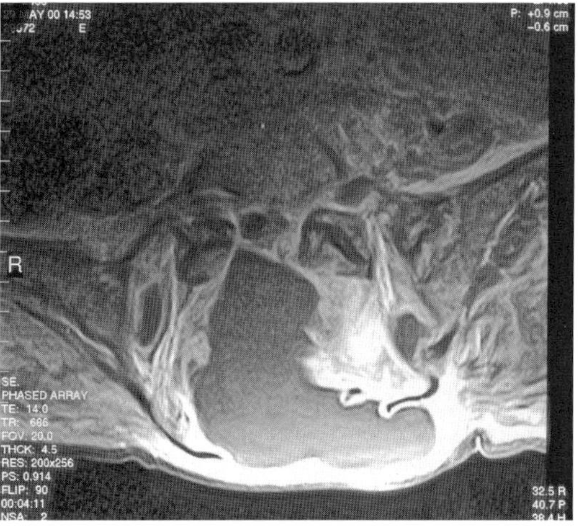

Fig. 7.21. Axial T1-weighted image after contrast administration depicting the large cystic lesion posterior to the L5-S1 interspace with no internal signal and no enhancement. The appearance is consistent with a large seroma after surgical decompression of L5-S1

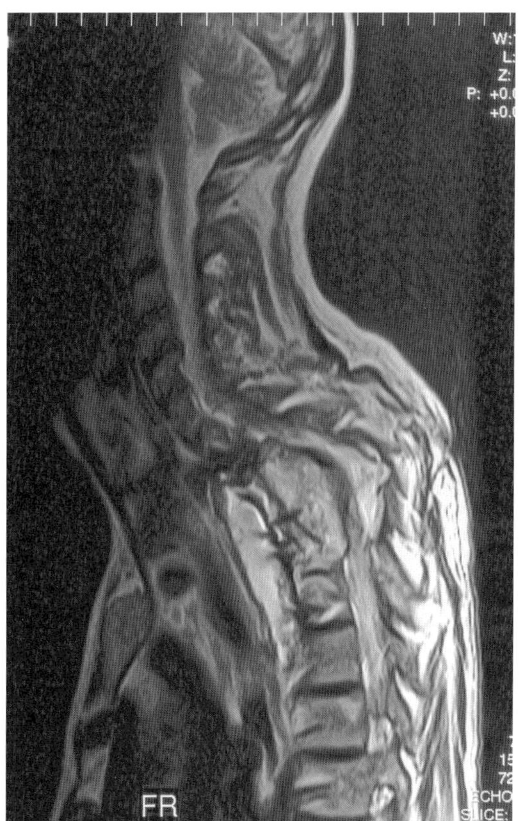

Fig. 7.22. Sagittal T2-weighted image of a postoperative seroma anterior to the spine and posterior to the spinal canal extending from T1 through T4 after anterior stabilization. The image shows a tongue-shaped high-signal-intensity lesion with a slightly irregular margin anterior to the spine. Susceptibility artifacts in the area of the upper thoracic spine

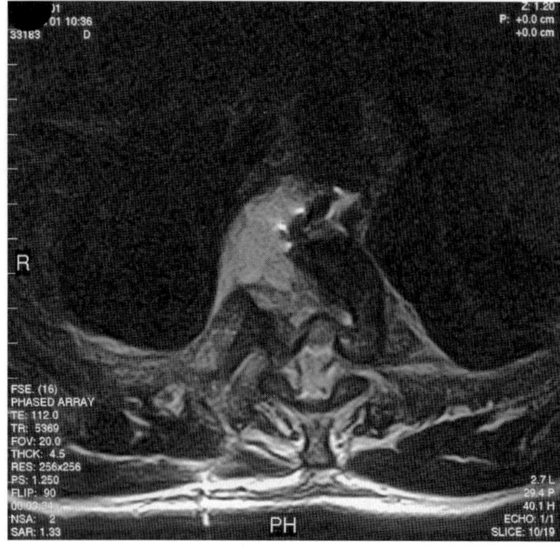

Fig. 7.23. Same patient. Axial T2-weighted image through the T2 level showing a small bone defect of the vertebral body and the right anterolateral seroma after anterior decompression

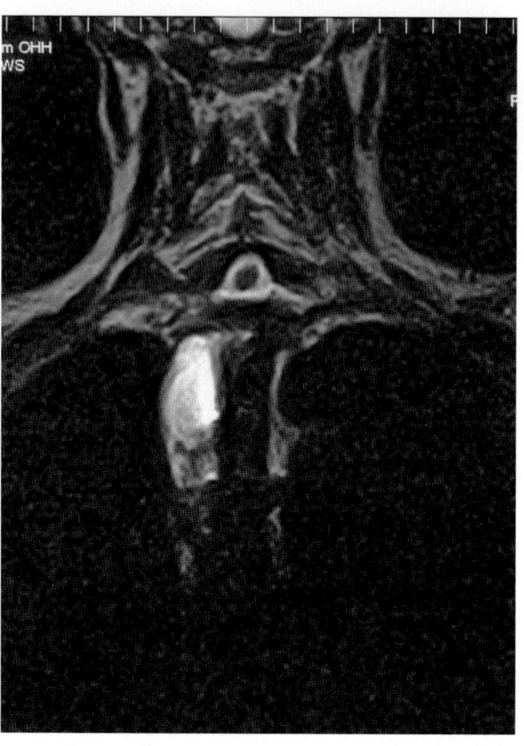

Fig. 7.24. Coronal T2-weighted image. Postoperative seroma depicted as a high-signal-intensity mass from T1 through T4 to the right of the spine

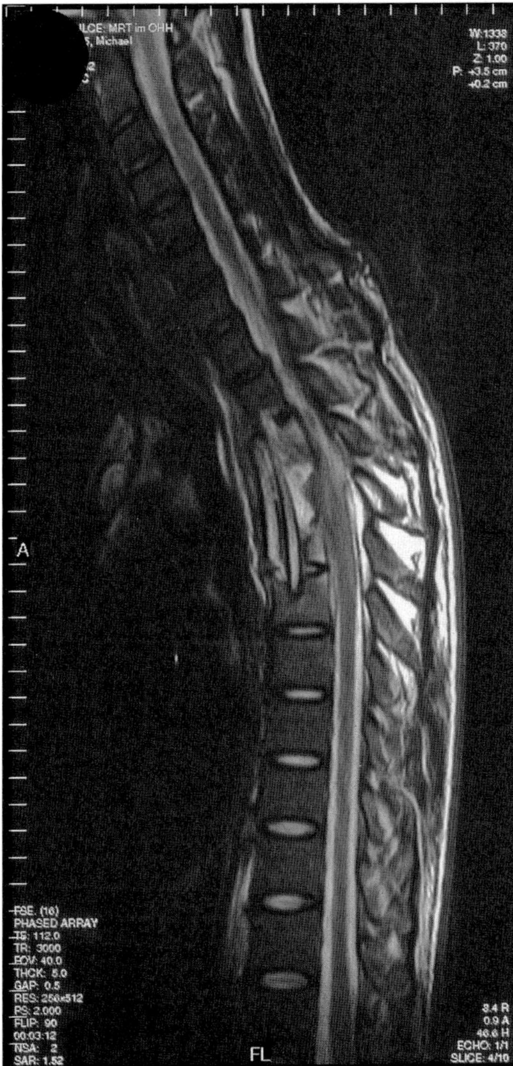

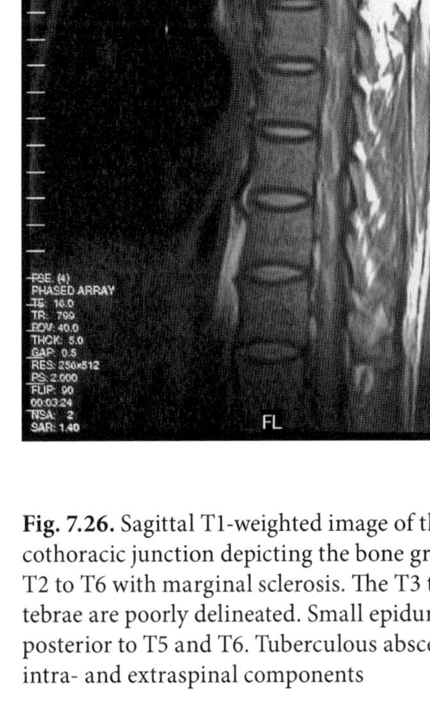

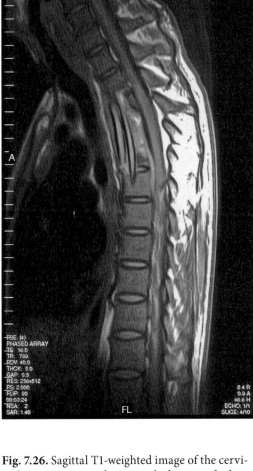

Fig. 7.25. Sagittal T2-weighted image after tuberculous spondylodiscitis. Insertion of two bone grafts from T2 to T6, which are depicted as longitudinally oriented structures of low signal intensity from T2 to T6. The bone grafts bridge the partially destroyed T4 vertebra, which has much higher signal intensity than the other vertebrae. In addition, partial destruction and slight hyperintensity of T3 and T5

Fig. 7.26. Sagittal T1-weighted image of the cervicothoracic junction depicting the bone grafts from T2 to T6 with marginal sclerosis. The T3 to T5 vertebrae are poorly delineated. Small epidural lesions posterior to T5 and T6. Tuberculous abscess with intra- and extraspinal components

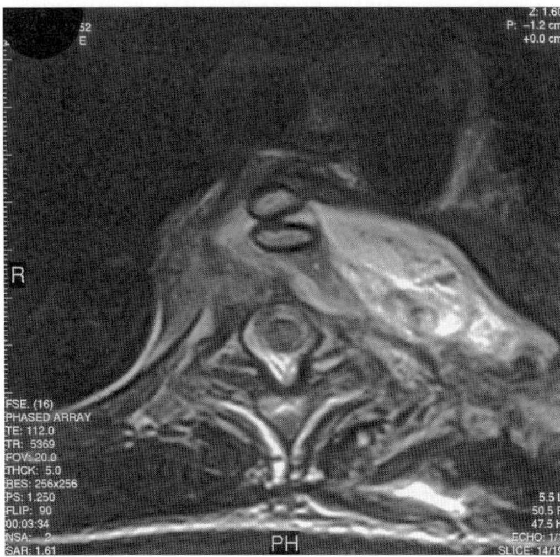

Fig. 7.27. Same patient. Axial T2-weighted image through the T5 level depicting the bone graft as an oval structure with marginal sclerosis in the area of the destroyed vertebral body. Larger fluid collection to the left of the spine

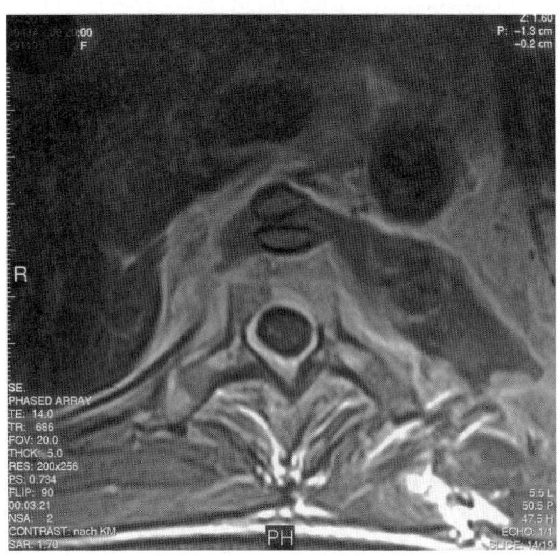

Fig. 7.28. Axial T1-weighted image after contrast administration showing marked abnormal contrast enhancement around the fluid collection to the left of the spine. No irritation of the two bone grafts

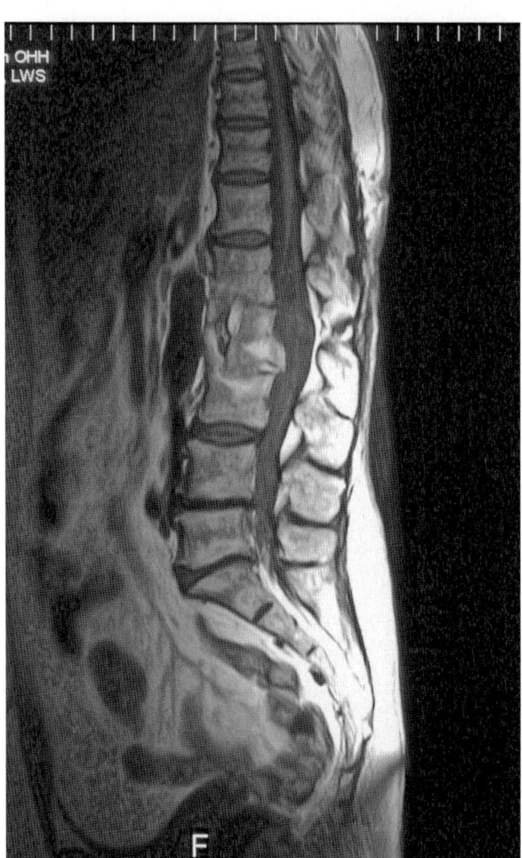

Fig. 7.29. Status after bone chip implantation following spondylodiscitis at L1-2 and L2-3. Sagittal T1-weighted image of the lumbar spine showing bony consolidation of these two disc spaces and the bone graft. There is partial narrowing of the spinal canal due to extension of the posterior edge of L2 into the spinal canal. The elongated bone chip is seen in the anterior portions of the destroyed L1 and L2 vertebral bodies

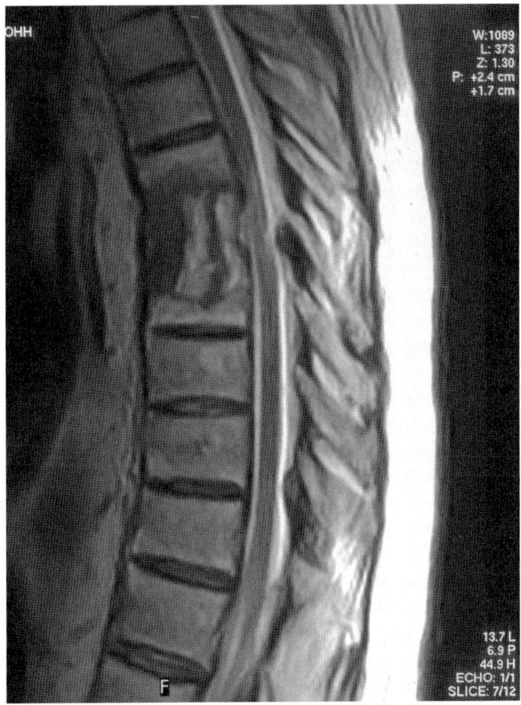

Fig. 7.30. Status after bone chip implantation in the mid-thoracic spine (T6 through T8) with partial destruction of T7, which has low signal intensity. The two longitudinal bone implants are very conspicuous. Thoracic cord segment showing signal changes consistent with myelomalacia after spondylodiscitis at T7

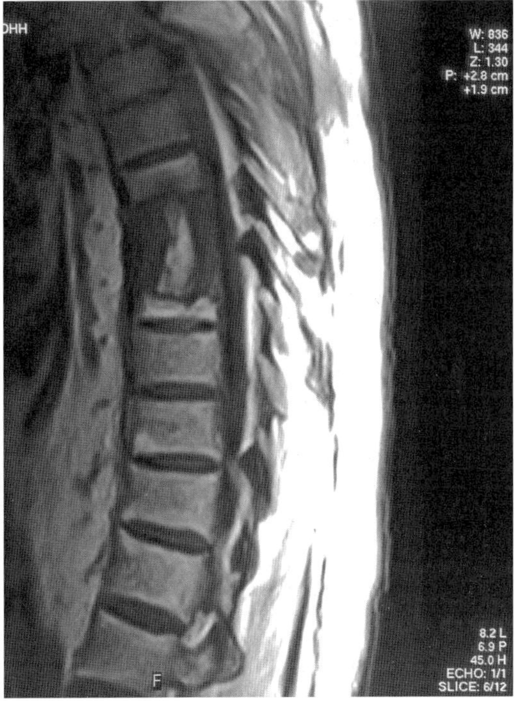

Fig. 7.31. Sagittal T1-weighted image of the mid-thoracic spine after bone chip implantation from T6 to T8

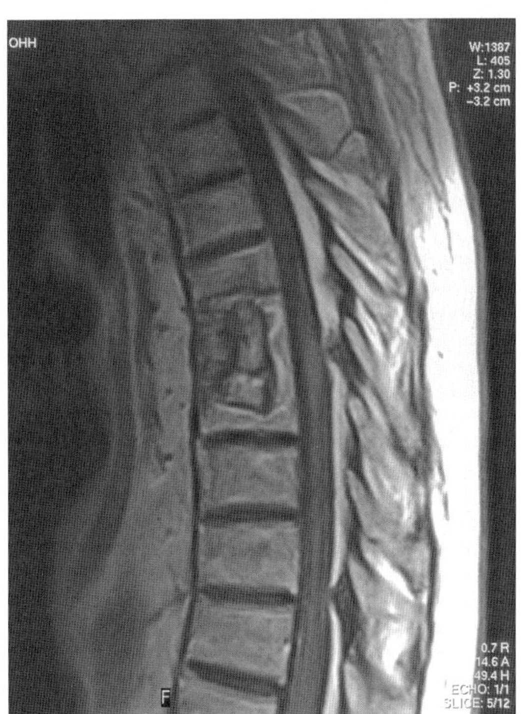

Fig. 7.32. Sagittal T1-weighted image of the same patient after contrast administration. Clear enhancement around the implanted bone. Status after spondylodiscitis with destruction of T7

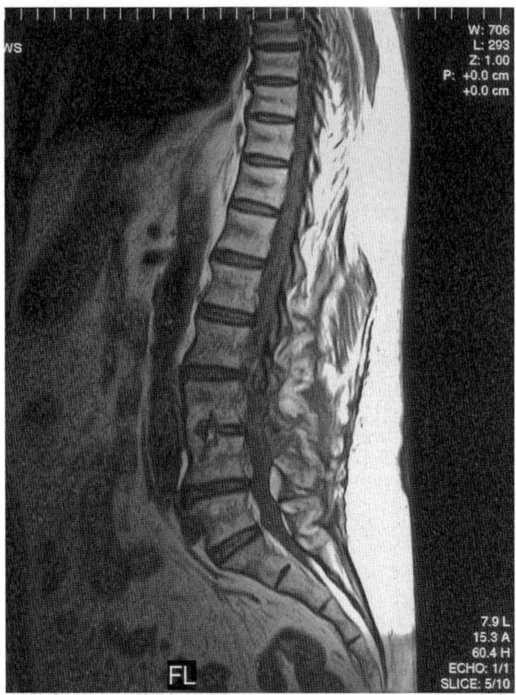

Fig. 7.33. Sagittal T1-weighted image after bone chip implantation and bony consolidation of the anterior portion of L4-5 following spondylodiscitis. The longitudinal bone chip bridging the former L3-4 disc space shows marginal sclerosis. Appearance suggesting nonirritable status after bone graft implantation

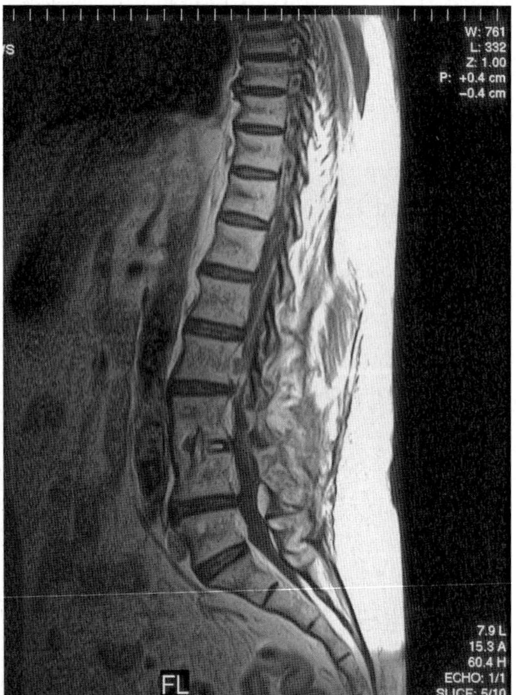

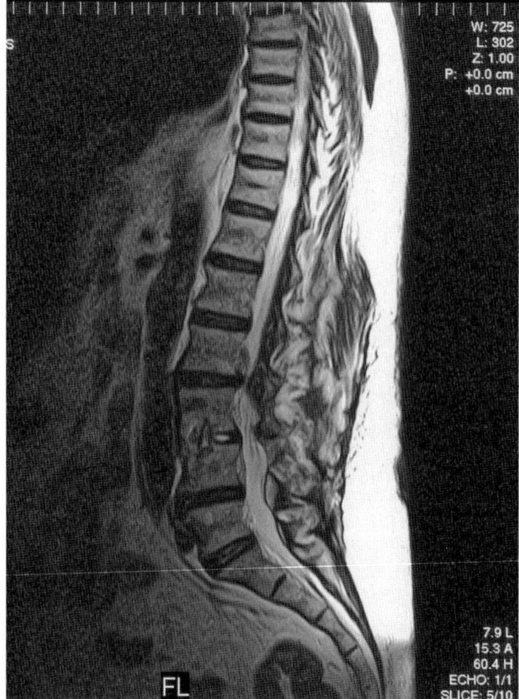

Fig. 7.34. Sagittal T1-weighted image of the lumbar spine after contrast administration. No signs of irritation around the implanted bone graft following L3-4 spondylodiscitis. Improved visualization of a nodular mass posterior to L2 representing a disc fragment arising from the L2-3 disc

Fig. 7.35. Sagittal T2-weighted image showing the L3-4 bone chip implant after spondylodiscitis. L2-3 herniation with a free disc fragment migrated cranially

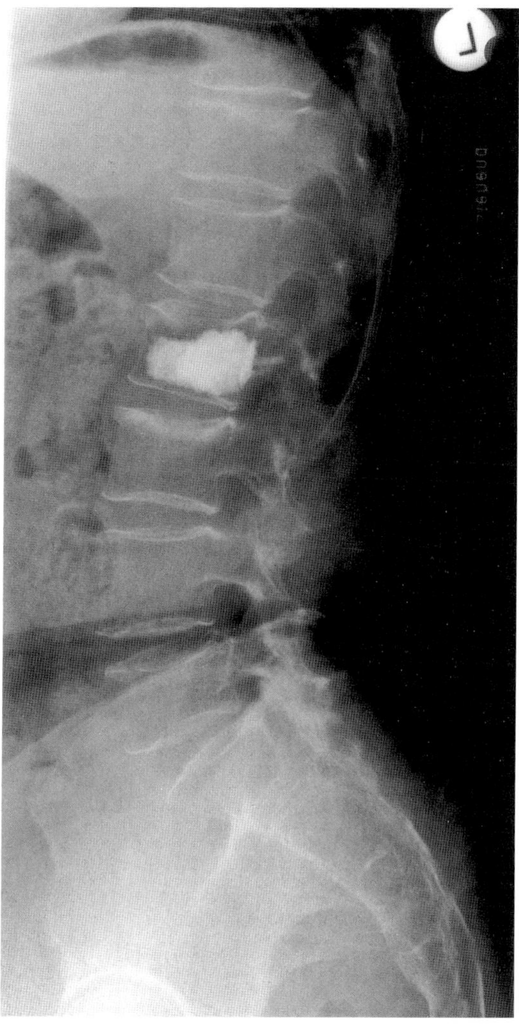

Fig. 7.36. Status after L2 vertebroplasty. Lateral radiograph of the lumbar spine showing a densification in the inferior and posterior aspects of the L2 vertebral body

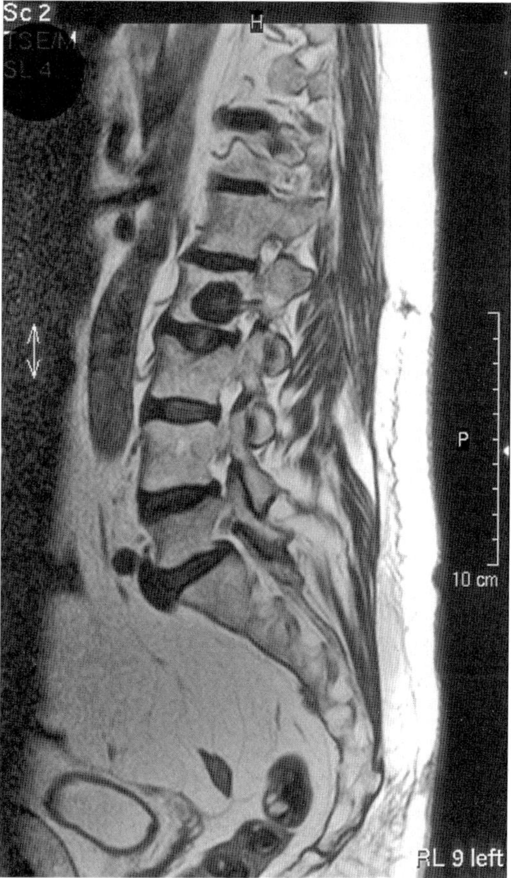

Fig. 7.37. Sagittal T2-weighted image of the same patient showing the appearance after L2 vertebroplasty on MRI. Focal low-signal-intensity area about 2 cm in diameter within the body of L2.

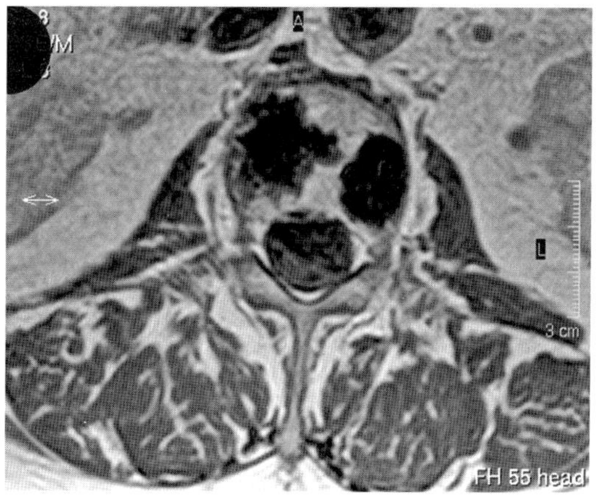

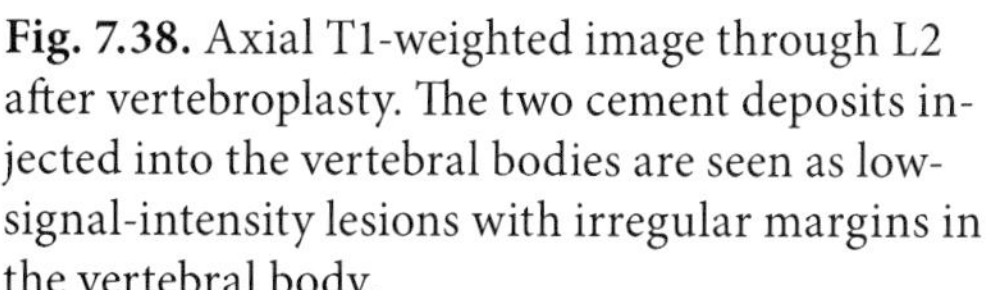

Fig. 7.38. Axial T1-weighted image through L2 after vertebroplasty. The two cement deposits injected into the vertebral bodies are seen as low-signal-intensity lesions with irregular margins in the vertebral body.

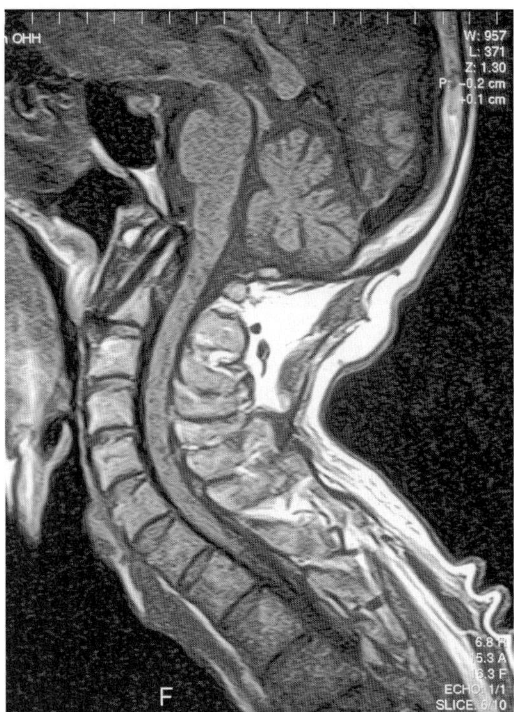

Fig. 7.39. Patient after screw osteosynthesis of the dens after dens fracture. Sagittal T1-weighted image depicting the screw with low signal intensity extending from the base to the tip of the dens. Only a few surrounding artifacts (titanium implant)

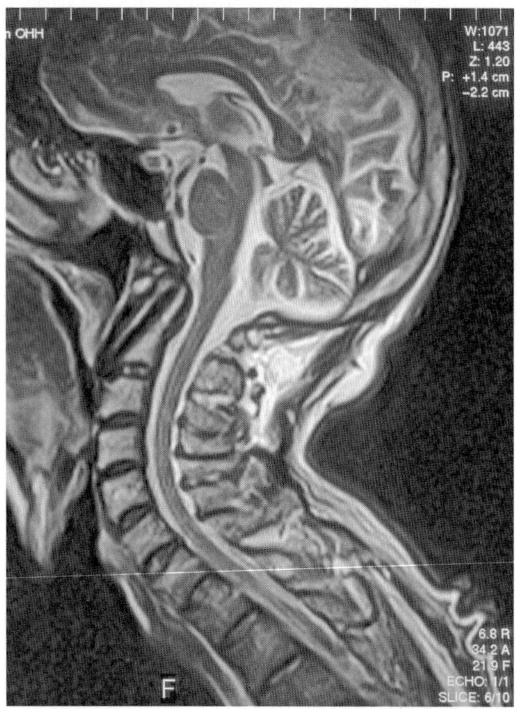

Fig. 7.40. Sagittal T2-weighted image of the craniocervical junction of the same patient depicting the screw within the dens as a low-signal-intensity structure

References

Further Reading
General

Abel R, Gerner HJ, Mariß G (1998) Wirbelsäule und Rückenmark, Klinischer Leitfaden. Blackwell, Oxford

Dihlmann W (1987) Gelenke – Wirbelverbindungen, Klinische Radiologie – Diagnose, Differentialdiagnose. Thieme, Stuttgart

Grumme T, Kluge W, Kretzschmar K, Roesler A (1998) Zerebrale und Spinale Computertomographie. Blackwell Wissenschafts-Verlag, Berlin

Krämer J, Schleberger R, Hedtmann A (1997) Bandscheibenbedingte Erkrankungen. Ursachen, Diagnose, Behandlung, Vorbeugung, Begutachtung. Thieme, Stuttgart

Lissner J, Seiderer M (1990) Klinische Kernspintomographie. Enke, Stuttgart

Modic MT, Ross JS, Mararyk TJ (1989) Magnetic resonance of the spine. Year Book, Chicago

Rummeny EJ, Reimer P, Heindel W (2002) Ganzkörper-MR-Tomographie. Referenz-Reihe-Radiologie. Thieme, Stuttgart

Runge VM, Bittner DF, Awh MH, Kirsch JE (1995) Magnetic resonance imaging of the spine. J.B. Lippincott, Philadelphia

Uhlenbrock D (1992) Radiologische Diagnostik: Kernspintomographie der Wirbelsäule und des Spinalkanals. Thieme, Stuttgart

Uhlenbrock D (2001) MRT der Wirbelsäule und des Spinalkanals. Referenz-Reihe Radiologie. Thieme, Stuttgart

Vahlensieck M, Reiser M (2002) MRT des Bewegungsapparats. Thieme, Stuttgart

Chapter 1: Normal Anatomy and Variants

Küper K (2001) MR/CT-Atlas der Anatomie. Version 5, CD-ROM with Booklet. Thieme, Stuttgart

Lustrin ES, Karakas SP, Ortiz AO et al. (2003) Pediatric cervical spine: normal anatomy, variants, and trauma. RadioGraphics 23:539

White AA, Panjabi MM (1978) The basic kinematics of the human spine. Spine 3:12–20

Zur Nedden D, Putz R (1985) Anatomie und Computertomographie des lumbalen Wirbelkanals. Röntgenprax 38:153–157

Chapter 2: Congenital and Developmental Anomalies

Acosta FL Jr, Quinones-Hinojosa A, Schmidt MH, Weinstein PR (2003) Diagnosis and management of sacral Tarlov cysts. Case report and review of the literature. Neurosurg Focus 15:E15

Bassiouni H, Hunold A, Asgari S, Hubschen U, Konig HJ, Stolke D (2004) Spinal intradural juxtamedullary cysts in the adult: surgical management and outcome. Neurosurgery 55:1352–1360

Beyer HK (2003) MRT der Gelenke und der Wirbelsäule. Radiologisch-orthopädische Diagnostik. Springer, Berlin Heidelberg, New York, Tokio

Bulsara KR, Zomorodi AR, Villavicencio AT, Fuchs H, George TM (2001) Clinical outcome differences for lipomyelomeningocele, intraspinal lipomas and lipomas of the filum terminale. Neurosurg Rev 24:192–194

Chang IC (2004) Surgical experience in symptomatic congenital intraspinal cysts. Pediatr Neurosurg 40:165–170

Christ B, Wilting J (1992) From somites to vertebral column. Ann Anat 174:23–32

Cohen E, Stuecker RD (2005) Magnetic resonance imaging in diagnosis and follow-up of impending spondylolysis in children and adolescents: early treatment may prevent pars defects. J Pediatr Orthop B 14:63:67

Dai L, Yuan W, Ni B, Jia L (2000) Os odontoideum: etiology, diagnosis and management. Surg Neurol 53:106–108

Davis PC, Hoffmann JC Jr, Ball TI et al. (1988) Spinal abnormalities in pediatric patients: MR imaging findings compared with clinical, myelographic, and surgical findings. Radiology 166:679 – 685

Dorward NL, Scatliff JH, Hayward RD (2002) Congenital lumbosacral lipomas. Pitfalls in analysing the results of prophylactic surgery. Child Nerv Syst 18:326–332

Forlin E, Herscovici D, Bowen JR (1992) Understanding the os odontoideum. Orthop Rev 21:1441–1471

French BN (1982) The embryology of spinal dysraphism. Clin Neurosurg 30:295–340

Gräulich W, Pyle S (1966) Radiography atlas of skeletal development of the hand and wrist. Oxford University Press, London, 1966

Hendrick EB, Hoffman HJ, Humphreys RP (1983) The tethered spinal cord. Clinical Neurosurg 30:457–463

Inoue M, Minami S, Nakata Y et al. (2005) Preoperative MRI analysis of patients with idiopathic scoliosis: a prospective study. Spine 30:108–114

Klekamp J (2002) The pathophysiology of syringomyelia –historical overview and current concept. Acta Neurochir (Wien) 144:649–664

Klekamp J, Samii M (Hrsg) (2001) Syringomyelia- diagnosis and treatment. Springer, Berlin Heidelberg New York Tokyo

Köhler A, Zimmer EA (1967) Grenzen des Normalen und Anfänge des Pathologischen im Röntgenbild des Skeletts, 11th edn. Thieme, Stuttgart

Krings T, Lukas R, Reul J, Spetzger U, Reinges MH, Gilsbach JM, Thron A (2001) Diagnostic and therapeutic management of spinal arachnoid cysts. Acta Neurochir (Wien) 143:227–234

Langdown AJ, Grundy JR, Birch NC (2005) The clinical relevance of Tarlov cysts. J Spinal Disord Tech 18:29–33

Liljenquist U (2004) The natural history of congenital defects and deformities of the spine (I). Versicherungsmedizin 56:174–177

Lonstein J, Bradford D, Winter R, Ogilvie J (Hrsg) (1995) Moe's textbook of scoliosis and other spinal deformities, 3rd edn. Saunders, Philadelphia

Marquardt E (1968) Entwicklungsstörungen der Wirbelsäule bei Dysmelien. In: Lange M, Motta C (Hrsg) Orthopädischer Gemeinschaftskongreß 1966. Enke, Stuttgart

McLone DG, Knepper PA (1889) The cause of Chiari II malformation: a unified theory. Paediatric Neurosci 15:1–12

Muraszko K, Youkilis A (2000) Intramedullary spinal tumors of disordered embryogenesis. J Neurooncol 47:271–281

Naidich TP et al. (2001) Congenital anomalies of the spine and spinal cord. In: Atlas SW (Hrsg) Magnetic imaging of the brain and spine, 3rd edn. Lippincott, Williams & Wilkins, Philadelphia, pp 1527–1631

McLone DI (2000) Congenital malformations of the central nervous system. Clin Neurosurg 47:346–377

Okumura R, Minami S, Asato R, Konishi J (1990) Fatty filum terminale: assessment with MR imaging. J Comput Assist Tomogr 14:571–573

Pang D, Dias MS, Ahab-Barmada M (1992) Split cord malformation. Part I. A unified theory of embryogenesis for double spinal cord malformations. Neurosurgery 31:451–480

Pang D, Wildberger JE (1982) Tethered cord syndrome in adults. J Neurosurg 57:32–47

Raghavan N, Barkovich AJ, Edwards M, Norman D (1989) MR imaging in the tethered spinal cord syndrome. AJNR 10:27–36

Scatliff JH, Kendall BE, Kingsley DPE, Britton J (1989) Closed spinal dysraphism: analysis of clinical, radiological and surgical findings in 104 consecutive patients. Am J Roentgenol 152:1049–1057

Sgouros S, Williams B (1996) Management and outcome of posttraumatic syringomyelia. J Neurosurg 85:197–205

Töndury G (1958) Entwicklungsgeschichte und Fehlbildungen der Wirbelsäule. Die Wirbelsäule in Forschung und Praxis, vol. 7. Hippokrates, Stuttgart

Uchino A, Mori T, Ohno M (1991) Thickened fatty filum terminale. Neuroradiology 33:331–333

Weber U, Schwetlick G (1994) Wirbelsäulenerkrankungen Wirbelsäulenverletzungen. Operative Therapie – Stabilisierungsverfahren. Thieme, Stuttgart

Williams B (1972) Pathogenesis of syringomyelia. Lancet ii: 969–970

Wittenberg RH, Willburger RE, Krämer J (1998) Spondylolyse und Spondylolisthese. Diagnose und Therapie. Orthopäde 27:51–63

Yu YL, Mosely IF (1987) Syringomyelia and cervical spondylosis: a clinicoradiological investigation. Neuroradiology 29:143–151

Chapter 3: Trauma and Fractures

Davis SJ, Terest LM, Bradley WG Jr et al. (1991) Cervical spine hyperextension injuries: MR Findings. Radiology 180:245

Dvorak J, Grob D (1999) Halswirbelsäule – Diagnostik und Therapie. Thieme, Stuttgart

Gergy BA, Jesselink JR (1994) MR imaging of the spine: recent advances in pulse sequences and special techniques. Am J Roentgenol 162:923–924

Giuliano V, Giuliano C, Pinto F, Scaglione M (2002) The use of flexion and extension MR in the evaluation of cervical spine trauma: initial experience in 100 trauma patients compared with 100 normal subjects. Emerg Radiol 9:249–253

Gundry CR, Fritts HM (1997) Magnetic resonance imaging of the musculoskeletal system. Spine Clin Orthop Rel Res 138:275–287

Hawighorst H, Berger MF, Moulin P, Zäch GA (2001) MRT bei spinaligamentären Verletztungen. Radiologe 41:307–322

Kathol MH (1997) Cervical spine trauma. What is new? Radiol Clin N Amer 3:507–532

Kress B, Bähren W (2001) Wertigkeit der MRT in der Akutdiagnostik von spinalen Traumen. Röntgenpraxis 54:71–76

Louis R (1982) Chirurgie du rachis: Anatomie chirurgicale et voies d'abord. Springer, Berlin Heidelberg New York

Magerl F, Aebi M, Gertzbein SD, Harms J, Nazarian S (1994) A comprehensive classification of thoracic and lumbar fractures. Eur Spine J 3:184–201

Quencer RM, Bunge RP, Egnor M et al. (1992) Acute traumatic central cord syndrome: MRI-pathologic correlation. Neuroradiology 34:85–94

Shellock FG, Morisoli S, Kanal E (1993) MR procedures and biomedical implants, materials, and devices: 1993 update. Radiology 189:587–599

Sliker CW, Mirvis SE, Shanmuganathan S (2005) Assessing cervical spine stability in obtunded blunt trauma patients: review of medical literature. Radiology 234:733–739

Teli M, De Roeck N, Horowitz MD, Saifuddin A, Green R, Noordeen H (2005) Radiographic outcome of vertebral bone bruise associated with fracture of the thoracic and lumbar spine in adults. Eur Spine J 14:541–545

Terk MR, Hume-Neal M, Fraipont M et al. (1997) Injury of the posterior ligament complex in patients with acute trauma: evaluation by MR imaging. Am J Roentgenol 168:1481–1486

Weber U, Schwetlick G (1994) Wirbelsäulenerkrankungen Wirb elsäulenverletzungen. Operative Therapie – Stabilisierungsverfahren. Thieme, Stuttgart

Chapter 4: Degenerative Disorders

Allgayer B, Frank A, Daller D, von Einsiedel H, Trappe A (1993) Die Magnetresonanztomographie in der Diagnostik des Failed Back Surgery Syndroms. Fortschr Röntgenstr 158:160–165

Amundsen T, Weber H, Lileas F et al. (1995) Lumbar spinal stenosis: clinical and radiologic features. Spine 20:1178

Annertz M, Jönsson B, Strömqvist B, Holtas S (1995) Serial MRI in early postoperative period after lumbar discectomy. Neuroradiology 37:177–182

Claussen C, Grumme T, Treitsch J, Lochner B, Kazner E (1982) Die Diagnostik des lumbalen Bandscheibenvorfalls. Fortschr Röntgenstr 136:1–8

Delank KS, Furderer S, Popken F, Eysel P (2004) Juxta-facet cysts as a differential diagnosis for lumbar neuralgia. Z Orthop/Grenzgeb 142:410–414

Dihlmann W (1987) Lumbaler Reprolaps oder Narbengewebe? Fortschr Röntgenstr 146:330–334

Freund M, Hutzelmann A, Steffens C et al. (1997) MR-Myelographie bei Spinalkanalstenosen. Fortschr Röntgenstr 167:474

Healy JF, Healy BB, Wong WHM, Olson EM (1996) Cervical and lumbar MRI in asymptomatic older male lifelong athletes: frequency of degenerative findings. J Comput Assist Tomogr 20:107–112

Kafer W, Cakir B, Richter M (2004) Osteoarthritis – a rare indication for atlantoaxial fusion. A case report and review of the literature. Acta Orthop Belg 70:380–385

Kahn T, Quaschling U. Engelbrecht V (2004) MRT diagnosis for degenerative changes in the spine. Radiologe 44:789–799

Khan AM, Synnot K, Cammisa FP, Girardi FP (2005) Lumbar synovial cysts of the spine: an evaluation of surgical outcome. J Spinal Disord Tech 18: 127–131

Lane JI, Koeller KK, Atkinson JDL (1996) MR imaging of the lumbar spine: enhancement of the radicular veins. Am J Roentgenol 166:181–186

Lang P, Genant HK, Chafetz N, Steiger P, Stoller D (1987) Mag netresonanztomographie bei der Beurteilung funktioneller Stabilität posterlateraler lumbaler Spondylodesen. Fortschr. Röntgenstr 147:420–426

Milette PC, Fontaine S, Lepanto L, Dery R, Breton G (1996) Clinical impact of contrast-enhanced MR imaging reports in patients with previous lumbar disk surgery. Am J Roentgenol 167:217–223

Modic MT, Masaryk TJ, Ross JS, Carter JR (1988) Imaging of degenerative disk disease. Radiology 168:177–186

Resnick D, Niwayama G (1988) Diagnosis of bone and joint disorders. Saunders, Philadelphia

Ulmer JL, Elster AD, Mathews VP, Allen AM (1995) Lumbar spondylosis: reactive marrow changes seen in adjacent pedicles on MR images. Am J Roentgenol 164:429–433

Verbiest H (1984) Stenose des knöchernen lumbalen Wirbelkanals. In: Hohmann D, Kügelgen B, Lübig K, Schirmer M (eds.)

Neuroorthopädie 2. Springer, Berlin Heidelberg New York Tokio, pp 231–270

Yu S, Haughton VM, Ho PSP, Sether LA, Wagner M, Ho KC (1980) Progressive and regressive changes in the nucleus pulposus. Part. II. The adult. Radiology 169:93–97

Chapter 5: Inflammatory Conditions

Andronikou S, Albuquerque-Jonathan G, Wilmshurst J, Hewlett R (2003) MRI findings in acute idiopathic transverse myelopathy in children. Pediatr Radiol 33:624–629

Baraliakos X, Landewe R, Hermann KG et al. (2005) Inflammation in ankylosing spondylitis: a systematic description of the extent and frequency of acute spinal changes using magnetic resonance imaging. Ann Rheum Dis 64: 730–734

Fangerau T, Multiple Sclerosis Study Group (2004) Diagnosis of multiple sclerosis: comparison of the Poser criteria and the new McDonald criteria. Acta Neurol Scand 109:385–389

Grob D (2004) Surgical aspects of the cervical spine in rheumatoid arthritis. Orthopäde 33: 1201–1212, quiz 1213–1214

Karhu JO, Parkkola RK, Koskinen SK (2005) Evaluation of flexion/extension of the upper cervical spine in patients with rheumatoid arthritis: an MRI study with a dedicated positioning device compared to conventional radiographs. Acta Radiol 46:55–66

Lycklama A Nijeholt GJ, Uitdehaag BM, Bergers E, Castelijns JA, Polman CH, Barkhof F (2000) Spinal cord magnetic resonance imaging in suspected multiple sclerosis. Eur Radiol 10:368–376

Miller DH, Filippi M, Fazekas F, Frederiksen JL, Matthews PM, Montalban X, Polman CH (2004) Role of magnetic resonance imaging within diagnostic criteria for multiple sclerosis. Ann Neurol 56:273–278

Mushlin AI, Detsky AS, Phelps CE et al. (1993) The accuracy of magnetic resonance imaging in patients with suspected multiple sclerosis. The Rochester-Toronto Magnetic Resonance Imaging Group. JAMA 269:3146–3151

Radue EW, Kappos L (2003) Vancouver Consortium of MS Centers'Magnetic Resonance Imaging Guidelines. Int MS 10:131–133

Rudwaleit M, Baraliakos S, Listing J, Brandt J, Sieper J, Braun J (2005) Magnetic resonance imaging of the spine and the sacroiliac joints in ankylosing spondylitis before and during therapy with etanercept. Ann Rheum Dis 64:1305–1310

Sommer OJ, Kladosek A, Weiler V, Czembirek H, Boeck M, Stiskal M (2005) Rheumatoid arthritis: a practical guide to state-of-the-art imaging, image interpretation, and clinical implications. RadioGraphics 25:381–398

Tullman MJ, Delman BN, Lublin FD, Weinberger J (2003) Magnetic resonance imaging of meningoradiculomyelitis in early disseminated Lyme disease. J Neuroimaging 13:264–258

Weber U, Rettig H, Jungbluth H (1985) Knochen- und Gelenktuberkulose. Perimed Fachbuch-Verlagsgesellschaft mbH, Erlangen

Chapter 6: Tumors and Tumor-like Lesions

Abbot R, Shiminski-Maher T, Epstein FJ (1996) Intrinsic tumors of the medulla: predicting outcome after surgery. Pediatr Neurosurg 25:41–44

Browne TR, Adams RD, Roberson GH (1976) Haemangioblastoma of the spinal cord. Review and report of five cases. Arch Neurol 33:435–441

De Verdelhan O, Haegelen C, Carsin-Nicol B, Riffaud L, Amlashi SF, Brassier G, Carsin M, Morandi X (2005) MR imaging features of spinal schwannomas and meningiomas. J Neuroradiol 32:42–49

Fine KJ, Kricheff II, Freed D, Epstein FJ (1995) Spinal cord ependymomas: MR imaging features. Radiology 197:655–658

Fourney DR, Gokaslan ZL (2003) Current management of sacral chordoma. Neurosurg Focus 15: E9

Guzey F, Seyithanoglu MH, Sencer A, Emei E, Alatas I, Izgi AN (2004) Vertebral osteoid osteoma associated with paravertebral soft-tissue changes on magnetic resonance imaging. Report of two cases. J Neurosurg 100 (Suppl Pediatrics): 532–536

Immenkamp M, Härle A (1994) Geschwülste der Wirbelsäule. Knochentumoren in: Orthopädie in Praxis und Klinik, Band V/2. A.N. Witt, M. Rettig, K.F. Schlegel. Thieme Stuttgart-New York

Jallo GI, Zagzag D, Lee M, Deletis V, Morota N, Epstein FJ (1997) Intraspinal sarcoidosis: diagnosis and management. Surg Neurol 48:514–520

Joerger M et al. (2005) Von Hippel-Lindau disease – a rare disease important to recognise. Onkologie 28:159–163

Klekamp J, Samii M (2005) Tumoren des Spinalkanals. In: Moskopp D, Wassmann H (eds.) Neurochirurgie. Schattauer, Stuttgart New York, pp 616–634

Li MH, Holtas S, Larsson EM (1992) MR imaging of intradural extramedullary tumors. Acta Radiol 33:207–212

Pans S, Brys R, Van Breuseghem I, Geusens E (2005) Benign bone tumours of the spine. JBR-BTR 88:31–37

Papagelopoulos PJ, Mavrogenis AF, Galanis EC, Savvidou OD, Boscainos PJ, Katonis PG, Sim FH (2004) Chordoma of the spine: clinicopathological features, diagnosis, and treatment. Orthopedics 27:1256–1263, quiz 1264–1265

Roux FX, Nataf F, Pinaudeau M, Borne G, Devaux B, Meder JF (1996) Intraspinal meningiomas: review of 54 cases with discussion of poor prognosis factors and modern therapeutic management. Surg Neurol 456:458–463

Sandalcioglu IE, Gasser T, Asgari S et al. (2005) Functional outcome after surgical treatment of intramedullary spinal cord tumors: experience with 78 patients. Spinal Cord 43:34–41

Schmidt GP, Baur A, Stabler A, Schoenberg SO, Steinborn M, Baltin V, Reiser MF (2005) Diffuse bone marrow infiltration of the spine in multiple myeloma: correlation of the MRI with histological results. Rofo 177:745–750

Shrivastava RK et al. (2005) Intramedullary spinal tumors in patients older than 50 years of age: management and outcome analysis. J Neurosurgery Spine 2:249–255

Sung MS, Lee GK, Kang HS et al. (2005) Sacrococcygeal chordoma: MR imaging in 30 patients. Skeletal Radiol 34:87–94

Chapter 7: The Postoperative Spine

Hochegger M, Radl R, Leithner A, Windhager R (2005) Spinal canal stenosis after vertebroplasty. Clin Radiol 60:397–400

Subject Index

A

Abscess formation 143
Acoustic neurinomas 195
Acquired stenosis 102
Acute fracture 62
Adamkiewicz
- artery of 199
Adolescent kyphosis 21
Adult scoliosis 19
AIDS 147
Anatomy 1
Andersson 1 lesions 145
Andersson 2 lesions 66
Aneurysmal bone cyst 201
Angiectatic nevus 22
Angioblastic meningioma 195
Angioma 22
Ankylosed spine 61
Ankylosing spondylitis 61, 65, 143, 145
Annulus fibrosus 99, 104
Anterior longitudinal ligament 99
Antimicrobial chemotherapy 144
Arachnoid cysts 11
Arachnoid membrane 66
Arnold-Chiari malformation 2
- type I 17
- type II 18
Arteriovenous malformations 199
Assimilation 1
- incomplete 1
Astrocytoma 197
Atlantoaxial arthrosis 104
Atlantoaxial distance 14
Atlantoaxial instability 14
Atlantodental distance 145
Atlas assimilation 2
Atlas fractures 63
Autoimmune response 147

B

Back surgery 106
Bacterial spondylitis 144
Barkhof criteria 147
Basilar impression 13, 14
Bifid vertebra 16
Bipolar manifestation 144
Blood sediment 230
Bone
- bruise 73
- chip 154
- defect 273
- destruction 143
- dystrophies 22
- grafting 273
- tumors 200
Bony avulsions 65
Bony consolidation 286
Breast cancer 200
Burst fracture 61
Butterfly vertebra 12

C

Café-au-lait spots 195
Calcification 107
Calcifying chondrodystrophy 14
Candida spondylitis 143
Cartilaginous endplates 99
Cartilaginous matrix 101
Cement deposits 287
Central canal 16
Cervical disc herniation 105
Cervicothoracic junction 130
Chamberlain's line 14
Chiari type II malformation 16, 18
Classification of Anderson and D'Alonzo 62
Chondrosis 100
Chordoma 201
Cisterna magna 17, 45
Cleft 12
Colloid osmotic system 99
Compensatory scoliosis 19
Compression fracture 65, 75
Condylar hyperplasia 12
Congenitally narrow spinal canal 107
Congenital block vertebrae 15
Congenital scoliosis 15
Congenital spinal stenosis 102
Conjoined nerve roots 1
Contrast administration 43, 134
Contrast enhancement 1
Conus medullaris 7
Convexity 19
Coronal plexus 199
Cranial asymmetry 13
Cranial shift 2

D

Dandy-Walker cysts 16
Demyelination 147
Dermal sinus 17
Dermoid cyst 198
Dermomyotome 12
Devic's syndrome 147
Diastema 12
Diastematomyelia 15
Diffusion-weighted imaging 147
Diplomyelia 15
Discitis 143
Disc
- atresia 15
- extrusion 105, 106
- height 104
- Herniation 104
- injury 64
- protrusion 105, 106
Displacement 86
Dumbbell-shaped neurinomas 196
Dural leak 98
Dynamic stenosis 102
Dysplastic spondylolisthesis 23
Dysraphism 17

E

Electrocardiography-triggered pulse sequence 17
Encephalocele 13
Endovascular embolization 200
Endplate 99
Enhancement 278
Eosinophilic granuloma 201
Ependymomas 195, 197
Epidermoid cyst 198
Epidural abscess 144

Erosive osteochondrosis 100
Exogenous infection 143
Extradural
meningeal cysts 11

F

Facet joints 99
Facet syndrome 102
Fat-suppressed
sequences 1
Fatty degeneration 141, 185
Fatty marrow 100
Fatty tissue 3
Fat saturation 63
Fibrosarcomas 201
Filum terminale 19, 21
Fish vertebra 61
Flow velocity 1
Foramen magnum 37
Foraminal stenosis 103
Fracture 62
Functional scoliosis 19

G

Gadolinium-DTPA 147
Gibbus deformity 20, 34
Gliomas 195
Gravitation abscess 169
Gunshot injury 93

H

Hanged man's fracture 61, 62
Hard disc herniation 105
Hemangioblastoma 198
Hemangioma
- intraosseous 22
Hemimetameric
segmental shift 12
Hemivertebra 12, 20
Hemorrhage 62
Herniation 105
Hippel-Lindau syndrome 198
HLA-B27 146
Hurler's syndrome 20
Hydrocephalus 16
Hydromyelia 16
Hyperextension 66
Hyperextension injuries 64
Hyperlordosis 59
Hypernephroma 201
Hypertrichosis 16
Hypolordosis 20
Hypomochlion 13

I

Idiopathic scolioses 19
Impaction fracture 61
Impression fracture 75
Inflammatory
enthesopathy 146
Intervertebral discs 104
Intradural
meningeal cysts 11
Intraforaminal cyst 25
Intraforaminal herniation 105
Isthmic spondylolisthesis 23

J

Jefferson fractures 63
Juvenile ankylosing spondylitis 144

K

Kinking 18
Klippel-Feil syndrome 13
Kyphoscoliosis 53
Kyphosis 20

L

Laminectomy defect 274
Lateral
hemivertebrae 13
Lazorthes
- artery of 199
Ligamentum flavum 99
Ligament disruption 61
Ligament injuries 65
Lipoma 13, 22
- intraosseous 22
Lipomyelomeningocele 21
Liquefaction 144
Lisch nodules 195
Lumbar disc herniation 106
Lumbosacral junction 39
Lung cancer 200
Lupus erythematosus 147
Luschka
- uncovertebral joints of 105

M

M. tuberculosis 143
Malalignment 101
Malformations 2, 12
Malignant fibrous
histiocytoma 201
Malignant lymphoma 201
Malsegmentation 13
Marfan's syndrome 19
Marrow 3
Marrow edema 62
Meningeal cysts 11
Meningioma 195
Mesencephalic tectum 18
Mesoderm 12
Metal artifacts 274
Metastatic spread 200
Meyerding classification 58
Modic type 20, 100
MR myelography 106
MR spectroscopy 147
MRI sequences
- T1-weighted 1
- T2 weighted 1
- fast spin echo 1
- fat-suppressed 1
Multiple sclerosis 147
Muscle atrophy 19
Muscular atrophy 108
Muscular dystrophy 107
Myelin sheaths 147
Myelography 41
Myelomalacia 14
Myelotomy 197
Myopathic scoliosis 19

N

Nerve roots 1, 9, 25
Nerve root avulsion 98
Nerve sheath tumors 195
Neural foramina 7
Neurenteric cysts 16, 198
Neurinoma 195
Neurocele 18
Neurofibromas 195
Neurofibromatosis
- type I 195
- type II 195
Neuropathic scoliosis 19
Neurotization 67
Neurulation 11, 17
Non-Hodgkin lymphoma 200
Notochord 99, 201
Nucleus pulposus 99, 104

O

Occipitalization 14
Occult intrasacral
meningoceles 11
Ossicle 15
Osteoblastoma 201
Osteochondrodysplasia 20
Osteochondroma 200
Osteochondrosis 99
Osteoid osteoma 20, 201
Osteoligamentous injuries 66
Osteonecrosis 54
Osteopathic scoliosis 19
Osteophytes 101
Osteoporotic fracture 65
Osteosynthesis 273

Osteotomy defect 276
Os odontoideum 14

P

Pac-1 gene 15
Pannus 104, 145
Papillary edema 197
Pars interarticularis 24
Pedicles 6
Pia mater 21
Placode 18
Platybasia 13
PNETs 195
Polyarthritis 144
Posterior hemivertebrae 13
Posterior column 63
Posterior longitudinal ligament 99
Posterior spondylitis 143
Postganglionic injury 66
Postoperative hematoma 279
Pseudobulbar basilar impression 181
Pseudomeningocele 66
Pseudospondylolisthesis 23
Psoas abscess 143, 144
Pulsation artifacts 199

R

Rectal dysfunction 19
Recurrent disc herniation 273, 276
Resegmentation 12
Rheumatoid arthritis 145
Rib hump 19

S

S. aureus 143
Sacralization 2
Sacrum
- dome-shaped 23
Sagittal diameter 102
Sarcoidosis 200
Scalloping 21
Scars 273
Scheuermann's disease 21
Schmorl's node 21
Schwannoma 195, 205
Scoliosis 19
Secondary stenosis 101
Sensory deficits 19
Sequester 105
Seroma 273
Sharpey fibers 99
Shock absorption 100
Signal intensity 1
Sintering 64
Skin stigmata 16
Slippage 58
Soft herniation 105
Somite 12
Spinal
- angiography 219
- canal stenosis 102
- contusion 63
- injuries 61
- junctions 1
- lipomas 21
- meningeal cysts 11
- stenosis 20
Spinal meningioma
- psammomatous type 195
Spindle-shaped lesion 27
Spinous processes 81
Split cord malformation 15, 39
Split fracture 61
Spondylitis 143
Spondyloarthrosis 101
Spondylodiscitis 100, 143
Spondylolisthesis 23
Spondylolysis 23
Spondylophytes 145
Spondyloptosis 24
Sprengel's deformity 13
Striated muscle 108
String of pearls 45
Structural scoliosis 19
Subarachnoid space 11, 131
Superselective angiography 199
Supra-aortic vessels 5
Susceptibility artifact 275
Syndesmophytes 145
Synosthosis 173
Synovial cysts 102
Syringobulbia 17
Syringohydromyelia 16

T

T1-weighted images 1
T2-weighted images 2
Tarlov cysts 11, 28, 198
Teardrop fracture 62
Tethered cord 18
Thecal sac 1, 9
Thoracic disc herniation 106
Titanium 273
Torticollis 2
Toxoplasmosis 147
Transitional vertebrae 1
Transverse diameter 104
Transverse myelitis 147
Transverse processes 6, 99
Trisomy 21 14
Tuberculous spondylitis 153

U

Uncinate processes 105
Uncovertebral spondylosis 100

V

Vacuum phenomenon 99
Venous channels 8
Vertebral artery 237
Vertebral segmentation 15
Vertebra plana 201
Vertebroplasty 273
Vertical instability 144
Von Recklinghausen's neurofibromatosis 195

W

Wedge vertebra 13, 34

Printing: Krips bv, Meppel
Binding: Stürtz, Würzburg